Textbook of Good Clinical Practice in Cold Plasma Therapy

Hans-Robert Metelmann • Thomas von Woedtke
Klaus-Dieter Weltmann • Steffen Emmert
Editors

Textbook of Good Clinical Practice in Cold Plasma Therapy

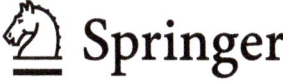 Springer

Editors
Hans-Robert Metelmann
Greifswald University Hospital
Greifswald, Germany

Klaus-Dieter Weltmann
Leibniz Institute for Plasma Science and
Technology (INP)
Greifswald, Germany

Thomas von Woedtke
Leibniz Institute for Plasma Science and
Technology (INP)
Greifswald, Germany

Steffen Emmert
University Medical Center Rostock
Rostock, Germany

ISBN 978-3-030-87856-6   ISBN 978-3-030-87857-3   (eBook)
https://doi.org/10.1007/978-3-030-87857-3

This Springer imprint is published by the registered company Springer Nature Switzerland AG
The registered company address is: Gewerbestrasse 11, 6330 Cham, Switzerland

Preface

Kind reader,

Welcome to the first textbook and manual for doctors in the field of a new specialty – plasma medicine.

How is it actually created and what makes a new specialty in medicine? There is a substantial, significant, and proven evolution in medical technology and treatment concept, a meaningful contribution for the benefit of patients that is calling for natural scientists, engineers, and medical doctors to link their competences and build an innovative scientific community. There are health problems frequently encountered in daily medical practice that can be solved with the new concept and technology. There is an innovative area of scientific and medical expertise not covered by just one established discipline in medicine. There is a structure and concerted workflow that keeps the new specialty standing freely and growing, grounded on national and international organizational bodies, on coordinated research, consented development of treatment guidelines, standard educational courses and specialist training, on scientific journals and academic background, and not at least on books like these. Roaming the chapters of this textbook you will recognize that clinical plasma medicine truly meets the aforementioned criteria of a new medical discipline.

A book does not develop on its own. The existence of this book became possible under the auspices of Ministerpräsidentin Manuela Schwesig, State Premier of Mecklenburg-Western Pomerania of the Federal Republic of Germanys, setting the goal "by offering a common forum for global players of plasma medicine ... [that] contributes to an even more effective cooperation and achievement of innovative objectives for the benefit of ... patients all over the world." We very much appreciate the high honor and the privilege to see the international development of plasma medicine so much supported.

We are very grateful for the idea and initiation of the project by Daniela Heller from the publishing house. We extend our sincere thanks for excellent supporting, mentoring, and coaching to Kerstin Böttger and Rakesh Kumar Jotheeswaran. Our profound gratitude goes to all authors for their substantial contributions and professional cooperation and to Dr. Philine Doberschütz as a medical writer involved. And we are especially grateful to our readers for personally getting involved with these reflections before starting to wander through the chapters. That looks like a keen and rewarding interest in clinical plasma medicine. We wish you success!

Hans-Robert Metelmann
Thomas von Woedtke
Klaus-Dieter Weltmann
Greifswald, Germany

Steffen Emmert
Rostock, Germany

Contents

I   Introduction

II   Concept

III   The Patient's View at Basic Clinical Principles

IV   Treatment Tailored to Indications

V   Devices

VI   Organization

Contributors

Robert Bansemer Leibniz Institute for Plasma Science and Technology (INP), Greifswald, Germany
robert.bansemer@inp-greifswald.de

Norbert Behnke, MD, DALM Private Dermatology Clinic, Panketal, Germany

Sander Bekeschus ZIK Plasmatis, Leibniz-Institute for Plasma Science and Technology (INP) Greifswald, Greifswald, Germany

ZIK plasmatis, Leibniz Institute for Plasma Science and Technology e.V., Greifswald, Germany
sander.bekeschus@inp-greifswald.de

Thoralf Bernhardt, M.Sc. Clinic and Polyclinic for Dermatology and Venereology, University Medical Center Rostock, Rostock, Germany
Thoralf.Bernhardt@med.uni-rostock.de

Lars Boeckmann Clinic and Polyclinic for Dermatology and Venereology, University Medical Center Rostock, Rostock, Germany
Lars.Boeckmann@med.uni-rostock.de

Thomas Borchardt University of Applied Sciences and Arts, Faculty of Engineering and Health Göttingen, Göttingen, Germany
thomas.borchardt1@hawk.de

Kerstin Böttger Department of Oral and Maxillofacial Surgery/Plastic Surgery, University Medicine Greifswald, Greifswald, Germany
kerstin.boettger@med.uni-greifswald.de

Ronny Brandenburg Leibniz Institute for Plasma Science and Technology, Greifswald, Germany
brandenburg@inp-greifswald.de

Benedikt Busse CINOGY GmbH, Duderstadt, Germany
benedikt.busse@cinogy.de

Maximilian Cantzler terraplasma GmbH, Garching, Germany
cantzler@terraplasma.com

Sylvia Cantzler terraplasma medical GmbH, Garching, Germany

terraplasma GmbH, Garching, Germany
sylvia.cantzler@terraplasma-medical.com

Eun Ha Choi   Applied Plasma Medicine Center and Plasma Bioscience Research Center, Kwangwoon University, Seoul, Republic of Korea

Plasma Bioscience Research Center, Kwangwoon University, Seoul, Republic of Korea
ehchoi@kw.ac.kr

Tania-Cristina Costea   Herz- und Diabeteszentrum NRW, Diabeteszentrum, Bad Oeynhausen, Germany

Ruhr-Universität Bochum, Bochum, Germany
tcostea@hdz-nrw.de

Philine H. Doberschütz   Department of Orthodontics, University Medicine Greifswald, Greifswald, Germany
philine.doberschuetz@uni-greifswald.de

Steffen Emmert, M.Sc.   Clinic and Policlinic for Dermatology and Venereology, University Medical Center Rostock, Rostock, Germany
steffen.emmert@med.uni-rostock.de

Tobias Fischer   Clinic and Polyclinic for Dermatology and Venereology, University Medical Center Rostock, Rostock, Germany
Tobias.Fischer@med.uni-rostock.de

Michael Fröhlich   Cranio-Maxdillo-Facial Surgeon, Dresden, Germany

Torsten Gerling   ZIK plasmatis, Leibniz Institute for Plasma Science and Technology (INP), Greifswald, Germany

Centre for Innovation Competency ZIK Plasmatis, Greifswald, Germany

Competency Centre for Diabetes KDK, Karlsburg, Germany

ZIK plasmatis, Leibniz Institute for Plasma Science and Technology e.V., Greifswald, Germany
gerling@inp-greifswald.de

Stefan Hammes   Oral & Maxillofacial Surgery/Plastic Surgery, University Medicine Greifswald, Greifswald, Germany

National Center of Plasma Medicine, Berlin, Germany

Deutsche Dermatologische Lasergesellschaft e.V, Konz, Germany

Laser Clinic Karlsruhe, Karlsruhe, Germany
stefan@hammes.de

Kristina Hartwig   Oral & Maxillofacial Surgery/Plastic Surgery, University Medicine Greifswald, Greifswald, Germany

Center for Low – Temperature Plasma Sciences, Nagoya University, Nagoya, Japan
kristina.hartwig@med.uni-greifswald.de

Andreas Helmke   Faculty of Engineering and Health, HAWK University of Applied Sciences and Arts, Göttingen, Germany
andreas.helmke@hawk.de

Lutz Hilker   Clinic for Cardiovascular Surgery, Klinikum Karlsburg, Heart and Diabetes Centre, Mecklenburg-Vorpommern, Karlsburg, Germany
hilker@drguth.de

Masaru Hori   Center for Low – Temperature Plasma Sciences, Nagoya University, Nagoya, Japan
hori@nuee.nagoya-u.ac.jp

Jeiram Jeyaratnam   Adtec Healthcare, London, UK
jeiram@adtecplasma.com

Alexander Kaminski   Clinic for Cardiovascular Surgery, Klinikum Karlsburg, Heart and Diabetes Centre, Mecklenburg-Vorpommern, Karlsburg, Germany
kaminski.alexander@drguth.de

Gyoo-Cheon Kim   Department of Oral Anatomy, School of Dentistry, Pusan National University, Yangsan-si, Republic of Korea
ki91000m@pusan.ac.kr

Jens Kirsch   terraplasma medical GmbH, Garching, Germany
jens.kirsch@terraplasma-medical.com

Anne Kirschner   Department of Oral and Maxillofacial Surgery/Plastic Surgery, University Medicine Greifswald, Greifswald, Germany

Regional Professional Education Centre in Health Sciences, Waren, Germany
Anne.Kirschner@rbb-mueritz.de

Stefanie Kirschner   Department of Oral and Maxillofacial Surgery/Plastic Surgery, University Medicine Greifswald, Greifswald, Germany

Department of Health Sciences, University of Applied Sciences, Neubrandenburg, Germany
Stefanie.Kirschner@rbb-mueritz.de

Jae-Sung Kwon   Department and Research Institute of Dental Biomaterials and Bioengineering, Yonsei University College of Dentistry, Seoul, Republic of Korea
jkwon@yuhs.ac

Michael Linner   terraplasma medical GmbH, Garching, Germany
michael.linner@terraplasma-medical.com

Tim Maisch   Department of Dermatology, University Hospital Regensburg, Regensburg, Germany
Tim.Maisch@klinik.uni-regensburg.de

Kai Masur   Leibniz-Institute for Plasma Science and Technology (INP), Greifswald, Germany
ZIK plasmatis, Leibniz Institute for Plasma Science and Technology e.V., Greifswald, Germany
kai.masur@inp-greifswald.de

Mary McGovern   Adtec Healthcare, London, UK
marymcgovern@adtec.eu.com

Hans-Robert Metelmann, MD, DMD, PhD, DALM   Department of Oral and Maxillofacial Surgery/Plastic Surgery, University Medicine Greifswald, Greifswald, Germany
National Center of Plasma Medicine, Berlin, Germany
Deutsche Dermatologische Lasergesellschaft e.V, Konz, Germany
metelman@uni-greifswald.de

Isabella Metelmann   Department of Visceral, Vascular, Transplant and Thoracic Surgery, University Medicine Leipzig, Leipzig, Germany
Department of Oral and Maxillofacial Surgery/Plastic Surgery, University Medicine Greifswald, Greifswald, Germany
isabella.metelmann@medizin.uni-leipzig.de

Vandana Miller   Department of Microbiology and Immunology, Drexel University College of Medicine, Philadelphia, PA, USA
vam54@drexel.edu

Nguyen Dinh Minh, MD, DMD   Department of Plastic, Aesthetic and Maxillofacial Surgery, E hospital, Cau Giay, Ha Noi, Vietnam

Seoul-Hee Nam   Department of Dental Hygiene, Kangwon National University, Samcheok, Republic of Korea
nshee@kangwon.ac.kr

Ajay Rana   Oral & Maxillofacial Surgery/Plastic Surgery, University Medicine Greifswald, Greifswald, Germany
National Center of Plasma Medicine, Berlin, Germany
Institute of Laser & Aesthetic Medicine (ILAMED), New Delhi, India
drajayrana@ilamed.org

Claudia C. Roskopf   terraplasma medical GmbH, Garching, Germany
claudia.roskopf@terraplasma-medical.com

Rico Rutkowski, MD, DMD Department of Oral and Maxillofacial Surgery, University Medical Center Hamburg Eppendorf, Hamburg, Germany
r.rutkowski@uke.de

Ulrike Sailer neoplas med GmbH, Greifswald, Germany
ulrike.sailer@neoplas-med.eu

Benjamin Schade Department of Oral and Maxillofacial Surgery/Plastic Surgery, University Medicine Greifswald, Greifswald, Germany
Benjamin.schade@med.uni-greifswald.de

Mirijam Schäfer, M.Sc. Clinic and Polyclinic for Dermatology and Venereology, University Medical Center Rostock, Rostock, Germany
Mirijam.Schaefer@med.uni-rostock.de

Anke Schmidt ZIK Plasmatis, Leibniz-Institute for Plasma Science and Technology (INP Greifswald), Greifswald, Germany
anke.schmidt@inp-greifswald.de

Christian Seebauer Department of Oral and Maxillofacial Surgery/Plastic Surgery, University Medicine Greifswald, Greifswald, Germany
National Center of Plasma Medicine, Berlin, Germany
christian.seebauer@med.uni-greifswald.de

Marie Luise Semmler Clinic and Polyclinic for Dermatology and Venereology, University Medical Center Rostock, Rostock, Germany
luise.semmler@med.uni-rostock.de

Karrer Sigrid Department of Dermatology, University Hospital Regensburg, Regensburg, Germany
sigrid.karrer@ukr.de

Katharina Stapelmann Department of Nuclear Engineering, NC State University, Raleigh, NC, USA
kstapel@ncsu.edu

Arndt Stephanie Department of Dermatology, University Hospital Regensburg, Regensburg, Germany
stephanie.arndt@ukr.de

Bernd Stratmann, M.D. Herz- und Diabeteszentrum NRW, Diabeteszentrum, Bad Oeynhausen, Germany
Ruhr-Universität Bochum, Bochum, Germany
bstratmann@hdz-nrw.de

Hiromasa Tanaka   Graduate School of Engineering, Nagoya University, Nagoya, Japan
htanaka@plasma.engg.nagoya-u.ac.jp

Vu Thi Thom, PhD   Department of Basic Science in Medicine and Pharmacy, School of Medicine and Pharmacy, Vietnam National University Hanoi, Cau Giay, Ha Noi, Vietnam

Eric Timmermann   Leibniz Institute for Plasma Science and Technology (INP), Greifswald, Germany
eric.timmermann@inp-greifswald.de

Runa Tschersche-Mondry   Department of Oral and Maxillofacial Surgery/Plastic Surgery, University Medicine Greifswald, Greifswald, Germany
runa.tschersche-mondry@med.uni-greifswald.de

Diethelm Tschoepe   Herz- und Diabeteszentrum NRW, Diabeteszentrum, Bad Oeynhausen, Germany

Ruhr-Universität Bochum, Bochum, Germany
diethelm.tschoepe@rub.de

Rico Unger   Ditabis Digital Biomedical Imaging Systems AG, Garching, Germany
r.unger@ditabis.de

Thomas von Woedtke   ZIK Plasmatis, Leibniz Institute for Plasma Science and Technology (INP), Greifswald, Germany

Leibniz-Institute for Plasma Science and Technology and Institute for Hygiene and Environmental Medicine, University Medicine Greifswald, Greifswald, Germany

Leibniz-Institute for Plasma Science and Technology (INP Greifswald), Greifswald, Germany

National Center of Plasma Medicine, Berlin, Germany

Department of Hygiene and Environmental Medicine, University Medicine Greifswald, Greifswald, Germany
woedtke@inp-greifswald.de

Philipp Wahl   Diaspective Vision, Pepelow, Germany
philip.wahl@diaspective-vision.com

Dirk Wandke   CINOGY GmbH, Duderstadt, Germany
dirk.wandke@cinogy.de

Hannes Weilemann   terraplasma GmbH, Garching, Germany
weilemann@terraplasma.com

Klaus-Dieter Weltmann   Leibniz-Institute for Plasma Science and Technology (INP), Greifswald, Germany
weltmann@inp-greifswald.de

Kristian Wende Leibniz Institute for Plasma Science and Technology, Greifswald, Germany
kristian.wende@inp-greifswald.de

Oksana Wladimirova Department of International Relations and Marketing, Stavropol State Medical University, Stavropol, Russia

Department of Surgery, Stavropol State Medical University, Stavropol, Russia

Hans-Georg Wollert Zarnekow, Germany
wollert@drguth.de

Martin Wunderl Ditabis Digital Biomedical Imaging Systems AG, Garching, Germany
m.wunderl@ditabis.de

Julia L. Zimmermann terraplasma medical GmbH, Garching, Germany

terraplasma GmbH, Garching, Germany
julia.zimmermann@terraplasma-medical.com

Introduction

Contents

From Leap Innovation to Integrated Medical Care

Hans-Robert Metelmann,
Thomas von Woedtke,
Klaus-Dieter Weltmann, Steffen Emmert,
Isabella Metelmann, Sander Bekeschus,
Kai Masur, Thomas Borchardt,
Katharina Stapelmann, Norbert Behnke,
and Michael Fröhlich

Contents

© Springer Nature Switzerland AG 2022
H.-R. Metelmann et al. (eds.), *Textbook of Good Clinical Practice in*
Cold Plasma Therapy, https://doi.org/10.1007/978-3-030-87857-3_1

⊜ Core Messages
- Plasma medicine based upon cold atmospheric pressure plasma (CAP) is indicated for chronic and infected wounds, suppurative focuses, wounds with a standstill of healing but no infection, acute wounds at high risk of infection, skin lesions at risk of serious progression, non-healing wounds by other reasons and skin and mucosa with certain local infections.
- Plasma medical devices exploit a leap innovation: Physical energy generates biochemical control of living human, animal, as well as microbial cells, giving way to utilization for medical purposes, for example, wound antisepsis combined with stimulation of soft tissue and skin.
- From a clinical point of view, this bivalent functionality is a unique selling proposition of plasma medical devices in comparison to conventional and established wound care measures.
- Integrated medical plasma care is a coordinated team performance of physicians, natural scientists, nurses, and other professionals.

1.1 Introduction

This book is intended to serve the practitioners of medicine in their general or specialist medical practice, in hospitals, in outpatient care service, or mobile nursing service, in health and care institutions, viz., whoever is involved in the therapy with cold physical atmospheric pressure plasma (CAP). Moreover, scientists in plasma medicine research and engineers are addressed, who would like to learn for their work about the practitioners´ point of view, the requirements and demands of applied plasma medicine for the benefit of patients.

Benefit of patients is the main intention of medicine and of good clinical practice. Good clinical practice in plasma medicine is based upon a leap innovation, profound basic research, evidence-based medicine, and finally becomes obvious in the daily medical work as a well-balanced ratio of benefit and risk for the informed and consenting patient.

Plasma medical devices are approved since 2013 for treating quite common and significant pathologies. Many patients suffer from wounds that are chronic, infected by pathogens or heal badly or from infected skin at all. Standard treatment of wounds is sometimes failing completely, or healing becomes delayed. Therefore, wound therapy to a large extent is in need for new opportunities, and plasma medicine contributes a leap innovation.

For appropriate clinical indication of plasma medicine, it has to be respected that a wound by itself is not a disease, and wound healing is just a natural process with no requirement of targeted treatment. Problems arise, when wounds become severely infected by pathogens while still open (curative indication), when wound healing is retarded and the risk of infection is climbing rapidly (preventive indication), when wounds cannot heal from consuming illness and show furthermore massive infection (palliative indication), when open wounds and infected skin have to convalesced as soon as possible because of pain or for risk prevention (acute

1

indication), when wounds are health-threatening suppurative focuses (acute as well as preventive indication). Plasma medicine covers all of these indications.

The purpose of this chapter is to start the book with a general overview of applied plasma medicine, a quick walkthrough before passing on to the following elaborated chapters for specialists´ differential interests as indicated by footnotes.

1.2 To Diagnose Problem Pathologies[1]

Good clinical practice puts diagnosis and identifying problem pathologies first. Many of these pathologies relevant for plasma therapy put a heavy burden on the health and well-being of patients. They are sometimes difficult to handle by established therapeutic procedures, calling for innovative treatment.

1.2.1 Chronic and Infected Wounds[2]

◘ Figure 1.1 gives a clinical example of poorly healing wounds occupying a large and flat area. This wound at the lower leg started with a minor injury and became infected by multi-resistant pathogens. The patient is severely compromised by co-morbidities and immunosuppressive medication. Complex cases like this one are considerably difficult to treat. Surgical deep debridement was needed to control a life-threatening sepsis and remove necrotic soft tissue. The resulting extended defect had to be covered by reconstructive surgery and a skin transplant, but the healing process failed. The figure shows the situation with some necrotic dark transplant remains and large areas of ulceration after three months of unsuccessful standard wound therapy.

The aim of treatment by now is to get wound healing going. Plasma medicine is indicated as curative treatment. Planar application of CAP is recommended.

◘ Figure 1.1b presents a clinical case of a poorly healing wound at the lower abdominal wall, caused by surgical site infection. This wound is of definitely a different morphology, being not large and flat, but like a crater, small and deep. Plasma medicine is urgently indicated as part of curative treatment to prevent further ingress of pathogens and peritonitis. Application of CAP in the depth of the crater demands a plasma jet.

◘ Figure 1.1c gives an example of a chronic and infected wound that is not urgently indicated for treatment by size or depth, but as a suppurative focus. As part of the pre-interventional management of major aseptic operations or immunosuppressive therapy, a suppurative focus should be cleared to prevent sepsis or a surgical site infection in the operation area. Clearing suppurative focuses can be a curative intervention for rheumatic diseases as well. CAP therapy is indicated for

---

1   For in-depth insight: Basic Principles of Treatment.
2   For in-depth insight: Chronic wounds; Surgical site infections.

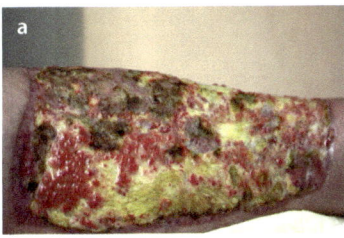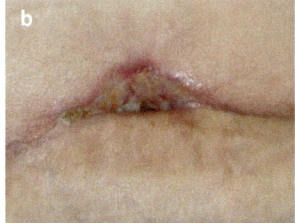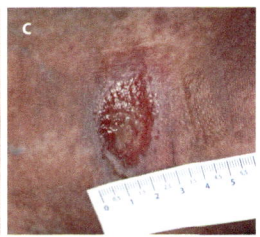

■ **Fig. 1.1**   **a** Chronic and infected wound, large area flat type. **b** Chronic and infected wound, crater type. **c** Chronic and infected wound as a possible suppurative focus

prevention, while being curative at the same time. CAP might be applied by jet or planar devices.

🛇 **Caution**

Make sure, if necessary by biopsy, not to mistake a skin cancer lesion for a wound with delayed healing.

1.2.2 Chronic Wounds, Not Infected[3]

The wound in ■ Fig. 1.2 has not been healing for three years. However, diagnostics of regular pathogenic microorganisms were negative, making an infection unlikely. The patient suffered from diabetic foot syndrome and lost his toes due to insufficient blood supply. Surgical amputation caused an open wound that was closed by displacement flap repair. Wound edges opened again because of still insufficient perfusion of the wound site's soft tissue and skin. Several standard procedures of wound treatment have failed.

Plasma medicine is indicated as another and innovative attempt at curative treatment.

1.2.3 Acute Wounds at Risk of Infection and Worsening[4]

The acute full-face wound in ■ Fig. 1.3 is a problem pathology of its own. It is a fresh wound resulting from laser skin ablation. The intention of this procedure is facial skin rejuvenation, a fully aesthetical and, therefore, extremely elective indication that cannot accept the slightest imperfection. The figure shows the typical wound situation three days after skin ablation. The wound is at risk of contamination and surgical site infection accompanied by pain and followed by absolutely unwanted scars.

The aim of treatment by now is to prevent infection. Plasma medicine is indicated as an acute and preventive treatment.

---

3   For in-depth insight: Chronic wounds. Surgical site at risk.
4   For in-depth insight: Acute wounds; Infected skin; Surgical site at risk; Aesthetic medicine.

1

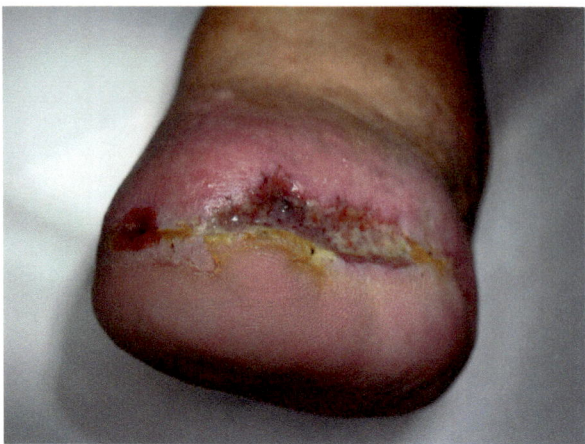

◘ **Fig. 1.2** Chronic and not infected wound

◘ Figure 1.3b is giving an example of an acute wound not caused by surgery or injury, but by constant bad conditions of the skin and soft tissue physiology. The visible skin lesion is a very common type of wound at the gluteal region, and a typical treatment problem mainly nurses are occupied with. The skin lesion is caused by permanent local pressure, for example, from long confinement to bed. Pressure reduces the blood perfusion, and skin cells and underlying tissue die off. The lesion is in danger of a decubital ulcer. Pressure relief is a main part of treatment, followed by keeping the wound free of pathogens and supporting re-epithelialization as soon as possible. Plasma medicine is indicated as a preventive treatment in combination with physiotherapy and mobilization of the patient.

1.2.4 Non-Healing Wounds by Other Reasons[5]

◘ Figure 1.4 is presenting a wound at the neck and cheek region, not resulting from surgery, laser impact injury, or pathophysiology of any kind, but from progress of cancer. Cancer cells of an advanced oral cavity carcinoma have infiltrated and destroyed the wall of the cheek. The ulceration is consisting of dead tissue heavily contaminated by pathogens. The rotting tissue causes a stench that is socially isolating the patient in his needy situation.

The patient is receiving full scope palliative care. The aim of treatment by now is to reduce the anaerobic pathogens responsible for bad odor, pain, and risk of sepsis. Plasma medicine is indicated as supplementary palliative treatment.

---

5   For in-depth insight: Contaminated cancer ulcerations.

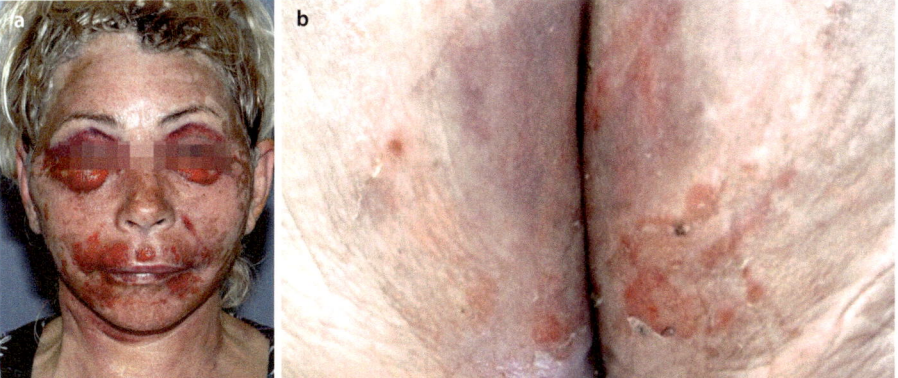

■ **Fig. 1.3** **a** Acute wound by surgery (Parts of this figure have been published in: Comprehensive Clinical Plasma Medicine – Cold Physical Plasma for Medical Application, Springer 2018, p. 356). **b** Acute wound by pathophysiology

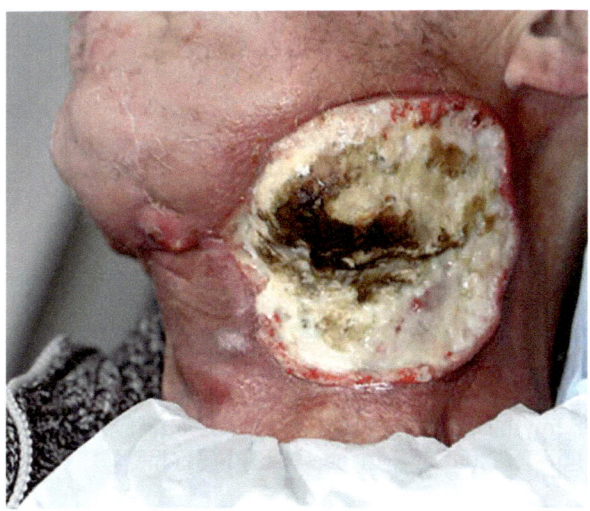

■ **Fig. 1.4** Cancer ulceration. (Parts of this figure have been published in: Comprehensive Clinical Plasma Medicine – Cold Physical Plasma for Medical Application, Springer 2018, p. 187)

1.2.5 Infected Skin[6]

■ Figure 1.5 is presenting a case of infected skin. Canker sores or aphthae do not mean a particular danger like the cases above, but a very nasty burden and restriction of well-being. They trigger a stabbing pain by the slightest touch, for example, during eating, and they do not heal easily.

---

6   For in-depth insight: Infected skin; Infected mucosa.

1

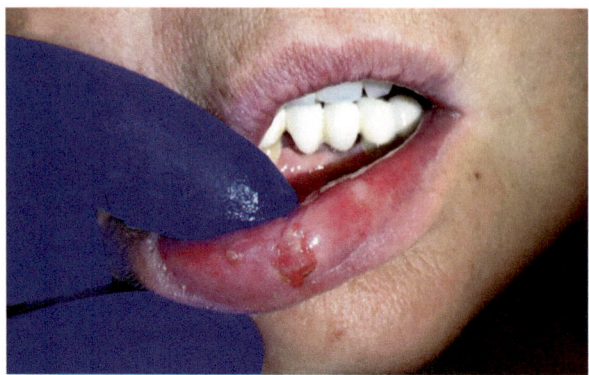

◻ Fig. 1.5 Infected skin lesion. (Parts of this figure have been published in: Der MKG-Chirurg. Klinik und Praxis der Plasmamedizin, Springer 2016, p. 264)

The aim of treatment by now is to reduce causal viruses and bacteria, to relieve pain, and to condition fast recovery of the mucosa. Plasma medicine is indicated as acute treatment.

❯ Important to know
CAP is medically prescribed for chronic and infected wounds, wounds with standstill of healing but no infection, acute wounds at high risk of infection, skin lesions at risk of serious progression, non-healing wounds by other reasons and skin with certain local infections and purulent focuses.

1.3   To Apply Clinical Plasma Research[7]

Good clinical practice requires an insight in current research to stay informed about the state of the art in clinical plasma medicine. This section is intended to lay the foundations for the understanding of plasma effects and mode of action of plasma medical devices and of evidence-based medicine.

1.3.1   Mode of Action[8]

Plasma medicine is exploiting physical plasmas that generate temperature not higher than 40 °C at the target site of treatment [1–5], which enables manipulation of living cells without thermal damage. The mode of action amounts to a leap innovation: physical energy generates ionized gas, this plasma cocktail induces biochemical reactions, the resulting molecules are controlling living human as well as

---

7   For in-depth insight: Concept.
8   For in-depth insight: What's this, cold physical plasma? How does plasma work in medicine? How safe is clinical plasma medicine?

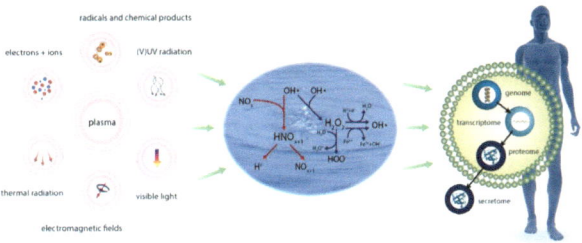

Fig. 1.6 Mode of action of plasma medicine in general [7]

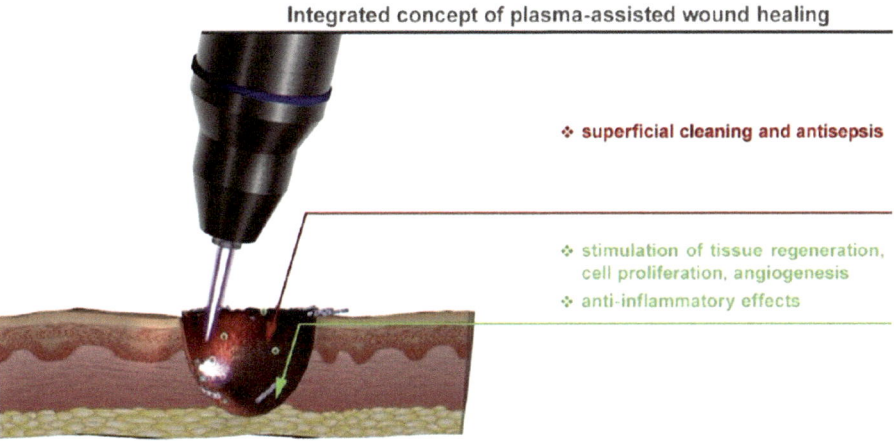

Fig. 1.7 Mode of action of plasma medicine in wound healing [7]

microbial cells [6], giving way to utilization for medical purposes as illustrated schematically in ◘ Fig. 1.6.

Plasma-assisted wound healing builds upon a two-step activity of CAP: antisepsis at the wound surface in combination with direct stimulation of tissue regeneration and microcirculation (◘ Fig. 1.7) [6, 8–13].

Any enhanced risk of genotoxic and mutagenic effects of CAP treatments has been excluded by well-established in vitro tests as well as by a long-term animal trial and long-term clinical observations [14–22].

1.3.1.1 Chronic Wounds

In the beginning, clinical plasma research was dealing with chronic wounds [23–24]. First clinical trials on the treatment of chronic ulcers have proven the plasma effect mainly on the reduction of bacterial load on wounds [25–29], then again, further clinical trials and animal studies have demonstrated a clear stimulating effect on wound healing independent of antisepsis.

1

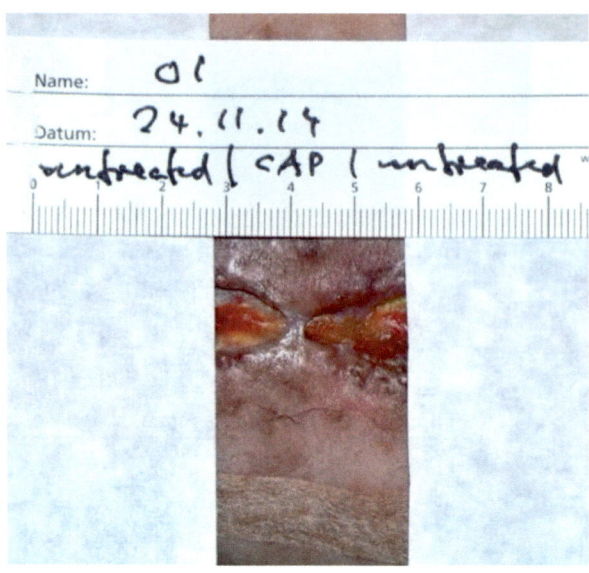

Name: O (

Datum: 24. 11. 14

            untreated | CAP | untreated "

Fig. 1.8 Chronic wound and effect of experimental plasma application. (This figure has been published in: Der MKG-Chirurg. Klinik und Praxis der Plasmamedizin, Springer 2016, p. 256)

To give an example, ▪ Fig. 1.8 shows a small part of a chronic wound with a history of unsuccessful standard treatment for months. Now, this open wound was treated experimentally with CAP in a middle strip ("CAP"), while the left and right side were left without plasma application ("untreated"). It is clearly visible that continuous local CAP treatment has stimulated a significant local healing effect, a scar-like bridge of skin between the gaping wound edges.

1.3.1.2 Acute Wounds

Cold plasma (CAP) is also effective in acute wounds of skin and mucosa. [14, 29–33].

CAP is in use to support healing of acute surgical wounds in cases where, for example, the patient's difficult health-status, biographic conditions, or medication push the risk of problem wounds [34]. The impact of acceleration of acute wound healing on scar formation is proven [14]. Together with possible preventive effects on wound infection, CAP treatment is a promising option to control the risk of surgical site infections in the field of plastic surgery and aesthetic medicine [35].

To give an example, ▪ Fig. 1.9 presents four acute adjacent experimental skin lesions at the same area (lower arm), of the same origin (ablative laser application ten days ago), same size ($1 cm^2$), and the same patient. The lesion in the lower right field remained untreated. The lesion in the upper right field received a short-time plasma application for one day (10 sec.). The lesion in the upper left field was

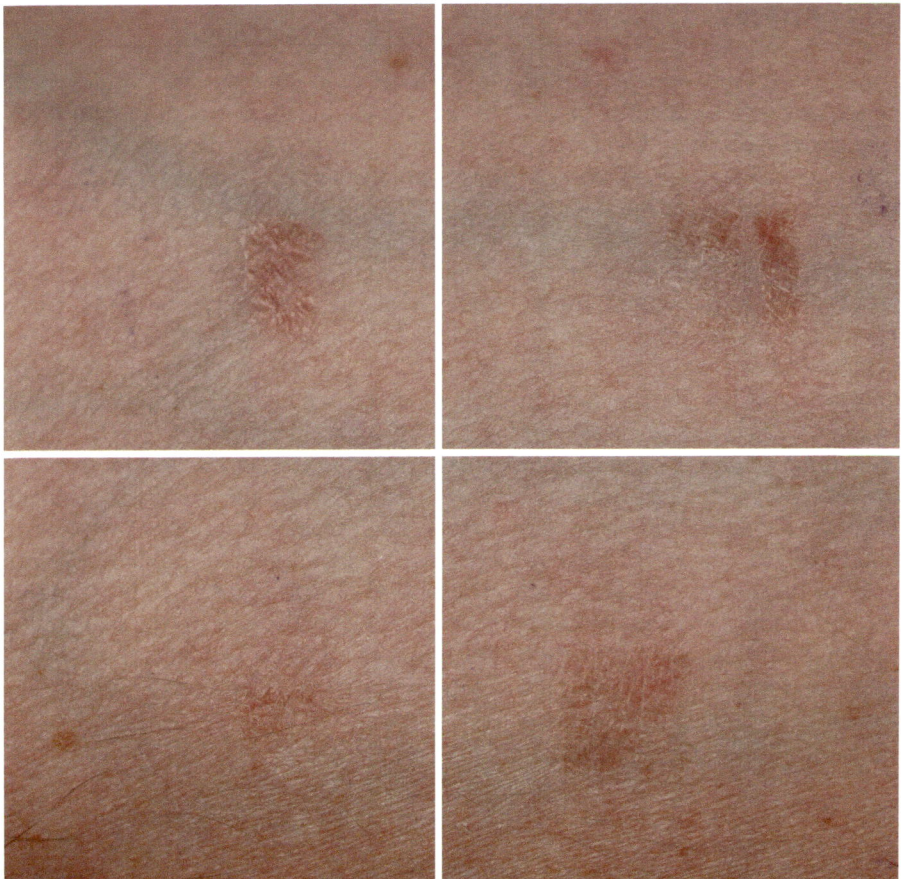

◘ **Fig. 1.9** Acute wound and effect of experimental plasma application

treated with long-time single plasma application (30 sec.). The lesion in the lower left field received a repeated short-time plasma treatment for three days with 10 sec. Every day. The figure represents the outcome of wound recovery after ten days of healing. It is quite obvious that the repeated plasma treatment with short single doses obtained the best result in terms of re-epithelialization and aesthetics.

Beyond wound healing as the most investigated CAP application in the clinical context, plasma devices are also used in the treatment of infective and inflammatory skin and mucosa diseases, like herpes zoster, atopic eczema, acne, athlete's foot, and others [28, 33, 36–40].

> **Important to know**
> From a clinical point of view, the direct combination of wound antisepsis with a stimulating effect on tissue regeneration is like a unique selling proposition of CAP in comparison to conventional and established wound care measures.

1

1.3.2 Approved Medical Devices[9]

Among the huge spectrum of technologies to generate cold plasma at atmospheric conditions, two basic types of CAP devices are dominating clinical plasma medicine: dielectric barrier discharges (DBD) and plasma jets. Usually driven by a high-frequency voltage or microwave power, atmospheric air, noble gases (argon, helium), as well as gas mixtures are used as working gases for plasma generation [5, 41–42].

Medical plasma devices for clinical application are the argon-driven HF plasma jet *kINPen® MED* (neoplas tools GmbH, Greifswald, Germany), the argon-driven microwave plasma torch SteriPlas (ADTEC, Hounslow, UK), the DBD-based devices *PlasmaDerm FLEX* and *Dress* (CINOGY GmbH, Duderstadt, Germany) and *plasma care®* (terraplasma medical GmbH, Garching, Germany), the latter two using atmospheric air as working gas. Their specific purpose is the treatment of chronic wounds as well as pathogen-associated skin diseases. Besides their CE certification as medical devices class-IIa according to the European Council Directive 93/42/EEC, all these devices are distinguished by comprehensive physical and biological characterization of the respective plasma source accompanied with detailed preclinical and clinical investigations [41–43]. ◘ Figure 1.10 is presenting the two medical plasma devices approved in 2013 as the first on the market. Jet plasma technology (left side) is recommended especially for wound craters, rugged tissue, and intraorally. Planar plasma technology (right side) is convenient for the treatment of large and flat areas.

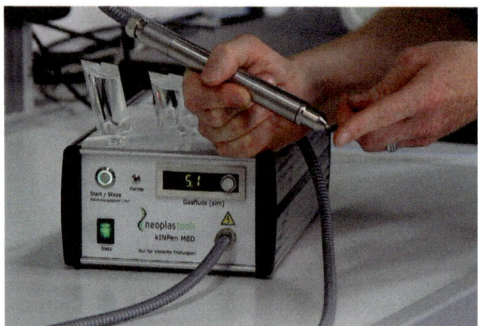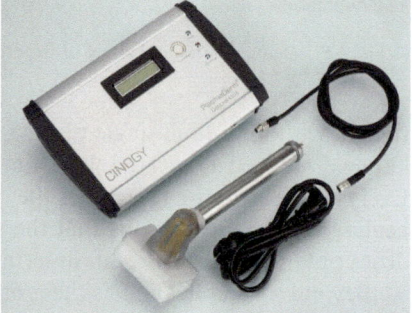

◘ **Fig. 1.10** The plasma jet kINPen® MED by Neoplas tools GmbH, Greifswald (left) and the DBD plasma source PlasmaDerm by Cynogy GmbH Duderstadt (right). (These figures have been published in: Comprehensive Clinical Plasma Medicine – Cold Physical Plasma for Medical Application, Springer 2018, p. 140)

---

9   For in-depth insight: Devices; Approved, unauthorized and fake plasma devices; Choice of plasma devices; What are the requirements of a plasma medicine clinic?

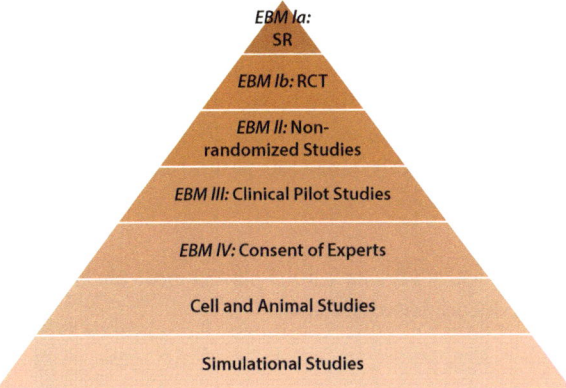

Fig. 1.11 Pyramid of evidence-based medicine (EBM) [U.S. Agency for Health Care Policy and Research 1992]

⏻ Caution
Good clinical practice insists on plasma devices that are distinguished by comprehensive physical and biological characterization of the respective plasma source accompanied by detailed preclinical and clinical investigations.

1.3.3 Evidence-Based Medicine[10]

Good clinical practice committed to quality is exercising effective and safe treatment procedures and employing well-trained staff. The scientific and expertise-based quality of a treatment concept according to Sackett [44] can be evaluated by the levels of evidence-based Medicine (EBM) (■ Fig. 1.11):

Introducing an innovative therapy like plasma medicine to be fully recognized as EBM has to start with simulation studies and investigations in cell cultures and animals (EBM-basic level), leading in summary to a consent of experts (EBM-level 4). This is giving way to clinical pilot studies (EBM-level 3) and non-randomized studies (EBM-level 2). The top-level of EBM-quality is reached with successfully evaluated randomized clinical trials (EBM-level 1b), concluded by a structured review and positive meta-analysis (EBM-level 1a).

Climbing up the pyramid from the basic level, genotoxic and mutagenic risks of plasma treatment could be excluded by several in vitro tests as well as by a long-term animal trial [15–21].

Corresponding to EBM-level 4, plasma devices are implemented by consent of scientific experts and medical practitioners in hospitals and private practices for the clinical treatment of wounds [6, 14, 26–29, 31–32, 35] as well as of infective and

---

10 For in-depth insight: How does plasma work in medicine? How safe is plasma medicine? How to assure good clinical practice.

1

inflammatory skin diseases like herpes zoster, atopic eczema, acne, athlete's foot, and others [28, 36–40].

Corresponding to EBM-level 3 and 2, clinical pilot studies and non-randomized on the treatment of chronic ulcers have proven the plasma effect by keeping an eye on the reduction of bacterial load on wounds [26–28]. Further clinical studies have demonstrated a clear stimulating effect on wound healing that is independent of antisepsis [14, 29, 31–32].

> **Important to know**
> First randomized clinical studies have lifted plasma medicine at present to the doorstep of level 1 of Evidence-based Medicine.

1.4   To Identify Wounds at Risk[11]

Good clinical practice includes the prognostic assessment of wound healing by identification of risk factors.

Medical evidence of poor healing or proof of pathogens leads to an easy assessment and a clear indication for curative or palliative CAP therapy.

Acute wounds, however, are difficult to assess in terms of healing prognosis and need for preventive plasma therapy. On principle, acute and well-handled surgical or traumatic wounds do not need additional targeted treatment because they are healing on their own under normal conditions. Nevertheless, there are some risk factors influencing healing conditions unfavorably and able to cause retarded healing time associated with infection and, for example, unwanted scarring.

1.4.1   Normal Healing Capability of Acute Wounds[12]

The most lifelike model to investigate clinical wound healing capability is the acute wound resulting from skin grafting [45–46]. The method is a common and standardized surgical shaving off the skin by a slicer (◘ Fig. 1.12) to gain a free transplant for reconstructive surgery.

The acute wound at the donor site of the transplant is standardized and reproducible for study protocols. Progress of wound healing can be easily observed and documented day by day with every change of dressings. ◘ Figure 1.13 is presenting the fresh wound still bleeding (left side) and the wound after 14 days of healing with the epithelial barrier 95% restored (right side).

The cumulative wound healing capability of 198 patients is given in ◘ Fig. 1.14 as a calibration curve of the standard time to wound closure [47]. The curve indicates how many of the wounds are already closed at certain days, running from no wound closed at day 0 to nearly all wounds closed at day 28.

---

11 For in-depth insight: Treatment Tailored to Indications.
12 For in-depth insight: Selection of patients; Surgical site at risk; Artificial fistula at risk; Aesthetic medicine; Dental aesthetics.

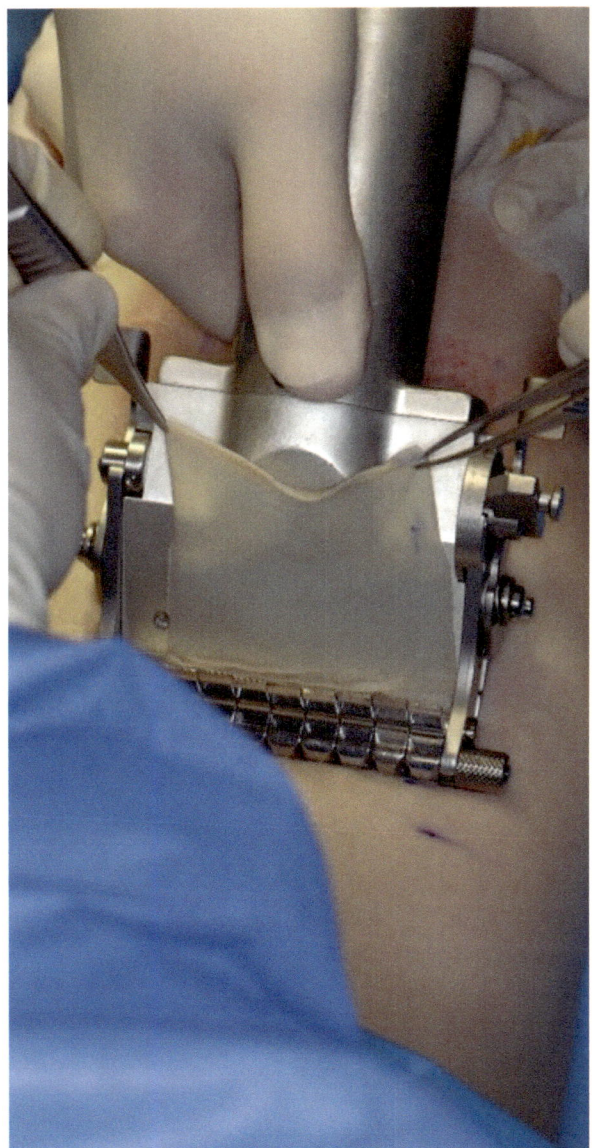

◘ Fig. 1.12   Generating an acute wound by harvesting a skin transplant

Completion of wound closure is taking at least about 7 days. In 50% of the patients, wound closure has been completed after 14 days of healing (◘ Fig. 1.13). Less than 5% of patients suffer from still incomplete wound closure after 28 days. They have to be considered at certain risk of chronic or non-healing wounds.

1

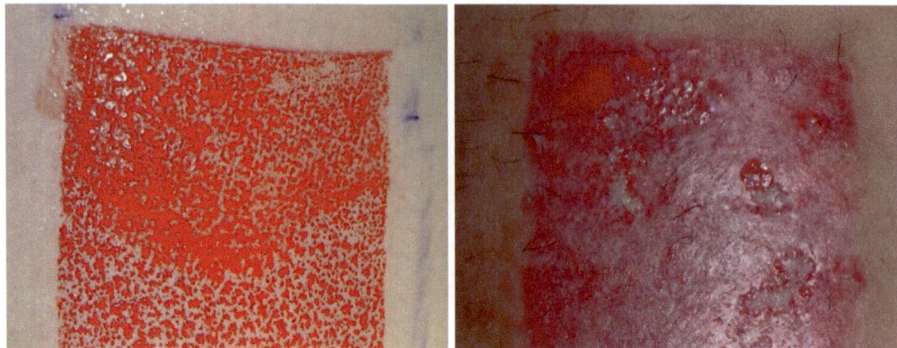

Fig. 1.13 Acute donor site wound, initial situation (left) and result after 14 days of healing without targeted treatment (right)

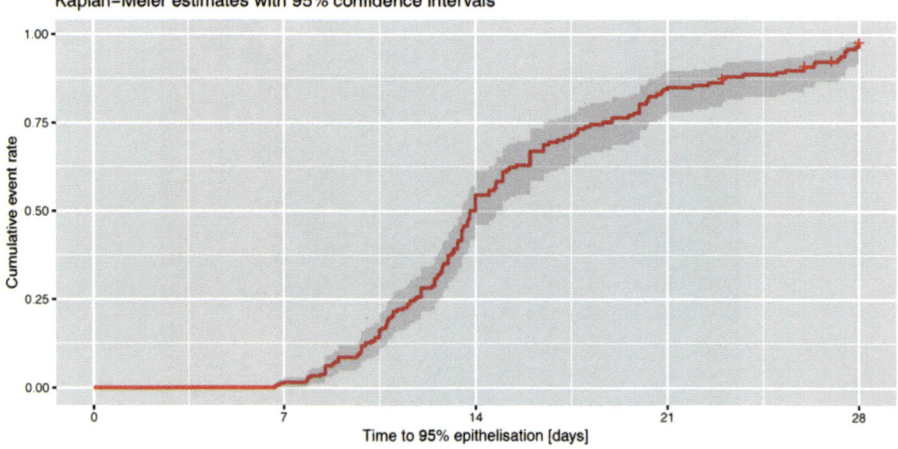

Kaplan–Meier estimates with 95% confidence intervals

Fig. 1.14 Normal distribution of wound healing capability [47]

> **Important to know**
> Patients with wounds still not closed after 28 days are at risk of poor healing and should be regarded from the perspective of plasma medicine.

1.4.2 Wound Healing Capability and Age[13]

When relating wound healing to age, wound closure is completed in 50% of adult patients by day 11 to 12, in middle-aged patients by day 13, and in elderly patients only after 18 days. Wound healing is significantly retarded with increasing age (**Fig. 1.15**).

---

13 For in-depth insight: Selection of patients; Surgical site at risk; Artificial fistula at risk; Aesthetic medicine; Dental aesthetics.

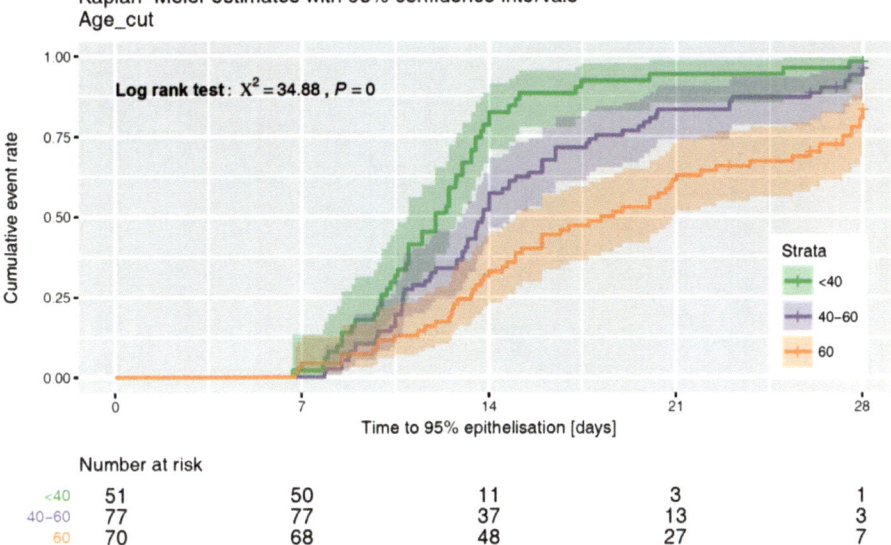

● **Fig. 1.15** Age-related time to wound closure [47]

Delayed wound healing in elder patients is due to the genetic constellation and hormone levels, as well as the relatively longer exposition to risk factors such as sun or smoke. While concomitant diseases and malnutrition are relevant conditions for retardation of wound closure, age over 60 years is an independent risk factor [48]. Retardation of wound healing does not implicate a worse quality of wound healing in the long run [49]. Differences in the early phases of tissue repair may be compensated in later stages [48].

In 15% of elderly patients, wound closure is not completed after 28 days of healing. Retardation of tissue repair mainly in elderly patients increases the risk of infection, immobilization, dehydration, and sometimes lethal outcome.

❯ **Important to know**

Patients with age over 60 years and wounds not closed after 28 days belong to the at-risk group of poorly healing wounds and might benefit from plasma medicine.

1.4.3 Wound Healing Capability and Gender[14]

Female gender in general seems to be a risk factor for prolonged and incomplete wound closure. However, women in the age of childbearing potential heal significantly faster than males in general (● Fig. 1.16).

---

14 For in-depth insight: Selection of patients; Surgical site at risk; Artificial fistula at risk; Aesthetic medicine; Dental aesthetics.

1

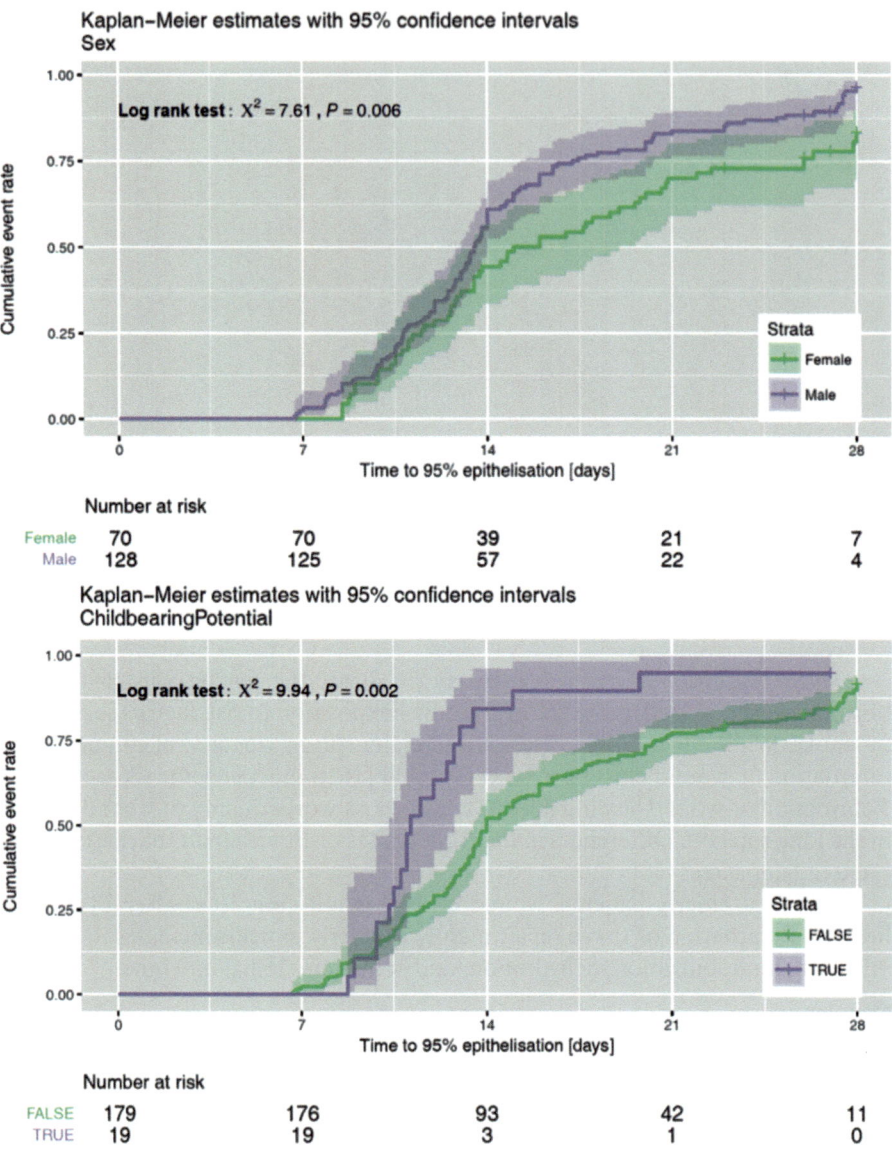

● **Fig. 1.16** Gender-related time to wound closure (left), and the influence of childbearing potential (right) [47]

This phenomenon is widely attributed to the effect of estrogen, which is signifi-cant for the production of growth factors, cell migration, and proliferation [50–53]. Various studies have shown that it hastens healing processes [54]. The decreased level of estrogen in post-menopausal women simultaneously explains the faster wound healing in younger and fertile women.

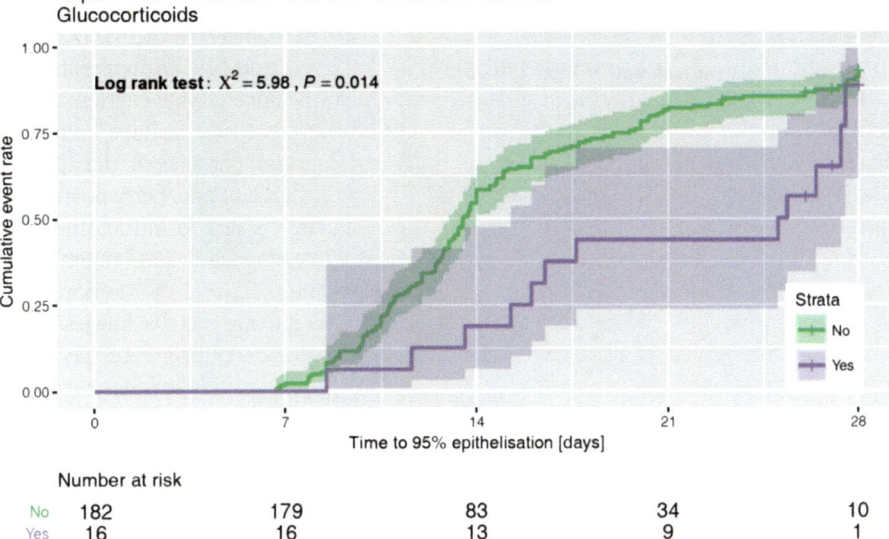

● **Fig. 1.17** Time to wound closure undergoing treatment with glucocorticoids [47]

> ❯ **Important to know**
> Women after menopause belong to an at-risk group with poorly healing wounds and should be considered for preventive plasma treatment.

1.4.4 **Wound Healing Capability and Concomitant Steroid Therapy[15]**

Wound patients with systemic steroid medication are not in danger of incomplete healing within 28 days, but healing seems to be apparently retarded (● Fig. 1.17).

The retardation is dose- and duration-dependent [55]. Glucocorticoids dampen the expression of cytokines, such as TGF-β, TNF, platelet-derived growth factor, and keratinocyte growth factor, in the early phase of inflammation and proliferation [55–56] and adversely affect collagen turnover [57–58] and accumulation therewith, reducing tensile strength [56].

> ❯ **Important to know**
> Wound patients with systemic steroid medication are at increased risk of retarded healing with intervening infection, and are therefore suitable candidates for preventive plasma medicine.

15 For in-depth insight: Selection of patients; Surgical site at risk; Artificial fistula at risk; Aesthetic medicine; Dental aesthetics.

1

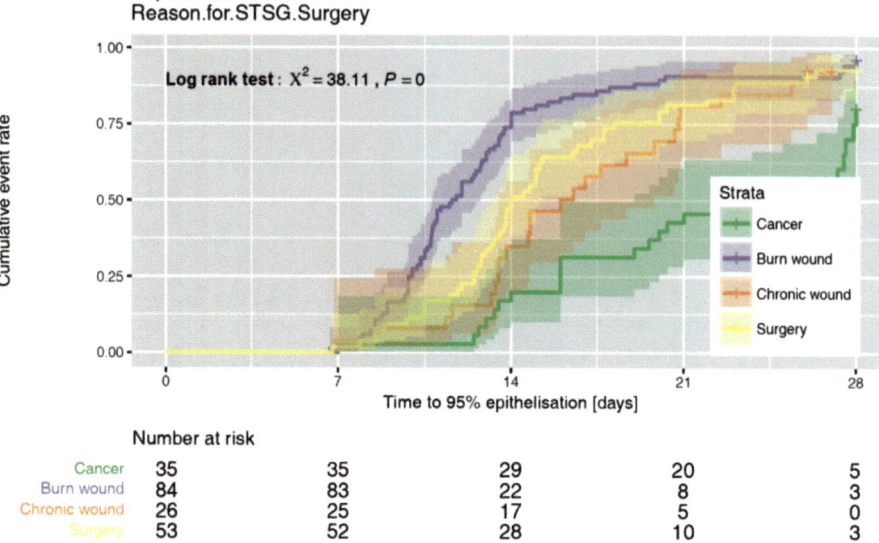

● **Fig. 1.18** Time to wound closure with a history of cancer, burns, chronic wounds and surgery [47]

1.4.5 Wound Healing Capability and Cancer[16]

Cancer patients show a very poor healing capability; 25% of them do not reach complete wound closure within 28 days. A history of previous chronic wounds predicts self-evidently further wound healing problems (● Fig. 1.18).

Immunosuppression, that is, immunosuppressive cancer medication, delays wound healing [59]. Impaired wound healing in malignant diseases can also arise from losses of bone marrow due to metastases. Radiotherapy is often named as a cancer-associated factor that leads to impaired wound healing [60–61].

❯ **Important to know**
   Patients with cancer or a history of previous impaired wound healing are obvious candidates for plasma medicine.

1.5 To Act in Concert with the Patient[17]

Good clinical practice is based on a qualified plasma medicine team and a well-organized plasma medicine clinic. An essential part of therapy is a balanced relationship with the patient. Plasma medicine treatment requires, as does every medical intervention, extensive information regarding the patient and consent to undergo

---

16 For in-depth insight: Selection of patients; Surgical site at risk; Artificial fistula at risk; Aesthetic medicine; Dental aesthetics.
17 For in-depth insight: How does plasma work in medicine? How safe is clinical plasma medicine? General aspects of treatment; Handling of complications.

the treatment. Most patients, for the time being, are not familiar with the innovative treatment opportunity. They have some frequently asked questions (☐ Table 1.1).

— Is clinical efficacy proven?

There is a number of plasma sources with detailed preclinical and clinical investigations to prove efficacy and with comprehensive physical and biological characterization. Their application for treatment purposes is authorized by CE certification as medical devices class IIa according to the European Council Directive 93/42/ EEC. They are approved for the treatment of chronic wounds and pathogen-associated skin diseases. First randomized clinical studies have lifted plasma medicine at present to the doorstep of level 1 of Evidence-based Medicine.

These plasma devices include, for example, the plasma jet kINPen MED, the DBD-based PlasmaDerm, the plasma torch SteriPlas, and the DBD-based plasma care.

These plasma devices do not include several other sources on the market that are offered to be useful for "plasma medicine," but have no or very inadequate physical, technical, biological, or clinical references that could prove this.

— No undesirable local or systemic side effects?

Approved plasma devices are in clinical use since 2013. There are no case observations or clinical studies available in the literature reporting severe side effects of any kind, including carcinogenesis or genetic damage.

Slight local effects have to be considered like a minor pinprick or irritation of hypersensitive dental neck areas related to the tip of the plasma plume when using plasma jets. In very rare cases and unclear connection, a brief and mild redness of the skin following unintended touch might occur.

— Medical effect reliable?

☐ Table 1.1	Ten questions to be solved individually before the start of treatment
1	Clinical efficacy proven?
2	No undesirable local or systemic side effects? (mutagenic, carcinogenic, toxic effects; pains, scars, pigmentation disorders…)
3	Medical effect reliable?
4	Medical effect well controllable?
5	Quick medical effect?
6	No development of resistances when treating infectious diseases as well as co-treating resident flora?
7	No inhibitory effect on normal flora?
8	Cost-effective?
9	No alternative solution (could it be done easier?)
10	High acceptance?

1

The effectiveness of CAP in wound healing and treatment of infected skin is well documented, but there are always a couple of patients not enjoying positive treatment results for unknown reasons. Especially in problem wounds, patients have to know that plasma medicine plays an important role, but is not the only player. Steady debridement, good dressings, restoration and perfusion of vessels, lymphatic drainage, and keeping relevant co-morbidities under control are important as well.

- Medical effect well controllable?

The medical effect at least in wound healing is easily controllable by measuring the re-epithelialization and shrinking of the wound surface. On-going photo documentation is important. Documents should include scale and date and follow the very basic requirements of scientific medical photography.

- Quick medical effect?

Wound healing is never quick. Patients have to know that it takes stamina by all persons involved and sometimes many weeks of repeated treatment to reach a reasonable result.

- No development of resistances when treating infectious diseases as well as co-treating resident flora?

One of the significant advantages of plasma medicine in comparison with other anti-microbial therapies is the in vitro and clinically observed wide susceptibility of multi-resistant skin and wound pathogens against planar plasma as well as jet plasma. From the opposite point of view, the development of resistances when treating pathogens with plasma has never been described either in clinical cases and studies or in pre-clinical and basic research.

- No inhibitory effect on normal flora?

Jet plasma devices are able to direct the plume precisely to the surface and extension of wounds and do not touch significantly unaffected skin and normal flora. Medical devices with a precast planar plasma source may have an overlapping field of action affecting skin with normal flora. However, in principle, there are no case reports or pre-clinical and basic research studies mentioning a problem of normal flora in clinical plasma medicine.

- Cost-effective?

A correct answer requires treatment-related economic and organizational studies and comparative analyses to standard procedures. There are no recent study results available for plasma medicine.

Clinical experience shows that material consumption does not cost much. However, staff costs are noteworthy because the treatment might be time-consuming due to the complexity and size of wounds and the optimal number of treatments. Several case reports mention a faster overall healing and shortening hospitalization by one quarter. The purchase price of medical plasma devices varies considerably, but is always well below medical laser devices.

- No alternative solution (could it be done easier)?

Patients suffering from problem wounds have usually experience with a lot of alternative but fruitless solutions. They do not ask whether it could be done easier. The question is, can it be done effectively?

— High acceptance?

By common clinical experience, patients are usually very grateful and appreciative for plasma medicine as an innovative and pleasant treatment procedure. However, there are no studies available in present literature dealing with a socio-medical and health economy view of this kind.

> ⓘ Caution
> An innovative treatment like cold plasma medicine (CAP) requires extended information of the patient.

1.6 To Evaluate Treatment[18]

Good clinical practice means to complete the therapy with evaluation and debriefing. The wound healing effectiveness of CAP is dependable, in some patients exceptional, as demonstrated in this section. However, there are always patients to keep in mind with insufficient treatment results for unknown reasons. Especially in chronic wounds, patients have to know that plasma medicine plays an important role, but is not the only player. Continuous debridement, proper wound dressings, and keeping relevant co-morbidities and current medication under control are important as well.

1.6.1 Chronic and Infected Wounds[19]

The case of this patient is known from <2.1>. The male patient belongs to the age group >60 and brings in a previous history of chronic wounds and current immunosuppressive medication.

After several months of unsuccessful standard wound therapy, the procedure changed to plasma medicine as a key component of treatment. ◘ Figure 1.19 allows a comparison of the wound situation before (◘ Fig. 1.22, left) and after two months of adding CAP application by jet plasma to the standard practice of cleaning or scraping away of dead cells and contaminated tissue out of a wound (◘ Fig. 1.22, right): The surface of the wound is covered by an almost completed layer of epithelial skin cells. The barrier of the skin is closed again.

The patient is very pleased with the result and feels confident for full recovery of the skin. CAP therapy has to continue. The patient still belongs to several risk groups of poor wound healing.

---

18 For in-depth insight: Treatment Tailored to Indications.
19 For in-depth insight: Chronic wounds; Surgical site infections.

1

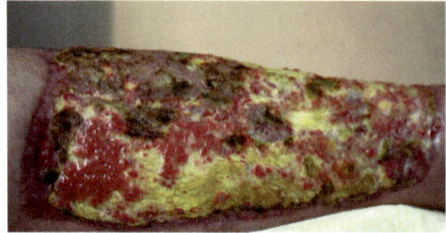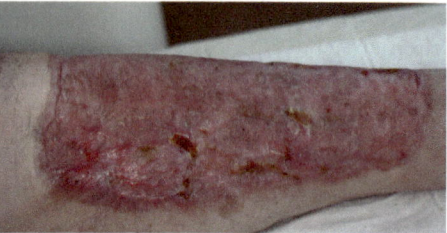

⬛ **Fig. 1.19** Chronic and infected wound, initial situation (left) and the result of CAP therapy (right)

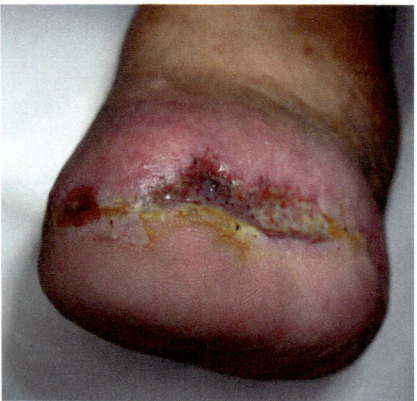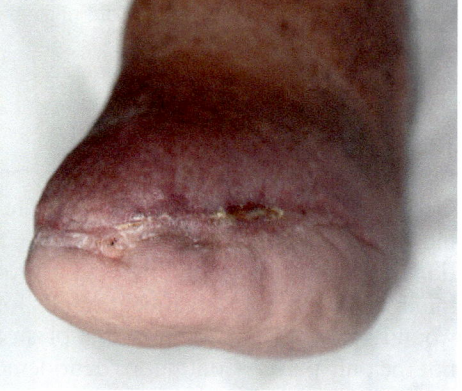

⬛ **Fig. 1.20** Chronic and not infected wound, initial situation (left) and the result of CAP therapy (right)

1.6.2 Non-Healing Wounds, Not Infected[20]

The case of this patient is known from <2.2>. The male patient belongs to the age group >60 and brings in a previous history of diabetes, chronic wounds, and current immunosuppressive medication.

Even though the area of the wound is smaller (⬛ Fig. 1.20, right) in comparison with the previous situation (⬛ Fig. 1.20, left), the edges are gapping after a long period of steady plasma treatment. The patient is still a diabetic with non-optimal medication. When carried out as standard procedures of wound treatment before, plasma therapy failed to some extent. This case exemplifies that plasma medicine plays an important role in wound healing, but is not the only player. Keeping an eye on relevant co-morbidities is important as well.

> **Tip**
>
> CAP no-touch-treatment is reducing the risk of unintentional injuries in numb wound areas typical for diabetic feet.

20 For in-depth insight: Chronic wounds; Surgical site at risk.

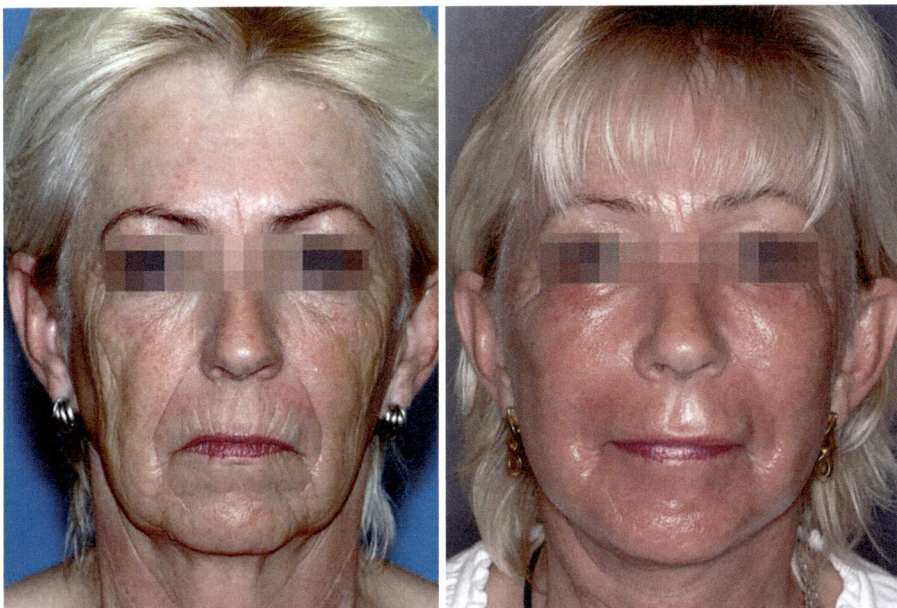

🔲 **Fig. 1.21** Acute wound, initial situation (left) and the result of CAP therapy (right). (Parts of this figure have been published in: Comprehensive Clinical Plasma Medicine – Cold Physical Plasma for Medical Application, Springer 2018, p. 356)

The patient accepts the result as the best possible outcome and values the benefit of less nursing care required. CAP therapy might go on to prevent late infection and to fight clinical worsening since the patient belongs to several risk groups associated with poor healing.

1.6.3 Acute Wounds at Risk of Infection and Worsening[21]

The case of this patient is known from <2.3>. The female patient belongs to the age group 40–60 years and is free of relevant co-morbidities or current medication.

The acute full-face wound resulting from recent laser skin ablation has been treated preventively for three days with CAP. 🔲 Figure 1.21 allows a comparison of the wound early after laser skin resurfacing (🔲 Fig. 1.21, left) and 22 days later (🔲 Fig. 1.21, right). Wound healing has proceeded in the typical time pattern without signs of disturbance. The skin is closed. The thread of infection and unwanted scars in aesthetic medicine is gone.

The patient is obviously very pleased with the undisturbed wound healing and the aesthetic outcome. Preventive CAP therapy was completed.

---

21 For in-depth insight: Acute wounds; Surgical site at risk; Aesthetic medicine.

1

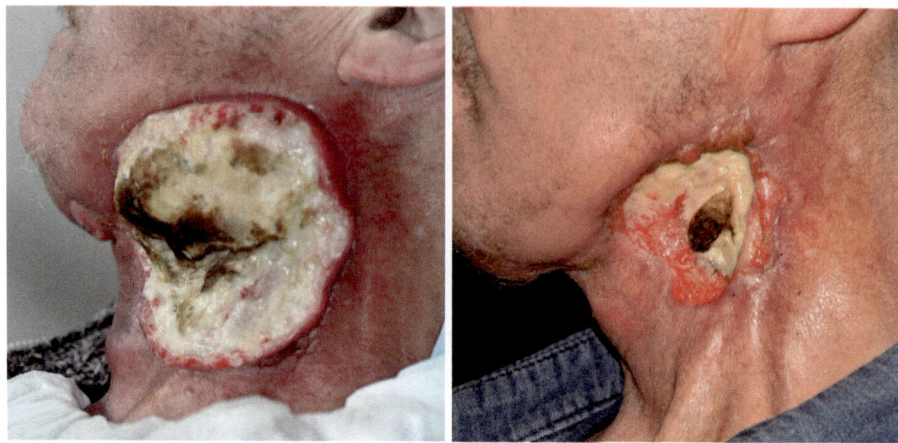

◘ Fig. 1.22   Cancer ulceration, initial situation (left) and the result of CAP therapy (right). (Parts of this figure have been published in: Comprehensive Clinical Plasma Medicine – Cold Physical Plasma for Medical Application, Springer 2018, p. 187)

1.6.4 Non-Healing Wounds by Other Reasons[22]

The case of this patient is known from <2.4>. The male patient belongs to the age group 40–60 years, suffers from cancer, and brings in current immunosuppressive medication.

Cancer ulcerations are problem wounds because of constantly growing malignant cells at the bottom and at the edges, and especially in certain areas of the body like the head and neck because of heavy contamination by pathogens. There is no chance for curative cancer treatment, that means healing of the disease. The aim of treatment in terms of benefit for the patient is palliative care to reduce the burden of the disease as long and as much as possible. Quality of life suffers from a socially isolating stench of rotten tissue, anaerobic microbial pathogens, and tumor cell debris. The patient has been treated continuously with CAP to reduce the pathogens.

◘ Figure 1.22 shows the tumor situation at the beginning of treatment (◘ Fig. 1.22, left) and after four months of steady and continuous CAP application (◘ Fig. 1.22, right). The treatment goal of palliation is achieved by eliminating the stench and reducing the pain. Furthermore, we can observe a remarkable shrinking of the tumor size suggesting a direct or indirect cancer cell reaction to plasma.

The patient has been very pleased about the absence of odor and pain and the shrinking of the tumor ulceration, but he passed away by cancer relapse nine months later.

---

22 For in-depth insight: Contaminated cancer ulcerations.

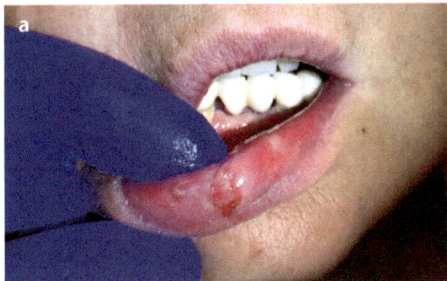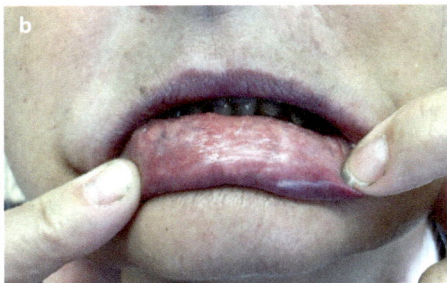

■ **Fig. 1.23**   Infected skin lesion, initial situation **a** and the result of CAP therapy **b** (This figure have been published in: Der MKG-Chirurg, Klinik und Praxis der Plasmamedizin, Springer 2016, p. 264)

1.6.5 Infected Skin[23]

The case of this patient is known from <2.5>. The male patient belongs to the age group <40 years and has no co-morbidities or medication.

The painful and easily bleeding lesion of the skin (■ Fig. 1.23a) is caused by local conditions and pathogens obviously sensitive to CAP application. Curative treatment of the wound took place only a few times and resulted in complete healing (■ Fig. 1.23b).

The patient is very pleased with the result and free of pain. CAP therapy was completed.

1.7 Conclusion

The benefit of patients is the main intention of medicine and good clinical practice. CAP therapy has found its way into good clinical practice. Plasma medicine is indicated for chronic and infected wounds, suppurative focuses, wounds with a standstill of healing, but no infection, acute wounds at high risk of infection, skin lesions at risk of serious progression, non-healing wounds by other reasons, and skin and mucosa with certain local infections.

Plasma medical devices exploit a leap innovation. Physical energy generates biochemical control of living human as well as microbial cells, giving way to utilization for medical purposes, for example, wound antisepsis combined with stimulation of soft tissue and skin. From a clinical point of view, this bivalent functionality is a unique selling proposition of plasma medical devices in comparison to conventional and established wound care measures.

Current research is extending the range of indications, for example, to cancer treatment and prevention of virus infections. Clinical plasma medicine will take the way of becoming a new specialty for physicians. Certain criteria are already coming about: an innovative area of expertise not covered by just one established

23 For in-depth insight: Infected skin Infected mucosa

discipline in medicine; a continuous growth of independent scientific and clinical research output; established national and international organizational bodies to serve the global scientific community; graduate and post-graduate university courses and specialist training; autonomous development of treatment guidelines on behalf of the Council of the Scientific Medical Societies in Germany; and last but not least, own scientific literature like the present textbook.

References

1. Stoffels E, Kieft IE, Sladek REJ, van der Laan EP, Slaaf DW. Gas plasma treatment: a new approach to surgery? Crit Rev Biomedical Engineering. 2004;32:427–60.
2. Fridman G, Friedman G, Gutsol A, Shekhter AB, Vasilets VN, Fridman A. Applied plasma medicine. Plasma Process Polym. 2008;5:503–33.
3. Laroussi M. Low-temperature plasmas for medicine? IEEE Transactions Plasma Scien. 2009;37:714–25.
4. Kong MG, Kroesen G, Morfill G, Nosenko T, Shimizu T, van Dijk J, Zimmermann JL. Plasma medicine: an introductory review. New J Phys. 2009;11:115012.
5. Weltmann KD, Kindel E, von Woedtke T, Haehnel M, Stieber M, Brandenburg R. Atmospheric-pressure plasma sources: prospective tools for plasma medicine. Pure Appl Chem. 2010;82:1223–37.
6. von Woedtke T, Schmidt A, Bekeschus S, Wende K, Weltmann KD. Plasma medicine: a field of applied redox biology. In Vivo. 2019;33:1011–26.
7. von Woedtke T, Schmidt A, Bekeschus S, Wende K. Introduction to plasma medicine. In: Metelmann HR, von Woedtke T, Weltmann KD, editors. Comprehensive clinical plasma medicine - cold physical plasma for medical application. Berlin, Heidelberg: Springer; 2018. p. 3–21.
8. Heuer K, Hoffmanns MA, Demir E, Baldus S, Volkmar CM, Röhle M, Fuchs PC, Awakowicz P, Suschek CV, Opländer C. The topical use of non-thermal dielectric barrier discharge (DBD): nitric oxide related effects on human skin. Nitric Oxide. 2015;44:52–60.
9. Kisch T, Helmke A, Schleusser S, Song J, Liodaki E, Stang FH, Mailaender P, Kraemer R. Improvement of cutaneous microcirculation by cold atmospheric plasma (CAP): results of a controlled, prospective cohort study. Microvasc Res. 2016;104:55–62.
10. Kisch T, Schleusser S, Helmke A, Mauss KL, Wenzel ET, Hasemann B, Mailaender P, Kraemer R. The repetitive use of non-thermal dielectric barrier discharge plasma boosts cutaneous microcirculatory effects. Microvasc Res. 2016;106:8–13.
11. Borchardt T, Ernst J, Helmke A, Tanyeli M, Schilling AF, Felmerer G, Viöl W. Effect of direct cold atmospheric plasma (di cap) on microcirculation of intact skin in a controlled mechanical environment. Microcirculation. 2017;24(8):e12399.
12. Rutkowski R, Schuster M, Unger J, Seebauer C, Metelmann HR, Woedtke TV, Weltmann KD, Daeschlein G. Hyperspectral imaging for in vivo monitoring of cold atmospheric plasma effects on microcirculation in treatment of head and neck cancer and wound healing. Clin Plasma Med. 2017;7:52–7.
13. Daeschlein G, Rutkowski R, Lutze S, von Podewils S, Sicher C, Wild T, Metelmann HR, von Woedtke T, Jünger M. Hyperspectral imaging: innovative diagnostics to visualize hemodynamic effects of cold plasma in wound therapy. Biomed Tech (Berl). 2018;63(5):603–8.
14. Metelmann HR, von Woedtke T, Bussiahn R, Weltmann KD, Rieck M, Khalili R, Podmelle F, Waite PD. Experimental recovery of CO2-laser skin lesions by plasma stimulation. Am J Cosmetic Surg. 2012;29:52–6.
15. Boxhammer V, Li YF, Koeritzer J, Shimizu T, Maisch T, Thomas HM, Schlegel J, Morfill GE, Zimmermann JL. Investigation of the mutagenic potential of cold atmospheric plasma at bactericidal dosages. Mutat Res Gen Tox En. 2013;753:23–8.
16. Wende K, Bekeschus S, Schmidt A, Jatsch L, Hasse S, Weltmann KD, Masur K, von Woedtke T. Risk assessment of a cold argon plasma jet in respect to its mutagenicity. Mutat Res Gen Tox En. 2016;798:48–54.

17. Kluge S, Bekeschus S, Bender C, Benkhai H, Sckell A, Below H, Stope MB, Kramer A. Investigating the mutagenicity of a cold argon-plasma jet in an HET-MN model. PLoS One. 2016;11:e0160667.
18. Maisch T, Bosserhoff K, Unger P, Heider J, Shimizu T, Zimmermann JL, Morfill GE, Landthaler M, Karrer S. Investigation of toxicity and mutagenicity of cold atmospheric argon plasma. Environ Mol Mutagen. 2017;58:172–7.
19. Schmidt A, von Woedtke T, Stenzel J, Lindner T, Polei S, Vollmar B, Bekeschus S. One year follow up risk assessment in SKH-1 mice and wounds treated with an argon plasma jet. Int J Mol Sci. 2017;18:868.
20. Bekeschus S, Schmidt A, Kramer A, Metelmann HR, Adler F, von Woedtke T, Niessner F, Weltmann KD, Wende K. High throughput image cytometry micronucleus assay to investigate the presence or absence of mutagenic effects of cold physical plasma. Environ Mol Mutagen. 2018;59:268–77.
21. Boehm D, Bourke P. Safety implications of plasma-induced effects in living cells – a review of in vitro and in vivo findings. Biol Chem. 2019;400:3–17.
22. Rutkowski R, Daeschlein G, von Woedtke T, Smeets R, Gosau M, Metelmann HR. Long-term risk assessment for medical application of cold atmospheric pressure plasma. Diagnostics. 2020;10(4):210.
23. Kramer A, Hübner NO, Weltmann KD, Lademann J, Ekkernkamp A, Hinz P, Assadian O. Polypragmasia in the therapy of infected wounds – conclusions drawn from the perspectives of low temperature plasma technology for plasma wound therapy. GMS Krankenhaushyg Interdiszip. 2008;3(1):Doc13.
24. Lloyd G, Friedman G, Jafri S, Schultz G, Fridman A, Harding K. Gas plasma: medical uses and developments in wound care. Plasma Process Polym. 2010;7:194–211.
25. Isbary G, Morfill G, Schmidt HU, Georgi M, Ramrath K, Heinlin J, Karrer S, Landthaler M, Shimizu T, Steffes B, Bunk W, Monetti R, Zimmermann JL, Pompl R, Stolz W. A first prospective randomized controlled trial to decrease bacterial load using cold atmospheric argon plasma on chronic wounds in patients. Brit J Dermatol. 2010;163:78–82.
26. Shimizu T, Ikehara Y. Benefits of applying low-temperature plasma treatment to wound care and hemostasis from the viewpoints of physics and pathology. J Phys D Appl Phys. 2017;50:503001.
27. Assadian O, Ousey KJ, Daeschlein G, Kramer A, Parker C, Tanner J, Leaper DJ. Effects and safety of atmospheric low-temperature plasma on bacterial reduction in chronic wounds and wound size reduction: a systematic review and meta-analysis. Int Wound J. 2019;16: 103–11.
28. Bernhardt T, Semmler ML, Schäfer M, Bekeschus S, Emmert S, Boeckmann L. Plasma medicine: applications of cold atmospheric pressure plasma in dermatology. Ox Med Cell Longev. 2019;3873928. eCollection 2019.
29. Arndt S, Unger P, Wacker E, Shimizu T, Heinlin J, Li YF, Thomas HM, Morfill GE, Zimmermann JL, Bosserhoff AK, Karrer S. Cold atmospheric plasma (CAP) changes gene expression of key molecules of the wound healing machinery and improves wound healing in vitro and in vivo. PLoS One. 2013;8:e79325.
30. Heinlin J, Zimmermann JL, Zeman F, Bunk W, Isbary G, Landthaler M, Maisch T, Monetti R, Morfill G, Shimizu T, Steinbauer J, Stolz W, Karrer S. Randomized placebo-controlled human pilot study of cold atmospheric argon plasma on skin graft donor sites. Wound Rep Reg. 2013;21:800–7.
31. Vandersee S, Richter H, Lademann J, Beyer M, Kramer A, Knorr F, Lange-Asschenfeldt B. Laser scanning microscopy as a means to assess the augmentation of tissue repair by exposition of wounds to tissue tolerable plasma. Laser Phys Lett. 2014;11:115701.
32. Schmidt A, Bekeschus S, Wende K, Vollmar B, von Woedtke T. A cold plasma jet accelerates wound healing in a murine model of full-thickness skin wounds. Exp Dermatol. 2017;26: 156–62.
33. Seebauer C, Freund E, Segebarth M, Hasse S, Miller V, Lucas C, Kindler S, Dieke T, Metelmann HR, Daeschlein G, Jesse K, Weltmann KD, Bekeschus S. Immunomodulation in premalignant oral lichen 3 planus via medical gas plasma treatment. Oral Dis. 2020, (in press).

1

34. Hartwig S, Doll C, Voss JO, Hertel M, Preissner S, Raguse JD. Treatment of wound healing disorders of radial forearm free flap donor sites using cold atmospheric plasma: a proof of concept. J Oral Maxillofac Surg. 2017;75:429–35.
35. Podmelle F, Alnebaari R, Shojaei RK, Rana A, Rutkowski R. Perspectives in aesthetic medicine. In: Metelmann HR, von Woedtke T, Weltmann KD, editors. Comprehensive clinical plasma medicine - cold physical plasma for medical application. Berlin/Heidelberg: Springer; 2018. p. 355–61.
36. Heinlin J, Morfill G, Landthaler M, Stolz W, Isbary G, Zimmermann JL, Shimizu T, Karrer S. Plasma medicine: possible applications in dermatology. J Dtsch Dermatol Ges. 2010;8: 968–76.
37. Heinlin J, Isbary G, Stolz W, Morfill G, Landthaler M, Shimizu T, Steffes B, Nosenko T, Zimmermann JL, Karrer S. Plasma applications in medicine with a special focus on dermatology. J Eur Acad Dermatol. 2011;25:1–11.
38. Isbary G, Zimmermann JL, Shimizu T, Li YF, Morfill GE, Thomas HM, Steffes B, Heinlin J, Karrer S, Stolz W. Non-thermal plasma - more than five years of clinical experience. Clin Plasma Med. 2013;1:19–23.
39. Emmert S, Brehmer F, Haenssle H, Helmke A, Mertens N, Ahmed R, Simon D, Wandke D, Maus-Friedrichs W, Daeschlein G, Schoen MP, Vioel W. Atmospheric pressure plasma in dermatology: Ulcus treatment and much more. Clin Plasma Med. 2013;1:24–9.
40. Tiede R, Hirschberg J, Daeschlein G, von Woedtke T, Vioel W, Emmert S. Plasma applications: A dermatological view. Contrib Plasma Physics. 2014;54:118–30.
41. von Woedtke T, Reuter S, Masur K, Weltmann KD. Plasmas for medicine. Phys Rep. 2013;530:291–320.
42. Tanaka H, Ishikawa K, Mizuno M, Toyokuni S, Kajiyama H, Kikkawa F, Metelmann HR, Hori M. State of the art in medical applications using non-thermal atmospheric pressure plasma. Rev Mod Plasma Phys. 2017;1:3.
43. Isbary G, Shimizu T, Li YF, Stolz W, Thomas HM, Morfill GE, Zimmermann JL. Cold atmospheric plasma devices for medical issues. Expert Rev Med Devices. 2013;10:367–77.
44. Sackett DL. Evidence-based medicine. Sem Perinatol. 1997;21(1):3–5.
45. Barret JP, Podmelle F, Lipovy B, Rennekampff HO, Schumann H, Schwieger-Briel A, Zahn TR, Metelmann HR. BSH-12 and BSG-12 study groups. Accelerated re-epithelialization of partial-thickness skin wounds by a topical betulin gel: results of a randomized phase III clinical trials program. Burns. 2017;43(6):1284–94.
46. Kindler S, Schuster M, Seebauer C, Rutkowski R, Hauschild A, Podmelle F, Metelmann C, Metelmann B, Mueller-Debus C, Metelmann HR, Metelmann I. Triterpenes for well-balanced scar formation in superficial wounds. Molecules. 2016;21(9):E1129.
47. Metelmann I. Velocity of clinical wound healing without targeted treatment - specified for age, gender, body weight, skin type, wound size and co-morbidities. Inaugural dissertation 2019; University Medicine Greifswald.
48. Sgonc R, Gruber J. Age-related aspects of cutaneous wound healing: a mini-review. Gerontology. 2013;59(2):159–64.
49. Gosain A, DiPietro LA. Aging and wound healing. World J Surg. 2004;28(3):321–6.
50. Gilliver SC, Wu F, Ashcroft GS. Regulatory roles of androgens in cutaneous wound healing. Thromb Haemost. 2003;90(6):978–85.
51. Kanda N, Watanabe S. 17beta-estradiol enhances heparin-binding epidermal growth factor-like growth factor production in human keratinocytes. Am J Physiol Cell Physiol. 2005;288(4): C813–23.
52. Emmerson E, Campbell L, Ashcroft GS, Hardman MJ. Unique and synergistic roles for 17beta-estradiol and macrophage migration inhibitory factor during cutaneous wound closure are cell type specific. Endocrinol. 2009;150(6):2749–57.
53. Perzelova V, Sabol F, Vasilenko T, Novotny M, Kovac I, Slezak M, Durkac J, Holly M, Pilatova M, et al. Pharmacological activation of estrogen receptors-α and -β differentially modulates keratinocyte differentiation with functional impact on wound healing. Int J Molecular Med. 2016;37(1):21–8.

54. Wehrens KM, Arnoldussen CW, Booi DI, van der Hulst RR. Clinical evaluation of wound healing in Split-skin graft donor sites using microscopic quantification of reepithelialization. Adv Skin Wound Care. 2016;29(6):254–60.

55. Wang A, Armstrong E, Armstrong A. Corticosteroids and wound healing: clinical considerations in the perioperative period. Am J Surg. 2013;206(3):410–7.

56. Ehrlich HP, Tarver H, Hunt TK. Effects of vitamin a and glucocorticoids upon inflammation and collagen synthesis. Ann Surg. 1973;177(2):222–7.

57. Cockayne D, Sterling KM, Shull S, Mintz KP, Illeyne S, Cutroneo KR. Glucocorticoids decrease the synthesis of type I procollagen mRNAs. Biochemist. 1986;25(11):3202–9.

58. Oishi Y, Fu ZW, Ohnuki Y, Kato H, Noguchi T. Molecular basis of the alteration in skin collagen metabolism in response to in vivo dexamethasone treatment: effects on the synthesis of collagen type I and III, collagenase, and tissue inhibitors of Metalloproteinases. Br J Dermatol. 2002;147(5):859–68.

59. Bootun R. Effects of immunosuppressive therapy on wound healing. Int Wound J. 2013;10(1):98–104.

60. Haubner F, Ohmann E, Pohl F, Strutz J, Gassner HG. Wound healing after radiation therapy: review of the literature. Radiol Oncol. 2012;7:162.

61. Jacobson L, Johnson M, Dedhia R, Niknam-Bienia S, Wong A. Impaired wound healing after radiation therapy: a systematic review of pathogenesis and treatment. JPRAS Open. 2017;13:92–105.

Concept

Contents

Cold Physical Plasma: A Short Introduction

Kristian Wende and Ronny Brandenburg

Contents

© Springer Nature Switzerland AG 2022
H.-R. Metelmann et al. (eds.), *Textbook of Good Clinical Practice in Cold Plasma Therapy*, https://doi.org/10.1007/978-3-030-87857-3_2

⬢ Core Messages

- Cold plasmas are gaseous multicomponent phenomena comprising chemical entities, light, and electrical fields that can be generated and controlled by various concepts.
- Plasma phenomena have been tested for medical use since the second half of the nineteenth century.
- The term and field of plasma medicine developed since the early twenty-first century.
- In medicine, cold plasmas are investigated and applied in inflammatory processes.
- Reactive species and UV light are the main contributors of biomedical plasma effects.
- Plasmas are used in a wide range of production and conversion processes, especially to treat surfaces, liquids, and exhaust gases.

2.1 Introduction

Plasmas are considered as the fourth state of matter (besides solid, liquid, gaseous) and are natural to the world we live in – the sun, stars, northern lights, or lightings are examples of matter in the plasma state. Many other plasmas are not so obvious, like the solar wind, a stream of charged particles released from the sun's atmosphere, or the rare St. Elmo's fire, a bright blue glow at sharp and tall objects at ships antedating severe thunderstorms. Altogether, 99% of the known and visible matter are in the plasma state. Consequently, plasmas found entrance into human myth, art, science, and technology (◘ Fig. 2.1). The term *plasma* is of ancient Greek origin (πλάσμα) meaning a moldable substance. Its use to describe a gas discharge goes back to Irving Langmuir, a chemist, physicist, and engineer, working on gas discharges in the 1920s, as a then colleague remembered later: "...the equilibrium part of the discharge ... reminded him of the way the blood plasma carries around red and white corpuscles and germs. So he proposed to call our *uniform discharge* a *plasma*" [1]. This term poses a risk for disambiguation, since in life science, blood plasma plays a fundamental role in both research and diagnostics. To circumvent this issue, a number of amendments have been introduced for plasma discharges used in the biomedical research or application that point at the physical origin of the appearance: non-thermal plasma, tissue-tolerable plasma, atmospheric pressure plasma, cold atmospheric plasma (CAP), cold physical plasma, and many more. Most terms are still in use, and when seeking for information on plasmas, this must be borne in mind. Physical plasmas denominate a physical phenomenon where the atoms or molecules of a gas, e.g., air, become ionized by the input of energy. In contrast to thermal plasmas, which are very hot (up to millions of Kelvins background gas and/or ion temperature), cold plasmas can be operated at room temperature or at least far below 1000 K. To achieve this at atmospheric pressure, cold plasma devices have a special design. The key aspect is that

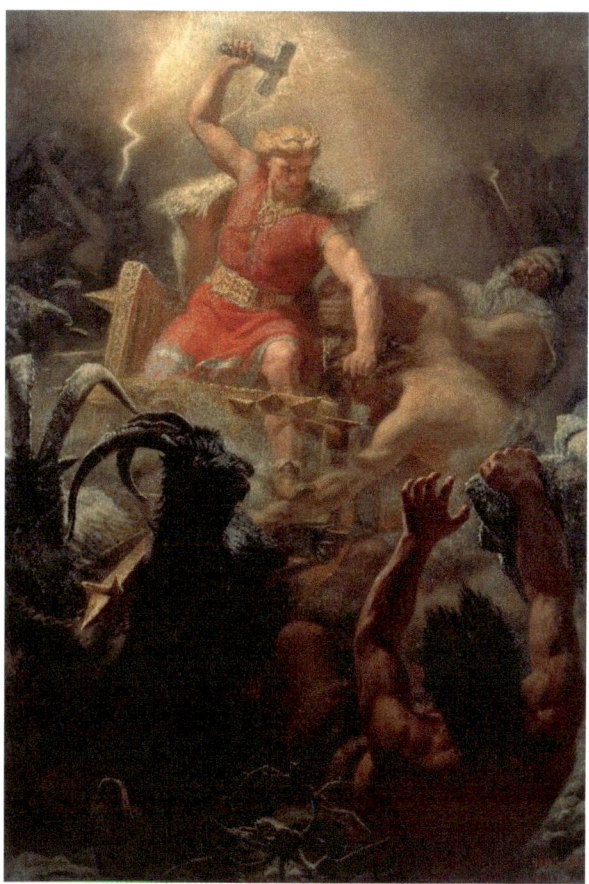

■ **Fig. 2.1** Mårten Eskil Winge: Tors strid med jättarna (Tor's Fight with the Giants), 1872, Nationalmuseum Sweden/Stockholm

only a small number of atoms or molecules is actually ionized – the lion's share of the gas remains in the normal ground state. Furthermore, most of the energy is coupled to the free electrons; thus, its mean energy or temperature is higher than the temperature of the ions and the neutral background gas as mentioned above. Such non-equilibrium state allows a precise control of the plasma activity. Consequently, cold plasmas are tools allowing the manipulation of delicate targets. For many decades, cold plasmas have been investigated and developed for technical and industrial applications. It serves for illumination purposes ("neon tubes," fluorescent tubes), provides the ability to produce nanometer-sized high aspect ratio structures for CPUs, allows the anti-reflexive, touch-sensitive coatings of their displays, and much more. Over the past 15 years, backed by an extensive biomedical research, cold plasmas made their way from the technical to the living world and subsequently medical application. Starting out from chronic wound management – where cold plasmas now represent a pari passu choice to classical interventions, the range of actual and potential applications covers numerous diseases that possess

2

an inflammatory component. This includes cancer and precancerous lesions or other application fields, e.g., in dentistry or ophthalmology. This chapter will address some fundamental and scientific aspects of cold plasmas: (1) a brief history emphasizing their medical use; (2) how cold plasmas are generated; (3) which principal components cold plasmas have; and (4) a brief survey of its current applications.

> **Box 3 Important Notes**
> - Cold plasmas are a natural phenomenon.
> - Cold plasmas comprise in part ionized (noble) gases.
> - Cold plasmas are utilized by humankind for industry, consumers, and healthcare.

2.2   A Brief History of Cold Plasmas

Electricity for medical purposes fascinated men since antiquity. In the first half of the nineteenth century, methods and devices were established for "franklinization" (pulsed static electricity), "galvanization" (direct currents), or "faradization" (alternating currents) [2]. The resulting effects remained mysterious, and the application was, from the medical point of view, more regarded as fraud and quackery than earnest therapy. Later in the same century (1860–70), legitimate scientific studies appeared, conducted by various European scientists. In the late nineteenth and the beginning of the twentieth centuries, pioneering work by Tesla, d'Arsonval, and Oudin led to devices that allowed the application of a cold plasma to the human body [3–5]. Using high voltage (10–300 kV) and high frequency ($\approx$10 kHz), stronger spark-like discharges or milder dielectric barrier discharges were applied to stimulate body functions or pain reduction during teeth pulling. In all cases, significant electrical power is delivered to larger areas of the human body, leading to non-specific generalized effects. In principle, the setup consisted of the energy source (a battery), an induction coil (Tesla coil), two capacitors (Leyden jars), spark gaps for wave formation, and an applicator – a coil (d'Arsonval), brush electrodes (Oudin), or plate electrodes (Tesla). The noisy devices were in use until the 1920s. The achieved medical effects were described as "creating … intense skin irritations and erythema by secondary capillary dilation, leading to decreased arterial blood pressure, among other things. Depending on the disposition of the patient, erythema lasting for hours was reported…" ([6] and citations therein). Microscopic alterations such as pyknosis and leucocytic infiltrations that can be interpreted as local cell death by apoptosis and inflammatory processes were described. The stage of the early research did not allow full understanding and attributed these effects to a de novo generation of proteins ("protein therapy") or simple "anionic" effects. Underlying the poorly understood medical effects, chemical, mechanical, and optical processes were discussed that tell of an early recogni-

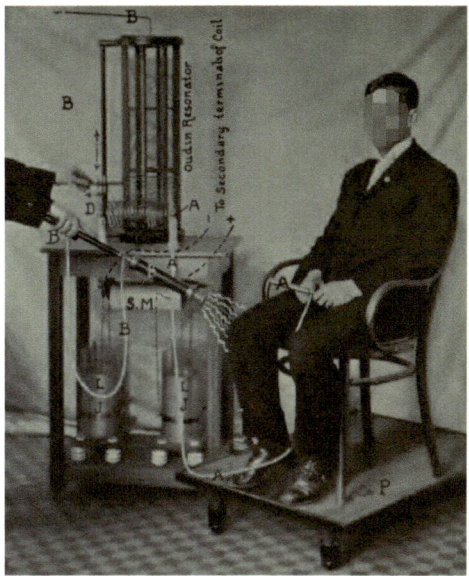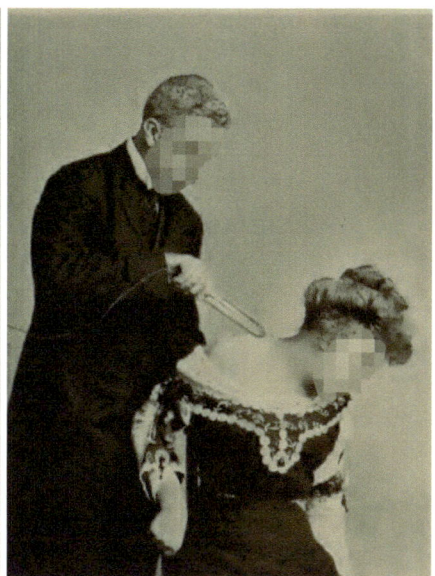

◻ Fig. 2.2 Early application of discharges for medical application. Effluviation using an Oudin resonator system, around 1900 (left) and early violet ray device (vacuum electrode) by Monell, around 1910 (right). (© IEEE, reprinted with permission from [2])

tion of the plasma compositions. Especially the splitting of electrons from nitrogen (N_2) and oxygen (O_2) molecules and the formation of molecules like ozone, nitric, and nitrous acid as well as the UV radiation were described and come close to modern interpretation of cold plasmas [7] (◻ Fig. 2.2).

The role of the assumed mechanical effects – the formation of ion winds by acceleration of air molecules – might be discussed controversially. The technology was early on further developed by the German physician and scientist Nagelschmidt around 1908 into the diathermy, a principle exploiting the production of heat by high frequency alternating currents flowing through a tissue [8] (◻ Fig. 2.3).

This therapy option is still open and used for pain reduction and suppression of inflammatory peaks in various rheumatoid disorders, but the modern devices lack the plasma aspect their ancestors had.

Box 3 Important Notes
- Cold plasmas are investigated for medical purposes since mid-nineteenth century.
- Experimental spark discharges yielded general effects, encouraging further work.
- Electrosurgery was invented as a spin-off in 1926, and since is in use.
- Violet ray devices (small light-emitting plasmas) were in use until the mid-1940s.
- Research on cold plasmas for medical purposes restarted in the late 1990s.

2

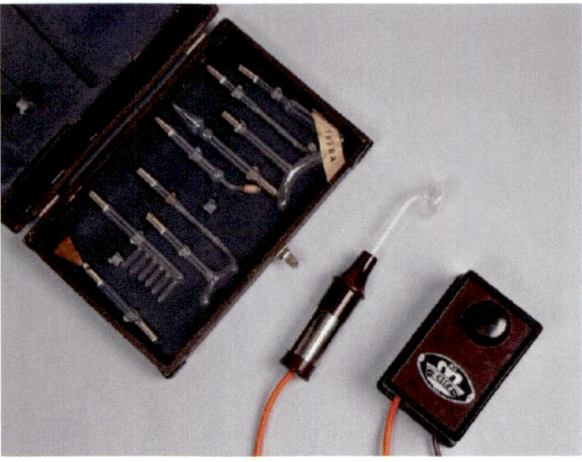

■ **Fig. 2.3** Violet ray plasma device, assortment of electrodes, hand-held wand, and control unit. (Reproduced with permission from [6]/CC BY 4.0)

Starting from 1926, surgical diathermy (electrosurgery) was established. The procedure involved the use of high-frequency electric current in surgery as either a cutting modality or else to cauterize small blood vessels to stop bleeding (cauterization). The devices possess characteristics of cold plasma devices; however, they are considerably hotter than most of the cold plasma sources under research today. The American physicians Strong and Monell promoted the use of vacuum electrodes with different shapes around 1910 [9]. Under reduced pressure, a glow discharge was ignited that functioned as a transmitter between the higher voltage electrode and the human body, reducing the energy densities significantly and allowing patients self-treatment without the physician's on-hand supervision. Emitting X-rays and/or UV light, these devices were used to "promote circulation, increase metabolism, optimize body function" (Strong), various skin diseases (Monell), and as disinfecting device due to its ozone formation. The UV emitting vacuum electrodes (termed "violet wand" or "violet ray" devices) were kept in service in the United States for a vast variety of applications, including lower back pain, carbuncles, or nasal catarrh. Due to limited – if not completely missing – evidence, legislation stopped its use from the 1940s. Approaches that are more recent strive to rehabilitate these devices [6]. Cold plasma devices started to reoccur in the interests of scientists and physicians in the mid-1990s, initially for "sterilization" procedures of tools and infectious waste [10]. Quickly, interest turned to human cells and tissues, with pioneering work from Stoffels and co-workers [11–17], Fridman and colleagues [18–24], Pouvesle and Robert [25–27], Weltmann/von Woedtke and colleagues [28–35], Lademann [36–40], and more (reviewed in part in [41–43]).

2.3 How to Generate a Cold Plasma?

Creating a plasma sounds easy: add energy to gaseous matter – et voilà – a spark or glow can be observed. Among chemical processes, heating, or compression, the generation via electric fields in electrical gas discharges or electromagnetic radiation are the most prominent methods for the generation of technical plasmas. In the simplest setup, two metal plate electrodes with a certain distance between each other and connected to a high voltage source are placed in a glass tube that is filled with a gas of desired composition and pressure. Air and all other gas mixtures or pure gases are electrical insulators at standard conditions. Its background ionization (by cosmic rays or radioactive radiation, or maybe, previous discharge cycles) is not sufficient to allow formation of an electrical gas discharge. However, if these initial electrons and ions are accelerated by outer electric or magnetic fields, they gain higher mean energies. If the energy of the electrons exceeds the threshold for ionization of the gas particles, electron avalanches are generated and the breakdown occurs. The voltage threshold or breakdown voltage is specific on the gas composition (electron shell configuration, purity of the gas) and solely depends on the product of gas pressure and electrode distance [44]. As shown in ◼ Fig. 2.6, the so-called Paschen-curves show a gas-specific minimum, i.e., the number of collisions between energetic electrons and background gas species has an optimum at which a so-called self-sustained gas discharge is formed. Counter-intuitively, at some distance and pressure settings, the breakdown voltages rises. At short interelectrode distances, the number of collisions is too low to generate sufficient secondary species at a given voltage. Thus, a higher voltage is needed to ensure that the electrons gain enough energy between two ionizing collisions. Of note, the noble gases, especially neon and neon-mixtures with argon or helium are most easily ignited (see neon tubes). Molecular gases, such as hydrogen, nitrogen, or oxygen need far higher voltages to form a plasma under these conditions. As an example to interpret the graph, take the atmospheric pressure (1021 mbar or 760 mm Hg) [45].

A vertical line corresponding to 76 on the x-axis gives the breakdown voltage for a gas between a pair of flat electrodes separated by 1 mm. For air, this gives a breakdown voltage of about 5 kV DC. However, electrode design such as surface roughness and sharp edges can reduce the breakdown voltage considerably. Of note, electrodes are not essential for gas breakdown – any method producing a strong electric field will also cause the gas tube (or regions therein) to glow: discharge tubes light up when placed near resonant radio antennas and coils. Once a glow discharge has been ignited, a low resistance current-path is formed that sustains the discharge. The glow will continue, until the current falls below a value called the "extinction point." The voltage at the extinction point is usually considerably lower than the breakdown voltage, i.e., the discharge is difficult to get going, and then difficult to stop once started. In a cold, non-equilibrium plasma, most of the present atoms or molecules remain in the lowest energy ground states. Beside ionization, atoms and molecules are electronically excited to higher states. The spontaneous de-excitation of these unstable excited states lead to emission of photons and generates the typical appearance of a plasma by the emission of light.

2

Box 3 Important Notes
- To ionize a gas, energy is needed – often, electrical energy is applied by an electrode.
- Most gases, including air, can be ionized, but noble gases (argon, helium) are ideal.
- Localization and movement of electrons are most important to generate/maintain a discharge.
- Cold plasmas can assume any shape; jets and sheet-like discharges dominate in medical applications.
- Modern devices are designed to deliver a stable, cold, and safe plasma discharge.

In ☐ Fig. 2.4, a typical current vs. voltage curve of a DC-operated discharge tube is shown. The voltages, currents, and relative length of the regions depend on the plasma sources design, but the general discharge events are universal. At low voltages and currents, a Townsend discharge (or dark discharge as it emits almost no light) is generated. Irradiating the electrode (more precisely the cathode) produces additional initial electrons by the photo-effect and thus, increases the current. Increasing the inter-electrode voltage enhances the number of ionizing collisions, and consequently leads to a point where the current increases significantly for minute increases in voltage – an unstable voltage plateau is reached. Upon further increase of the current, more and more ions – which are by orders of magnitude less mobile than the electrons – will remain in the discharge gap and form a space charge. The maximum of the space charge potential shifts towards the cathode with increasing current. In this situation, the electrons will gain most of its energy in the region between the cathode surface and the space charge potential maximum, the so-called cathode fall. This is the most important feature of the so-called glow-discharge, which is characterized by alternating dark spaces and light emitting areas ("glows" and "columns"). The glow discharge regime is stable over a wide range of currents. With a further increase of the current, the electrode area will be covered more and more and finally the full electrode will be glowing. Then, a further increase of the current leads to an increase of the conductivity, accompanied by an increase of the running voltage, and the glow discharge is called anomalous. This phase transits almost abruptly to the arc discharge if the current is further increased. In this mode, high currents pass through the plasma, while the potential between the plates falls. In arcing mode, the particle temperatures increase and the discharge is constricted to a small volume, resulting in potential damage of the device. Furthermore, thermionic emission of electrons becomes important. Thus, heating the electrode externally or by bombardment with particle beams favors arcing at lower currents. In clinical application, some surgery tools (e.g., coagulators) use this regime. Due to the atmospheric operational pressure, a rapid thermalization between electrons and the background gas takes place; thus, such plasmas are hot plasmas (some 1000 K gas temperature). In all other biomedi-

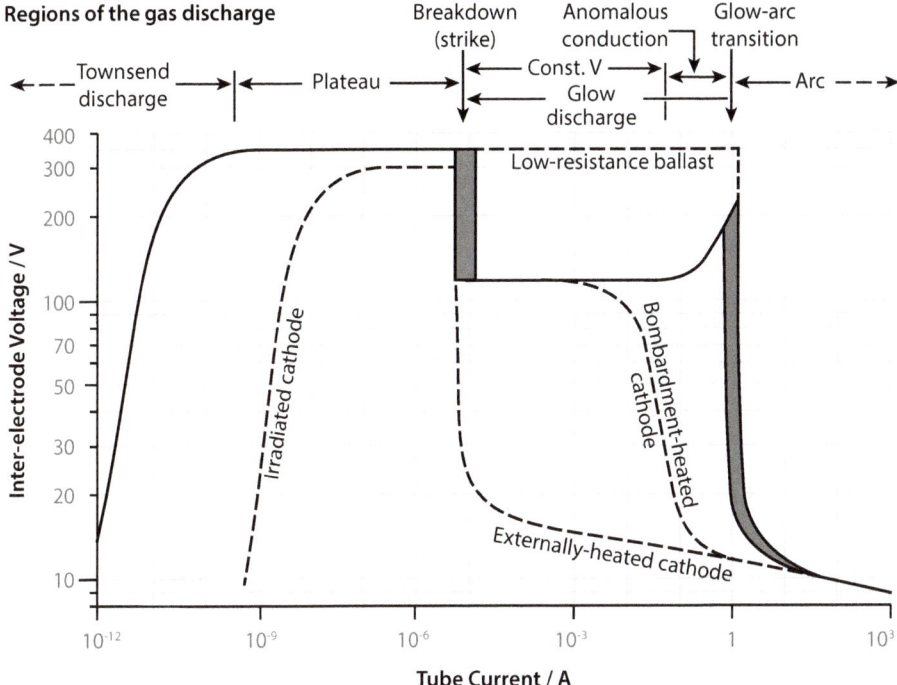

Regions of the gas discharge

Fig. 2.4 Idealized current vs. voltage characteristic for a gas discharge tube. (Reprinted with friendly permission of David Knight from ▶ http://g3ynh.info/disch_tube/intro.html)

cal applications, gas discharges are operated as cold, non-equilibrium plasmas similar to the glow discharge mode. The main challenge devices have to take is to control, sustain, and modulate the discharge in a way that is safe, reliable, and reproducible. To achieve this, cold plasma devices operate typically at low energy input, have a special electrode configuration, and may use a gas flow for cooling, and limit power dissipation [46–49]. An extremely rich variety of non-equilibrium atmospheric pressure plasmas exists ranging from Townsend discharges to spark discharges that span a range of ionization degrees of ten orders of magnitude. The most important in the scope of biomedical applications are dielectric barrier discharges (DBDs) and plasma jets (■ Fig. 2.5). As the name suggests, the main feature of the DBD is the presence of a dielectric barrier in the discharge path, e.g., by covering at least one of the electrodes. This can be any insulating material, but quartz, glass, or ceramics are favorable. Polymers, which would allow lightweight and sturdy plasma sources, must be carefully tested for suitability since plasmas can etch them, leading to a loss of function or impurities in the discharge [50].

The dielectric surface is charged during the breakdown. This reduces the local electric field that leads to the extinction of the discharge activity within nano- to microseconds. Consequently, it limits the current density and local energy dissipation.

2

Dielectric barrier discharge   **Plasma jet**   **Flexible barrier discharge**

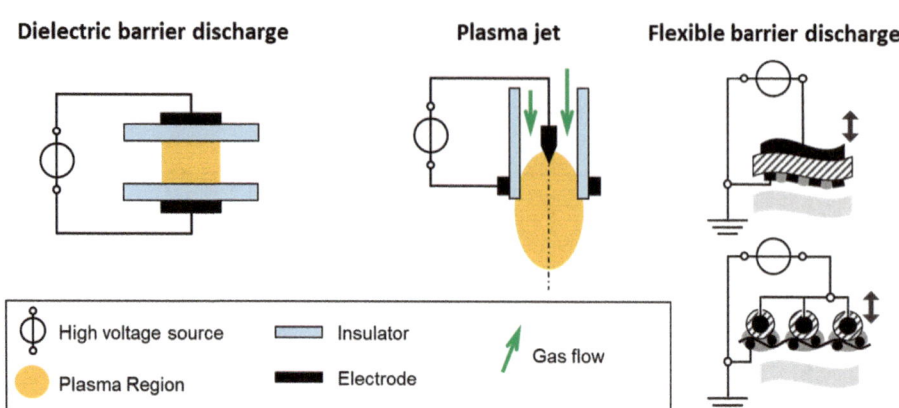

☐ **Fig. 2.5** Principle setup of a dielectric barrier discharge (left), a plasma jet (center), and recent flexible dielectric barrier discharges (silicone, fabric). Notice the presence of a powered electrode and a counter electrode, an insulator, and a high voltage source. (Figure adapted by K. Wende basing on drawings from R. Brandenburg)

Due to the capacitive character of the discharge arrangement, DBDs are operated with alternating voltage, usually in the kHz-range or by short high-voltage pulses. In most molecular gases, but also in argon or mixtures of noble gases with molecular gases, the streamer mechanism leads to so-called microdischarges that visually appear as filaments. Usually, several discharge channels are ignited and decay within each half-cycle of the high-voltage period. In case of higher frequencies in the MHz range, current limitation by the dielectric barriers is less effective and breakdown voltage is lower [51]. The discharge operation changes significantly since charge carriers in the volume do not completely diminish between two subsequent high voltage half-periods. The mobility of the ions is too small to follow the rapid changes of the applied electric field. The ions will be trapped at the discharge barriers and be deposited as surface charges there. In other words, the role of barrier is not to induce the self-pulsing character described above. The discharge operates in steady state regime and it can be characterized as a capacitively coupled plasma. The role of the barrier is mainly the protection of the electrode material. Plasma jets are gas discharges operated in a non-sealed electrode arrangement and projected outside the electrode arrangement into the environment [48]. The plasma region outside the inner electrode configuration ("effluent" or "plume") is generated from the core plasma by a gas flow. Gas flow contributes to the removal of heat away from the discharge and, at the same time, the enhancement of the transport of plasma species away from the discharge and onto the substrate. In many cases, noble gas (Ar, He) is used as a carrier gas because of the much lower breakdown voltage compared with air or other molecular gases (see the Paschen curves, ☐ Fig. 2.6). With the noble gas flow, a channel in which ionization takes place preferentially is generated. This effluent is most often composed of so-called guided streamers confined in the gas channel. Plasma jets are well suited for the delivery of localized treatments, e.g., wounds. Plasma jets have been realized with different electrode configurations and can be operated with DC and AC high voltage of different frequencies (from Hz to GHz).

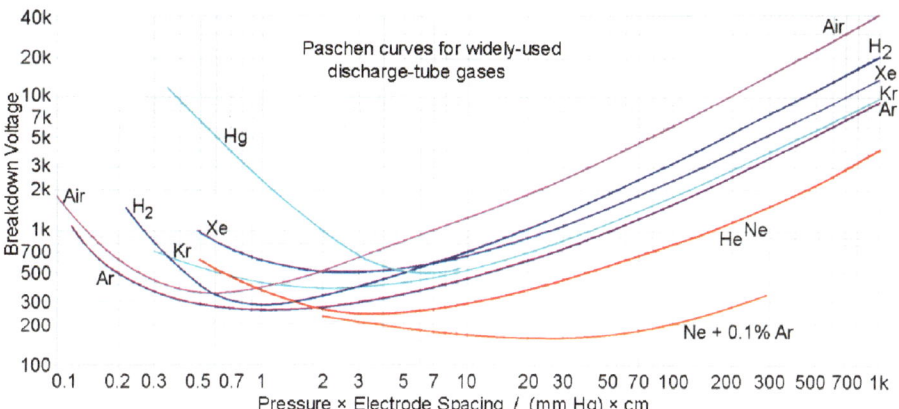

◻ Fig. 2.6 Breakdown voltage of various gases in relation to electrode distance and pressure (Paschen curve). Observe bathtub shape of the curves (see text). (Adapted based on Wittenberg [52] by Dave Knight (▶ http://g3ynh.info/disch_tube/intro.html). Reprinted with permission)

2.4 Principal Composition of a Cold Plasma

Cold physical plasmas are multi-component systems, similar to its namesake, the blood plasma and inherently not in equilibrium. The principal components are ultra-violet, visible, and infrared light, electrical fields, free electrons, ions, radicals, and excited gas atoms/molecules, dispersed in the bulk of slow gas atoms or molecules in ground state. These slow particles keep the average temperature of the system low. Although the electrons have, in certain areas of the plasma, energies of a few electron volts (eV), relating to a temperature of several 10,000 K, the whole plasma remains significantly cooler ($T_e \gg T_{gas}$). Depending on the intended application and the design of the plasma source, temperatures of the visible plume of plasma jet devices range close to room or body temperature. In normal application mode, plasma sources for the biomedical application are designed in a way that thermal damage of the tissue can be excluded. In addition, thermal load to the skin can be minimized assuming a brush-type treatment regimen with a velocity of about 10 mm/s [39] (◻ Fig. 2.7).

2.4.1 Radiation

The radiation emitted by cold physical plasmas is classified as vacuum ultraviolet (VUV) light (<200 nm), UVC, UVB, and UVA light (200–280 nm, 280–320 nm, and 320–400 nm, respectively), visible light (mainly below 450 nm), and infrared light of the NIR range (700–1000 nm) [53–55]. The spectrum of the plasma and, thus the contributions to the different spectral ranges strongly depends on the gas composi-tion and the energy density of the plasma. An example is given below (◻ Fig. 2.8).

By the ultraviolet radiation, photochemical processes can be initiated. Depending on the wavelength, photon energies range between 12.4 eV or 1200 kJ mol^{-1} (100 nm) and 3.1 eV or 300 kJ mol^{-1} (400 nm). Accordingly, the

■ **Fig. 2.7** Cold plasmas are multi-component systems. Current research identified reactive species as the major carrier of bioactivity. (Image: Johanna Striesow, INP Greifswald)

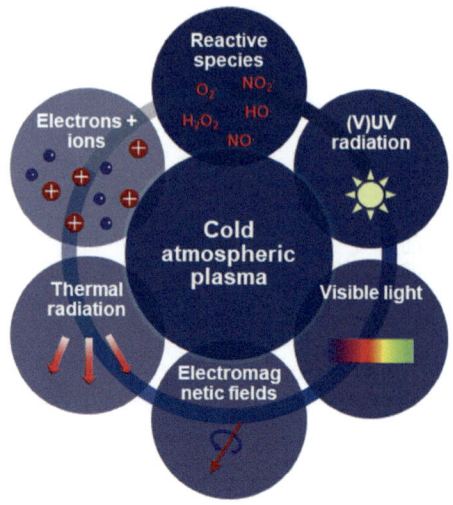

fission of chemical bonds is possible: many single bonds in organic molecules have bond energies starting from 305 kJ mol^{-1} (C–N) and 347 kJ mol^{-1} (C–C).[1] Chemical modifications by plasma-derived photons have been described but are more of scientific than of clinical interest [56, 57]. The penetration of the energy-rich VUV and UVC into cells or tissues is limited, as the photons are absorbed immediately, e.g., by the *Stratum corneum's* keratohyalin and urocaninic acid, interstitial liquids, or epithelial cells. When adhering to the suggested maximum treatment times, the overall radiation energy delivered does not exceed the accepted limits of the International Commission on Non-Ionizing Radiation Protection (ICNIRP) recommendations (30 J$_{eff}$ m^{-2})[2] [58]. For the argon plasma jet kINPen, only 1/30 of this dose is delivered [59]. In other applications, predominantly when using low-pressure plasmas, e.g., the inactivation of bacteria and spores, UV light contribute significantly to the effect [60–62]. The infrared light emitted by the discharge can penetrate tissues and cells significantly better than the short-wavelength counterparts. The observed increase in blood circulation and tissue oxygenation after plasma treatment of chronic wounds may in part be induced by the near-infrared radiation, as observations using plasma treatment and research focusing infrared light in wound management suggest [26, 63–65].

> **Box 3 Important Notes**
> — Cold plasmas are cocktails of reactive components.
> — Small reactive oxygen and nitrogen species (ROS/RNS), ultraviolet light, and electrical fields are most important in medical use.

---

1 ► https://chem.libretexts.org/Core/Physical_and_Theoretical_Chemistry/Chemical_Bonding/Fundamentals_of_Chemical_Bonding/Bond_Energies.
2 ► http://www.icnirp.org/en/frequencies/uv/index.html.

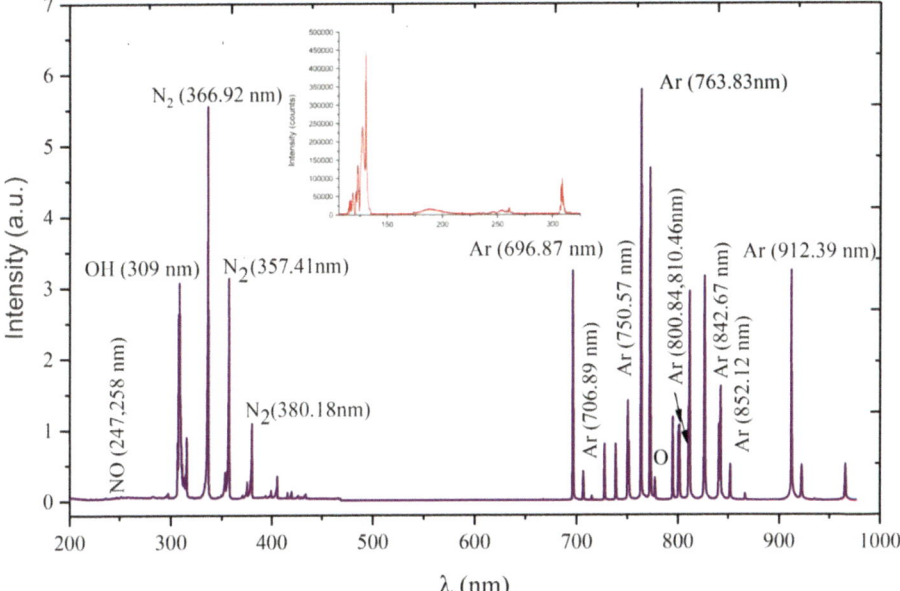

● **Fig. 2.8** Qualitative emission spectrum of an argon plasma jet (200–1000 nm). Below 200 nm (vacuum-UV) argon excimers radiate (small insert). Note the significant emission in the near-infrared range above 700 nm and in the UVB/UVA range (300–400 nm). (Figure adapted by K. Wende from Mahdikia and Jablonowski [54])

- Generated ROS/RNS mimic those occurring naturally in cells, allowing interference/modulation.
- Species in gas phase and liquid phase differ due to short lifetimes.

2.4.2 Electrical Fields

The role of the electric fields is discussed ambivalently in the recent years. It is generally accepted, that cold physical plasma discharges create electrical fields around them. The intensity and temporal and spatial changes along with the ignition process and/or the development in the discharge are under investigation [66–68]. It may be assumed that the electrical field may reach three to ten times higher strength at condensed (and short-lived) phenomena, such as streamers and bullets, in the discharge than the field necessary to create the discharge in the first place. Although these high electric fields can exert significant impact in biological systems, their role in plasma medicine is not fully elucidated yet. Due to the applied alternating currents to ignite the plasma, the generated electric fields fluctuate in the millisecond (kHz plasmas), microsecond (MHz plasmas), or nanosecond range (ns-pulsed plasmas). The fields can be extremely inhomogeneous, and their strength change with time, direction, surrounding gas, and discharge cycle, making the investiga-

2

tions difficult. Theoretically, they can be strong enough to allow the manipulation of cell membranes (kHz, MHz plasmas) or cell organelle membranes (ns-pulsed plasmas), as research using pulsed electric fields suggest [69]. However, to form a pore in a cell membrane, a potential of $1\ kV\ cm^{-1}$ is needed, for a mitochondrion at least $20\ kV\ cm^{-1}$. Whether standard plasma sources can deliver such high electrical fields outside the electrode area, e.g., at the tip of an effluent, is under debate, but a number of recent publications foster this notion [70–72]. Some substantial hypotheses assume a synergistic effect of the electric fields with small reactive species that are a major component of cold physical plasmas [73, 74]. An oxidation of the cell membrane lipids would yield in an increased membrane fluidity and fragility, facilitating pore formation [75].

2.4.3 Reactive Species

Small chemical entities like neutrals, ions, and radicals are a major fraction of the plasma. They are often referred to as *species*, circumscribing a (dynamic) mixture of short-lived and fast-reacting small chemicals, predominantly composed of single atoms or ions thereof (e.g., O*, O+), radicals (e.g., hydroxyl radicals OH, nitric oxide NO), or neutrals (e.g., hydrogen peroxide, H_2O_2).

2.4.3.1 In the Gas Phase

Composition and proportions of these species vary massively in dependence of plasma source design, working gas, presence of modifiers (e.g., molecular gas admixtures such as oxygen or nitrogen), power consumption, location in respect to the electrodes, and time. Numerous diagnostic methods like two-photon absorption laser-induced fluorescence (TALIF), Fourier-transformed infrared spectroscopy (FTIR), cavity-enhanced ring-down spectroscopy (CRDS), some offering spatio-temporal resolution in combination with computational models have been developed and deployed to investigate gas phase composition of cold physical plasmas. With time, an extensive hoard of knowledge has been compiled that cannot be reflected in full in this textbook chapter. The interested reader is referred to primary knowledge sources such as the following reviews [46, 76–80].

In the active plasma zone, close to the igniting electrode, primary species are formed by collisions and electron impact and collision with other reactive species. In jet plasmas driven by a noble gas (argon, helium, neon, or mixes thereof) excited states, ions, and excimers (excited dimers) or molecular ions of the respective noble gas atoms form. In the case of an argon jet (kINPen), argon excimers ($Ar_2\ (a^3\ \Sigma_u^+)$) and various excited argon states are present in the active plasma zone. These species have high energies and are mostly short-lived, and their presence strictly correlates with the electric field providing the energy for the discharge. In ◻ Fig. 2.9, the spike-like appearance of higher energy states of argon (e.g., Ar^+, $Ar(4s, {}^3P_1)$) corresponds to the plasma sources alternating current delivering the necessary energy in a megahertz frequency. The de-excitation processes are almost as quick as the formation (e.g., for the Ar^+ ions) and in the order of one microsecond and even faster. De-excitation can be linked with the emission of (UV) light (argon

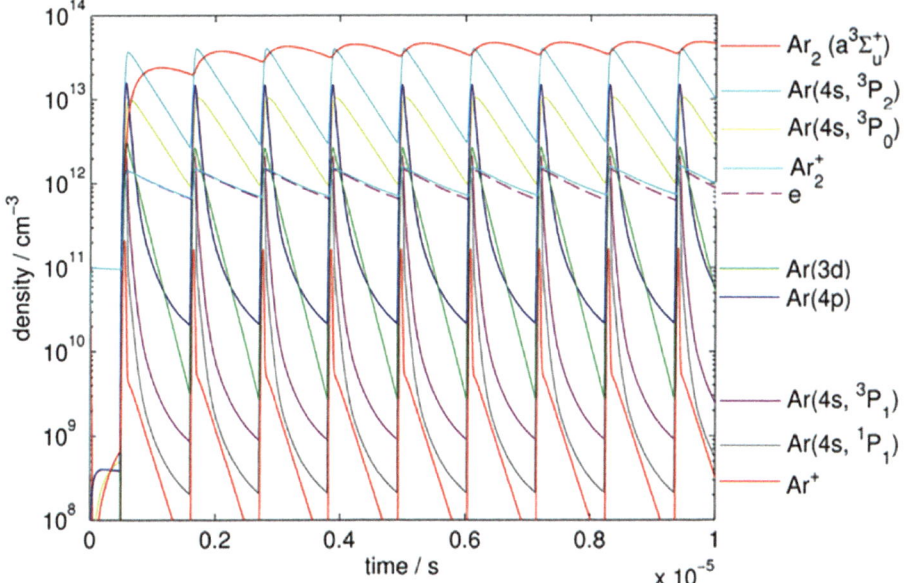

□ Fig. 2.9 Densities of argon species in the kINPen (model). (Reproduced with permission from [81]/CC BY 4.0)

excimer radiation –126 nm), the collision with walls, or the inelastic collision with atomic or molecular species (quenching). If energy supply is cut, the plasma extinguishes.

In addition, primary reactive oxygen or nitrogen species are generated by electron impact if suitable molecules such as oxygen (O_2), nitrogen (N_2), or water are present in the active plasma zone. For example, oxygen molecules are cleaved by fast electrons (3.9 eV) to form atomic oxygen:

Nitrogen molecules are fragmented to atomic nitrogen; water molecules yield hydroxyl radicals (OH) and hydrogen atoms (H). In addition, excited molecule states are formed, e.g., singlet oxygen, a molecule where in contrast to the ground state oxygen the electrons in antibonding molecular π-orbitals flip spin and orbital occupation. This results in an unstable molecule that has a higher oxidative potential than oxygen in the ground state. It, e.g., quickly reacts with the essential amino acid histidine, leading to a loss or gain of function of proteins in dependence of the histidine position. In the photodynamic therapy (PDT), where a photosensitizer and intense light are used to produce singlet oxygen, similar effects are exploited [82, 83].

The short-lived primary species, especially the noble gas excited states form in collision with molecular gases in the plasma core, but also at the intersection between the active plasma zone or an effluent with ambient gas molecules, secondary species:

This example uses molecular oxygen, but all other gas molecules can be attacked to form radicals or excited states. The extent and location of the reaction between

2

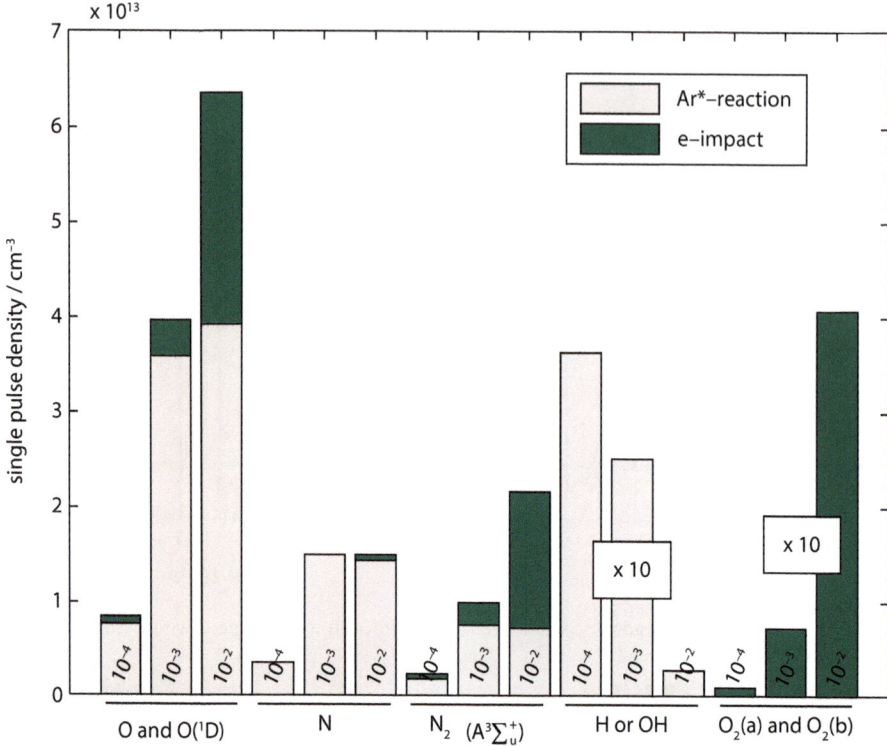

excited noble gas species and ambient gas molecules (e.g., O_2, N_2, H_2O of the air) are determined by the design of a plasma source and the respective gas flow dynamics. In the kINPen plasma jet, using argon with a higher gas flow velocity, and turbulences at the effluent, ambient air interface result in its significant enrichment with molecular gas species. As a result, this plasma source shows a desired high basal production of reactive oxygen and nitrogen species (ROs/RNS). ● Figure 2.10 illustrates the different reactive species present in the discharge, and their respective origin (either via electron impact or reaction with argon ions; also see ● Fig. 2.9). In the case of the argon-driven plasma jet kINPen (see ▶ Chap. 16), the generation of reactive species via secondary reactions of excited argon species dominate the profile.

In the case of a helium jet plasma source that has been designed specifically for research purposes (µAPPJ or COST-Jet) [84–87], species output is low when no molecular gas has been added to the working gas flow. The lower gas flow rate and significantly smaller specific weight of helium cause laminar gas flow dynamics and reduce the mixing with ambient air and with that the formation of secondary reactive species. Secondly, the very high energy of excited helium states (e.g., He*(2^3S_1),

He$_2$* helium excimers, He$^+$ ions) is less well transferred to molecular gases as in the case of the excited argon species. When molecular gases, especially oxygen, are added to the helium gas flow, this source is very effective in the production of atomic oxygen [88]. Cell experiments using this condition revealed a high toxicity towards cancer cells [89]. Atomic oxygen is also a major component in other (experimental) plasma sources [90–92].

By further elastic and inelastic collision of primary and secondary species with ambient molecules and themselves, downstream (tertiary) species are created. By the reaction of higher energy nitrogen species (N$_2$ (a)) with molecular oxygen, a number of nitrogen oxides occur (dinitrogen oxide N$_2$O, nitric oxide NO, nitrogen dioxide NO$_2$, nitrogen trioxide NO$_3$, and dinitrogen pentoxide N$_2$O$_5$). Having a different lifetime and reactivity, interconversion or reaction with other species present yield in highly dynamic non-equilibrium chemistry. The long-lived nitrogen species nitric and nitrous acid (HNO$_2$, HNO$_3$), and N$_2$O$_5$ are the major products. By tertiary reaction of (excited) oxygen species among themselves or with hydrogen atoms (H), long-lived reactive oxygen species like ozone (O$_3$) or hydrogen peroxide (H$_2$O$_2$) are formed along the metastable hydroperoxide radical (HO$_2$•).

2.4.3.2 In the Liquid Phase

The interaction between a plasma and a liquid became a target of interest with the increasing use of cold plasmas in biomedical applications in the recent 20 years only. The liquid phase is by far less well investigated than the gas phase. A number of reasons contributed to this imbalance: most plasmas are single-phase gaseous phenomena, and fundamental research concentrated on its description. The investigation of chemical and mass flow processes in liquids is hampered by the physics of itself: a gas-liquid interface confines the body of the liquid (the bulk). This interface, a few nanometers in width, is an extremely inhomogeneous environment. Local concentrations and species lifetimes are significantly different compared to the liquid bulk due to the molecular structures at the interface that affects how solute molecules are adsorbed or solvated into the liquid. Due to high dynamics, the investigation of the interface is demanding and limited by the current technical development of scientific instrumentation. At the gas-liquid interphase, the generation of tertiary species is assumed. Among these are nitric oxide radicals (•NO) [93], peroxynitrite ions (ONOO-) [94–96], and hypochlorite (from atomic oxygen reacting with chloride ions) [89, 92, 97]. While NO is also generated in the gas phase of cold plasmas, its transport through the interface into the liquid bulk is not favored due to its bad solubility in water. Data indicate that it is formed at the gas-liquid interface by the reaction of nitrogen dioxide radicals and atomic oxygen. Peroxynitrite can be formed by different reactions, e.g., between nitrite and hydrogen peroxide. This reaction takes place only in rather acidic conditions below pH 3.5 (blood pH is 7.4). The necessary low pH is reached at the thin interface between the gas phase and the liquid phase, in the bulk of distilled water treated for moderate to long times, but not in physiologic liquids that typically contain buffer systems (e.g., phosphate buffered saline, cell culture media, or blood). Atomic oxygen is a primary species, formed in the active plasma zone. It is

2

short-lived, and penetration into the bulk of a liquid has not been observed so far. At the interface, it may be scavenged by chloride ions (Cl^-), common to all biological systems yielding hypochlorite (OCl-). Hypochlorite is a moderate oxidant, and preserves the chemical activity of atomic oxygen that otherwise would be lost. It undergoes an aging process, with stable chlorate (ClO_3^-) as the final product. When deionized water is treated, atomic oxygen reacts with water to give hydroxyl radicals that recombine to form H_2O_2 and are quenched by the reaction with impurities and walls.

The liquid bulk, acting as a reservoir for the plasma-generated species, is a 1000-fold denser material than a gas at normal pressure. While 1 L of water contains $\approx 3.3 \times 10^{25}$ H_2O molecules, 1 L of oxygen (at normal pressure) contains only $\approx 2.7 \times 10^{22}$ molecules (1 mol of gas $\approx$ 22.4 L). This reduces species lifetimes due to a significantly higher number of collision than in gas phase, and the water molecule, a dipol, is very reactive.

2.4.3.3 In the Solid Phase

For many decades, targets of plasmas were solids – metals, glass, or similar materials [98–100]. The interaction with such surfaces has been investigated thoroughly, but the transferability of the results to human or animal tissue is very limited.

2.5 Applications of Cold Plasmas

Along with the versatility of cold plasmas, its spectrum of uses is too broad to be covered in this chapter except for a brief outlook predominantly introducing literature for further reading (e.g., compiled in [101, 102]). The following paragraph will focus only on applications outside plasma medicine to provide an overview on relevant application fields of cold plasma technology. Besides the direct use of an open or hidden plasma source like in plasma medicine or in illumination technology, plasmas are predominantly applied in numerous production processes. In automotive, surfaces, especially of the window glass, are refined to increase surface tension with the effect that water droplets run off the glass without the need for wiping. Dominating percentages of the facades of recent buildings are made of glass – yielding to the need of special glass properties such as heat and light reflection, insulation, or endurance against harsh conditions. Thin surface coatings made of metal oxides and metal nitrides are generated on the glass by industrial cold plasma processes (plasma sputtering). In addition, etching of hard and/or delicate surfaces can be achieved by plasma guns, yielding ultra-precise optical surfaces. The heart piece of the world's largest optical telescope to be, the extremely large telescope (ELT) built by the European Southern Observatory on Cerro Amazones in the Atacama Desert of northern Chile (Antofagasta, Chile), is a 39 m diameter segmented primary mirror. Each of its 798 pieces with 1.45 m edge length will be refined by a plasma ion beam polishing process to reduce surface roughness down to a few nanometers

[103]. Polymers and plastics, inevitable items of modern technology, are etched by plasma to improve bonding strength of glues or to facilitate imprinting. Here, the surface of the respective material is chemically modified, e.g., to contain polar chemical groups such as amino or carboxyl groups. Surplus to the general improvement of the polymers wettability, these groups can be used as chemical anchors to immobilize proteins or other biomolecules, opening the field of bio-sensors and other functional surfaces [104]. Further, metals and ceramics intended for implantation into the human or animal body may be modified to foster osseointegration, both in dentistry (dental implants) [105–107] and in trauma or salvage surgery (e.g., joint replacements) [108, 109]. Plasma sputter processes achieve a surface suitable for cell attachment, and release antimicro-bial agents such as silver ions to reduce the risk of infections [110, 111]. Also in the energy industry, plasmas are of relevance. Switching a few hundred thousand volts is a demanding task needed in power plants – the simple disconnection of two pieces of conducting metal that works well to switch off the light at home does not yield the desired result: a plasma arc forms between the two pieces, and since the plasma is a decent conductor, the current is not stopped. A whole research field has formed around this phenomenon, and modern high circuit breakers use a combination of suitable enduring materials, electrode shapes, hard to ionize gas fillings, and timing to disconnect the energy supply safely [112]. Research is needed in the case of direct current circuit breakers that are of interest in terms of photovoltaic energy generation and direct current energy grids [113]. This also applies towards the use of plasma processes for the produc-tion of new materials, for hydrogen technologies, energy conversion and storage, where efficiency increases and upscaling are required in addition to providing unique material properties [101]. Welding is still the most important technique to join metals and, more recently, used on thermoplastics. (Electrical) welding pro-cesses make use of the same phenomenon with inverted algebraic signs; research on electrode material, supply gases, and current waveforms is performed to improve the bonding between the welded materials and to reduce energy con-sumption. Plasma discharges are used for cleaning processes – both in liquids (wastewater treatments) or gas phase (exhaust gases, air conditioning, and deodorization), combating environmental pollution [114]. Large-scale plasma-reactors can remove NO_x, SO_x, and dust in the flue gas emissions of industrial incinerators (50,000 m^3/h) [115]. More recently, the conversion of greenhouse gases mainly carbon dioxide (CO_2) and methane (CH_4) into value-added chemi-cals and liquid fuels gained increasing attention, and research targets the efficacy of the process [116]. In agriculture, also the fixation of nitrogen from air for soil fertilization is an emerging plasma process that is of interest, where transport is the limiting factor and energy can be generated locally from renewable energies [117]. Overall, optimization of pre- and post-harvesting processes in agriculture and food industry is an emerging field of plasma technology [102]. The disinfec-tion of food containers and fresh produce is a major, near-to-market application in this respect [118, 119].

2

Box 3 Important Notes
- Cold plasmas are versatile:
- Main fields of cold plasma application are: illumination technology, surface editing and refinement, cleaning purposes (including liquids and gases), welding, chemical conversions.

Conclusion

Cold physical plasmas of natural and artificial origin are common to the environment we live in. They represent an enabling technology that can be adapted by engineering to a multitude of applications, both in the technical and the biomedical world. Being an attractive research target, cold plasmas entered biomedical application in the later nineteenth century. Their use subsided due to the lack of scientific background in the middle of the twentieth century, and since the beginning of the current millennium, a substantial increase in knowledge supported their successful return to clinical application. Cold plasmas comprise a mix of potentially bioactive components, with reactive oxygen and nitrogen species, ultraviolet light, and electrical fields as major effectors. Acting jointly, biological processes relevant in various inflammatory events such as cell-cell-communication, cell proliferation, cell migration, and others are modulated. Subsequently, a precise stimulation of tissue functions allows the application of plasmas in conditions like acute and chronic wounds, precancerous and cancerous lesions, and to stop bleeding (e.g., after surgical interventions).

Literature

1. Mott-Smith HM. History of plasmas. Nature. 1971;233(5316):219.
2. Graves DB. Lessons from tesla for plasma medicine. IEEE Trans Radiat Plasma Med Sci. 2018;2(6):594–607.
3. Brenni P. Les courants à haute-fréquence apprivoisés à travers la darsonvalisation et les spectacles publics (1890-1930). Annales historiques de l'électricité. 2010;8(1):53.
4. Collins AF. An easily-made high-frequency apparatus. Sci Am. 1907;63(1618supp):25929.
5. Reif-Acherman S. Jacques Arsene d'Arsonval: his life and contributions to electrical instrumentation in physics and medicine. Part iii: high-frequency experiences and the beginnings of diathermy [scanning our past]. Proc IEEE. 2017;105(2):394–404.
6. Napp J, Daeschlein G, Napp M, von Podewils S, Gumbel D, Spitzmueller R, et al. On the history of plasma treatment and comparison of microbiostatic efficacy of a historical high-frequency plasma device with two modern devices. GMS Hyg Infect Control. 2015;10:Doc08.
7. Schnee A. Kompendium der Hochfrequenz in ihren verschiedenen Anwendungsformen einschliesslich der Diathermie. O. Nemnich; 1920.
8. Rhees DJ. Electricity – "the greatest of all doctors": an introduction to "high frequency oscillators for electro-therapeutic and other purposes". Proc IEEE. 1999;87(7):1277–81.
9. Monell SH. High frequency electric currents in medicine and dentistry: their nature and actions and simplified uses in external treatments. New York: William R. Jenkins Company; 1910.
10. Laroussi M. Sterilization of contaminated matter with an atmospheric pressure plasma. IEEE Trans Plasma Sci. 1996;24(3):1188–91.

11.   Stoffels E, Flikweert AJ, Stoffels WW, Kroesen GMW. Plasma needle: a non-destructive atmospheric plasma source for fine surface treatment of (bio)materials. Plasma Sources Sci Technol. 2002;11(4):383–8.

12.   Stoffels E, Kieft IE, Sladek REJ. Superficial treatment of mammalian cells using plasma needle. J Phys D Appl Phys. 2003;36(23):2908–13.

13.   Kieft IE, Broers JL, Caubet-Hilloutou V, Slaaf DW, Ramaekers FC, Stoffels E. Electric discharge plasmas influence attachment of cultured CHO K1 cells. Bioelectromagnetics. 2004;25(5):362–8.

14.   Sosnin EA, Stoffels E, Erofeev MV, Kieft IE, Kunts SE. The effects of UV irradiation and gas plasma treatment on living mammalian cells and bacteria: a comparative approach. IEEE Trans Plasma Sci. 2004;32(4):1544–50.

15.   Stoffels E, Sladek REJ, Kieft IE. Gas plasma effects on living cells. Phys Scr. 2004;T107(5):79–82.

16.   Kieft IE, Kurdi M, Stoffels E. Reattachment and apoptosis after plasma-needle treatment of cultured cells. IEEE Trans Plasma Sci. 2006;34(4):1331–6.

17.   Stoffels E, Gonzalvo YA, Whitmore TD, Seymour DL, Rees JA. A plasma needle generates nitric oxide. Plasma Sources Sci Technol. 2006;15(3):501–6.

18.   Fridman G, Friedman G, Gutsol A, Shekhter AB, Vasilets VN, Fridman A. Applied plasma medicine. Plasma Process Polym. 2008;5(6):503–33.

19.   Kalghatgi SU, Fridman G, Fridman A, Friedman G, Clyne AM. Non-thermal dielectric barrier discharge plasma treatment of endothelial cells. Conf Proc IEEE Eng Med Biol Soc. 2008;2008:3578–81.

20.   Dobrynin D, Fridman G, Friedman G, Fridman A. Physical and biological mechanisms of direct plasma interaction with living tissue. New J Phys. 2009;11(11):115020.

21.   Kalghatgi SU, Fridman A, Friedman G, Clyne AM. Cell proliferation following non-thermal plasma is related to reactive oxygen species induced fibroblast growth factor-2 release. Conf Proc IEEE Eng Med Biol Soc. 2009;1:6030–3.

22.   Kalghatgi S, Friedman G, Fridman A, Clyne AM. Endothelial cell proliferation is enhanced by low dose non-thermal plasma through fibroblast growth Factor-2 release. Ann Biomed Eng. 2010;38(3):748–57.

23.   Dobrynin D, Fridman G, Friedman G, Fridman A, editors. Physical mechanisms of plasma assisted wound healing: production and delivery of active species. Slovakia: Demanovska dolina; 2011.

24.   Kalghatgi S, Kelly CM, Cerchar E, Torabi B, Alekseev O, Fridman A, et al. Effects of non-thermal plasma on mammalian cells. PLoS One. 2011;6(1):e16270.

25.   Robert E, Sarron V, Ries D, Dozias S, Vandamme M, Pouvesle JM. Characterization of pulsed atmospheric-pressure plasma streams (PAPS) generated by a plasma gun. Plasma Sources Sci Technol. 2012;21(3):34017.

26.   Collet G, Robert E, Lenoir A, Vandamme M, Darny T, Dozias S, et al. Plasma jet-induced tissue oxygenation: potentialities for new therapeutic strategies. Plasma Sources Sci Technol. 2014;23(1):012005.

27.   Pouvesle JM, Robert E, editors. Non thermal atmospheric plasma jets: a new way for cancer treatment? GD2008 Conference Proceedings; 2014.

28.   von Woedtke T, Kramer A, Weltmann K-D. Plasma sterilization: what are the conditions to meet this claim? Plasma Process Polym. GD2008 Conference Proceedings. 2008;5(6):534–9.

29.   Bender C, Matthes R, Kindel E, Kramer A, Lademann J, Weltmann KD, et al. The irritation potential of nonthermal atmospheric pressure plasma in the HET-CAM. Plasma Process Polym. 2010;7(3–4):318–26.

30.   Wende K, Landsberg K, Lindequist U, Weltmann KD, von Woedtke T. Distinctive activity of a nonthermal atmospheric-pressure plasma jet on eukaryotic and prokaryotic cells in a cocultivation approach of keratinocytes and microorganisms. IEEE Trans Plasma Sci. 2010;38(9):2479–85.

31.   Haertel B, Wende K, von Woedtke T, Weltmann KD, Lindequist U. Non-thermal atmospheric-pressure plasma can influence cell adhesion molecules on HaCaT-keratinocytes. Exp Dermatol. 2011;20(3):282–4.

32. Bekeschus S, von Woedtke T, Kramer A, Weltmann K-D, Masur K. Cold physical plasma treatment alters redox balance in human immune cells. Plasma Med. 2013;3(4):267–78.
33. Bundscherer L, Bekeschus S, Tresp H, Hasse S, Reuter S, Weltmann K-D, et al. Viability of human blood leukocytes compared with their respective cell lines after plasma treatment. Plasma Med. 2013;3(1–2):71–80.
34. Schmidt A, Wende K, Bekeschus S, Bundscherer L, Barton A, Ottmuller K, et al. Non-thermal plasma treatment is associated with changes in transcriptome of human epithelial skin cells. Free Radic Res. 2013;47(8):577–92.
35. Winter J, Wende K, Masur K, Iseni S, Dunnbier M, Hammer MU, et al. Feed gas humidity: a vital parameter affecting a cold atmospheric-pressure plasma jet and plasma-treated human skin cells. J Phys D Appl Phys. 2013;46(29):295401.
36. Lademann O, Richter H, Meinke MC, Patzelt A, Kramer A, Hinz P, et al. Drug delivery through the skin barrier enhanced by treatment with tissue-tolerable plasma. Exp Dermatol. 2011;20(6):488–90.
37. Lademann O, Richter H, Kramer A, Patzelt A, Meinke MC, Graf C, et al. Stimulation of the penetration of particles into the skin by plasma tissue interaction. Laser Phys Lett. 2011;8(10):758–64.
38. Lademann O, Richter H, Patzelt A, Alborova A, Humme D, Weltmann KD, et al. Application of a plasma-jet for skin antisepsis: analysis of the thermal action of the plasma by laser scanning microscopy. Laser Phys Lett. 2010;7(6):458–62.
39. Lademann J, Richter H, Alborova A, Humme D, Patzelt A, Kramer A, et al. Risk assessment of the application of a plasma jet in dermatology. J Biomed Opt. 2009;14(5):054025.
40. Teichmann A, Heuschkel S, Jacobi U, Presse G, Neubert RH, Sterry W, et al. Comparison of stratum corneum penetration and localization of a lipophilic model drug applied in an o/w microemulsion and an amphiphilic cream. Eur J Pharm Biopharm. 2007;67(3):699–706.
41. von Woedtke T, Schmidt A, Bekeschus S, Wende K, Weltmann KD. Plasma medicine: a field of applied redox biology. In Vivo. 2019;33(4):1011–26.
42. Weltmann KD, von Woedtke T. Plasma medicine-current state of research and medical application. Plasma Phys Controlled Fusion. 2017;59(1):014031.
43. Graves DB. Mechanisms of plasma medicine: coupling plasma physics, biochemistry, and biology. IEEE Trans Radiat Plasma Med Sci. 2017;1(4):281–92.
44. Meichsner J, Schmidt M, Schneider R, Wagner HE. Nonthermal plasma chemistry and physics. Boca Raton: CRC Press; 2013.
45. Loveless AM, Garner AL. A universal theory for gas breakdown from microscale to the classical Paschen law. Phys Plasmas. 2017;24(11):113522.
46. Reuter S, von Woedtke T, Weltmann KD. The kINPen-a review on physics and chemistry of the atmospheric pressure plasma jet and its applications. J Phys D Appl Phys. 2018;51(23):233001.
47. Weltmann KD, von Woedtke T. Basic requirements for plasma sources in medicine. Eur Phys J Appl Phys. 2011;55(1):13807.
48. Winter J, Brandenburg R, Weltmann KD. Atmospheric pressure plasma jets: an overview of devices and new directions. Plasma Sources Sci Technol. 2015;24(6):064001.
49. Bruggeman PJ, Iza F, Brandenburg R. Foundations of atmospheric pressure non-equilibrium plasmas. Plasma Sources Sci Technol. 2017;26(12):123002.
50. Winter J, Nishime TMC, Bansemer R, Balazinski M, Wende K, Weltmann KD. Enhanced atmospheric pressure plasma jet setup for endoscopic applications. J Phys D Appl Phys. 2019;52(2):024005.
51. Kunhardt EE. Generation of large-volume, atmospheric-pressure, nonequilibrium plasmas. IEEE Trans Plasma Sci. 2000;28(1):189–200.
52. Wittenberg HH. Gas tube design. Electron tube design. Harrison: Radio Corporation of America; 1962. p. 792–817.
53. Wattieaux G, Yousfi M, Merbahi N. Optical emission spectroscopy for quantification of ultraviolet radiations and biocide active species in microwave argon plasma jet at atmospheric pressure. Spectrochim Acta B At Spectrosc. 2013;89:66–76.

54. Jablonowski H, Bussiahn R, Hammer MU, Weltmann KD, von Woedtke T, Reuter S. Impact of plasma jet vacuum ultraviolet radiation on reactive oxygen species generation in bio-relevant liquids. Phys Plasmas. 2015;22(12):122008.

55. Lange H, Foest R, Schafer J, Weltmann KD. Vacuum UV radiation of a plasma jet operated with rare gases at atmospheric pressure. IEEE Trans Plasma Sci. 2009;37(6):859–65.

56. Fingerhut BP, Herzog TT, Ryseck G, Haiser K, Graupner FF, Heil K, et al. Dynamics of ultraviolet-induced DNA lesions: Dewar formation guided by pre-tension induced by the backbone. New J Phys. 2012;14(6):065006.

57. Stinson CA, Xia Y. Radical induced disulfide bond cleavage within peptides via ultraviolet irradiation of an electrospray plume. Analyst. 2013;138(10):2840–6.

58. Protection ICoN-IR. Guidelines on limits of exposure to ultraviolet radiation of wavelengths between 180 nm and 400 nm (incoherent optical radiation). Health Phys. 2004;87(2):171–86.

59. Jablonowski H, Bussiahn R, Hammer MU, Weltmann K-D, von Woedtke T, Reuter S. Impact of plasma jet vacuum ultraviolet radiation on reactive oxygen species generation in bio-relevant liquids. Phys Plasmas. 2015;22(12):122008.

60. Lackmann JW, Schneider S, Edengeiser E, Jarzina F, Brinckmann S, Steinborn E, et al. Photons and particles emitted from cold atmospheric-pressure plasma inactivate bacteria and biomolecules independently and synergistically. J R Soc Interface. 2013;10(89):20130591.

61. von Woedtke T, Julich WD, Thal S, Diederich M, Stieber M, Kindel E. Antimicrobial efficacy and potential application of a newly developed plasma-based ultraviolet irradiation facility. J Hosp Infect. 2003;55(3):204–11.

62. Judee F, Wattieaux G, Merbahi N, Mansour M, Castanie-Cornet MP. The antibacterial activity of a microwave argon plasma jet at atmospheric pressure relies mainly on UV-C radiations. J Phys D Appl Phys. 2014;47(40):405201.

63. Hoffmann G, Hartel M, Mercer JB. Heat for wounds - water-filtered infrared-a (wIRA) for wound healing - a review. Ger Med Sci. 2016;14:Doc08.

64. Daeschlein G, Rutkowski R, Lutze S, von Podewils S, Sicher C, Wild T, et al. Hyperspectral imaging: innovative diagnostics to visualize hemodynamic effects of cold plasma in wound therapy. Biomed Tech (Berl). 2018;63(5):603–8.

65. Kisch T, Schleusser S, Helmke A, Mauss KL, Wenzel ET, Hasemann B, et al. The repetitive use of non-thermal dielectric barrier discharge plasma boosts cutaneous microcirculatory effects. Microvasc Res. 2016;106:8–13.

66. Darny T, Pouvesle JM, Puech V, Douat C, Dozias S, Robert E. Analysis of conductive target influence in plasma jet experiments through helium metastable and electric field measurements. Plasma Sources Sci Technol. 2017;26(4):045008.

67. Schmidt-Bleker A, Norberg SA, Winter J, Johnsen E, Reuter S, Weltmann KD, et al. Propagation mechanisms of guided streamers in plasma jets: the influence of electronegativity of the surrounding gas. Plasma Sources Sci Technol. 2015;24(3):035022.

68. Gaborit G, Jarrige P, Lecoche F, Dahdah J, Duraz E, Volat C, et al. Single shot and vectorial characterization of intense electric field in various environments with pigtailed electrooptic probe. IEEE Trans Plasma Sci. 2014;42(5):1265–73.

69. Nuccitelli R. Application of pulsed electric fields to cancer therapy. Bioelectricity. 2019;1(1):30–4.

70. Griseti E, Kolosnjaj-Tabi J, Gibot L, Fourquaux I, Rols MP, Yousfi M, et al. Pulsed electric field treatment enhances the cytotoxicity of plasma-activated liquids in a three-dimensional human colorectal cancer cell model. Sci Rep. 2019;9(1):7583.

71. Steuer A, Wolff CM, von Woedtke T, Weltmann KD, Kolb JF. Cell stimulation versus cell death induced by sequential treatments with pulsed electric fields and cold atmospheric pressure plasma. PLoS One. 2018;13(10):e0204916.

72. Keidar M, Shashurin A, Volotskova O, Stepp MA, Srinivasan P, Sandler A, et al. Cold atmospheric plasma in cancer therapy. Phys Plasmas. 2013;20(5):057101.

73. Yusupov M, Van der Paal J, Neyts EC, Bogaerts A. Synergistic effect of electric field and lipid oxidation on the permeability of cell membranes. Biochim Biophys Acta. 2017;1861(4):839–47.

2

74. Wolff CM, Kolb JF, Weltmann KD, von Woedtke T, Bekeschus S. Combination treatment with cold physical plasma and pulsed electric fields augments ROS production and cytotoxicity in lymphoma. Cancers (Basel). 2020;12(4):845.

75. Azan A, Gailliègue F, Mir LM, Breton M. Cell membrane Electropulsation: chemical analysis of cell membrane modifications and associated transport mechanisms. In: Transport across natural and modified biological membranes and its implications in physiology and therapy. Cham: Springer; 2017. p. 59–71.

76. Golda J, Held J, Redeker B, Konkowski M, Beijer P, Sobota A, et al. Concepts and characteristics of the 'COST reference microplasma jet'. J Phys D Appl Phys. 2016;49(8):084003.

77. Adamovich I, Baalrud SD, Bogaerts A, Bruggeman PJ, Cappelli M, Colombo V, et al. The 2017 plasma roadmap: low temperature plasma science and technology. J Phys D Appl Phys. 2017;50(32):323001.

78. Bruggeman PJ, Kushner MJ, Locke BR, Gardeniers JGE, Graham WG, Graves DB, et al. Plasma-liquid interactions: a review and roadmap. Plasma Sources Sci Technol. 2016;25(5):053002.

79. Graves DB. Reactive species from cold atmospheric plasma: implications for cancer therapy. Plasma Process Polym. 2014;11(12):1120–7.

80. Graves DB. Low temperature plasma biomedicine: a tutorial review. Phys Plasmas. 2014;21(8):080901.

81. Schmidt-Bleker A, Winter J, Bosel A, Reuter S, Weltmann KD. On the plasma chemistry of a cold atmospheric argon plasma jet with shielding gas device. Plasma Sources Sci Technol. 2016;25(1):015005.

82. Callaghan S, Senge MO. The good, the bad, and the ugly – controlling singlet oxygen through design of photosensitizers and delivery systems for photodynamic therapy. Photochem Photobiol Sci. 2018;17(11):1490–514.

83. Fan W, Huang P, Chen X. Overcoming the Achilles' heel of photodynamic therapy. Chem Soc Rev. 2016;45(23):6488–519.

84. Reuter S, Niemi K, Schulz-von der Gathen V, Dobele HF. Generation of atomic oxygen in the effluent of an atmospheric pressure plasma jet. Plasma Sources Sci Technol. 2009;18(1):015006.

85. Schulz-von der Gathen V, Schaper L, Knake N, Reuter S, Niemi K, Gans T, et al. Spatially resolved diagnostics on a microscale atmospheric pressure plasma jet. J Phys D Appl Phys. 2008;41(19):194004.

86. Knake N, Reuter S, Niemi K, Schulz-von der Gathen V, Winter J. Absolute atomic oxygen density distributions in the effluent of a microscale atmospheric pressure plasma jet. J Phys D Appl Phys. 2008;41(19):6.

87. Schulz-von der Gathen V, Buck V, Gans T, Knake N, Niemi K, Reuter S, et al. Optical diagnostics of micro discharge jets. Contrib Plasma Physics. 2007;47(7):510–9.

88. Waskoenig J, Niemi K, Knake N, Graham LM, Reuter S, Schulz-von der Gathen V, et al. Atomic oxygen formation in a radio-frequency driven micro-atmospheric pressure plasma jet. Plasma Sources Sci Technol. 2010;19(4):045018.

89. Bekeschus S, Wende K, Hefny MM, Rodder K, Jablonowski H, Schmidt A, et al. Oxygen atoms are critical in rendering THP-1 leukaemia cells susceptible to cold physical plasma-induced apoptosis. Sci Rep. 2017;7(1):2791.

90. Park GY, Hong YJ, Lee HW, Sim JY, Lee JK. A global model for the identification of the dominant reactions for atomic oxygen in He/O-2 atmospheric-pressure plasmas. Plasma Process Polym. 2010;7(3–4):281–7.

91. Georgescu N, Lungu CP, Lupu AR, Osiac M. Atomic oxygen maximization in high-voltage pulsed cold atmospheric plasma jets. IEEE Trans Plasma Sci. 2010;38(11):3156–62.

92. Wende K, Williams P, Dalluge J, Gaens WV, Aboubakr H, Bischof J, et al. Identification of the biologically active liquid chemistry induced by a nonthermal atmospheric pressure plasma jet. Biointerphases. 2015;10(2):029518.

93. Jablonowski H, Schmidt-Bleker A, Weltmann KD, von Woedtke T, Wende K. Non-touching plasma-liquid interaction - where is aqueous nitric oxide generated? Phys Chem Chem Phys. 2018;20(39):25387–98.

94. Breen C, Pal R, Elsegood MRJ, Teat SJ, Iza F, Wende K, et al. Time-resolved luminescence detection of peroxynitrite using a reactivity-based lanthanide probe. Chem Sci. 2020;11(12):3164–70.

95. Girard F, Badets V, Blanc S, Gazeli K, Marlin L, Authier L, et al. Formation of reactive nitrogen species including peroxynitrite in physiological buffer exposed to cold atmospheric plasma. RSC Adv. 2016;6(82):78457–67.

96. Lukes P, Dolezalova E, Sisrova I, Clupek M. Aqueous-phase chemistry and bactericidal effects from an air discharge plasma in contact with water: evidence for the formation of peroxynitrite through a pseudo-second-order post-discharge reaction of H2O2and HNO2. Plasma Sources Sci Technol. 2014;23(1):015019.

97. Jirásek V, Lukeš P. Formation of reactive chlorine species in saline solution treated by non-equilibrium atmospheric pressure He/O2 plasma jet. Plasma Sources Sci Technol. 2019;28(3):035015.

98. d'Agostino R, Favia P, Oehr C, Wertheimer MR. Low-temperature plasma processing of materials: past, present, and future. Plasma Process Polym. 2005;2(1):7–15.

99. Foest R, Kindel E, Ohl A, Stieber M, Weltmann KD. Non-thermal atmospheric pressure discharges for surface modification. Plasma Phys Control Fusion. 2005;47(12B):B525–B36.

100. Cvelbar U, Walsh JL, Černák M, de Vries HW, Reuter S, Belmonte T, et al. White paper on the future of plasma science and technology in plastics and textiles. Plasma Process Polym. 2019;16(1):1700228.

101. Weltmann KD, Kolb JF, Holub M, Uhrlandt D, Šimek M, Ostrikov K, et al. The future for plasma science and technology. Plasma Process Polym. 2018;16(1):1800118.

102. Brandenburg R, Bogaerts A, Bongers W, Fridman A, Fridman G, Locke BR, et al. White paper on the future of plasma science in environment, for gas conversion and agriculture. Plasma Process Polym. 2018;16(1):1–18.

103. Schulze C, Nestler M, Zeuner M. Ion-beam figuring of x-ray mirrors. SPIE; 2019.

104. Makhneva E, Barillas L, Farka Z, Pastucha M, Skládal P, Weltmann K-D, et al. Functional plasma polymerized surfaces for biosensing. ACS Appl Mater Inter. 2020;12(14):17100–12.

105. Duske K, Koban I, Kindel E, Schroder K, Nebe B, Holtfreter B, et al. Atmospheric plasma enhances wettability and cell spreading on dental implant metals. J Clin Periodontol. 2012;39(4):400–7.

106. Le Guehennec L, Soueidan A, Layrolle P, Amouriq Y. Surface treatments of titanium dental implants for rapid osseointegration. Dent Mater. 2007;23(7):844–54.

107. Naujokat H, Harder S, Schulz LY, Wiltfang J, Florke C, Acil Y. Surface conditioning with cold argon plasma and its effect on the osseointegration of dental implants in miniature pigs. J Craniomaxillofac Surg. 2019;47(3):484–90.

108. Liang H, Shi B, Fairchild A, Cale T. Applications of plasma coatings in artificial joints: an overview. Vacuum. 2004;73(3–4):317–26.

109. Naresh Kumar N, Yap SL, Bt Samsudin FND, Khan MZ, Pattela Srinivasa RS. Effect of argon plasma treatment on tribological properties of UHMWPE/MWCNT nanocomposites. Polymers. 2016;8(8):295.

110. Chen Y-H, Hsu C-C, He J-L. Antibacterial silver coating on poly(ethylene terephthalate) fabric by using high power impulse magnetron sputtering. Surf Coat Technol. 2013;232:868–75.

111. Kratochvíl J, Kuzminova A, Kylián O. State-of-the-art, and perspectives of, silver/plasma polymer antibacterial nanocomposites. Antibiotics. 2018;7(3):78.

112. Schade E. Physics of high-current interruption of vacuum circuit breakers. IEEE Trans Plasma Sci. 2005;33(5):1564–75.

113. Tahata K, Oukaili SE, Kamei K, Yoshida D, Kono Y, Yamamoto R, et al. HVDC circuit breakers for HVDC grid applications. IET Conference Proceedings [Internet]. 2015;[044(9.)-(9.) pp.]. Available from: https://digital-library.theiet.org/content/conferences/10.1049/cp.2015.0018.

114. Timmermann E, Prehn F, Schmidt M, Hoft H, Brandenburg R, Kettlitz M. Indoor air purification by dielectric barrier discharge combined with ionic wind: physical and microbiological investigations. J Phys D Appl Phys. 2018;51(16):164003.

115. Kim HH. Nonthermal plasma processing for air-pollution control: a historical review, current issues, and future prospects. Plasma Process Polym. 2004;1(2):91–110.
116. Bogaerts A, Kozak T, van Laer K, Snoeckx R. Plasma-based conversion of CO2: current status and future challenges. Faraday Discuss. 2015;183:217–32.
117. Graves DB, Bakken LB, Jensen MB, Ingels R. Plasma activated organic fertilizer. Plasma Chem Plasma Process. 2018;39(1):1–19.
118. Bourke P, Ziuzina D, Boehm D, Cullen PJ, Keener K. The potential of cold plasma for safe and sustainable food production. Trends Biotechnol. 2018;36(6):615–26.
119. Schnabel U, Niquet R, Schlüter O, Gniffke H, Ehlbeck J. Decontamination and sensory properties of microbiologically contaminated fresh fruits and vegetables by microwave plasma processed air (PPA). J Food Process Preserv. 2015;39(6):653–62.

Further Reading

Adamovich I, et al. The 2017 plasma roadmap: low temperature plasma science and technology. J Phys D Appl Phys. 2017;50(32):323001.

Becker KH, et al. Non-equilibrium air plasmas at atmospheric pressure. Boca Raton: CRC press; 2004.

Brandenburg R. Dielectric barrier discharges: progress on plasma sources and on the understanding of regimes and single filaments. Plasma Sources Sci Technol. 2017;26(5):053001.

Fridman A. Plasma chemistry. Cambridge, Cambridge university press; 2008.

Graves DB. Low temperature plasma biomedicine: a tutorial review. Phys Plasmas. 2014;21(8):080901.

Graves DB. Lessons from tesla for plasma medicine. IEEE Trans Radiat Plasma Med Sci. 2018;2(6):594–607.

Laroussi M, et al. Perspective: the physics, diagnostics, and applications of atmospheric pressure low temperature plasma sources used in plasma medicine. J Appl Phys. 2017;122(2):020901.

Lu X, et al. On atmospheric-pressure non-equilibrium plasma jets and plasma bullets. Plasma Sources Sci Technol. 2012;21(3):034005.

Meichsner J, et al. Nonthermal plasma chemistry and physics. Boca Raton: CRC Press; 2012.

Metelmann H-R, et al. Plasmamedizin. Berlin/Heidelberg: Springer; 2016. (in German)

Metelmann H-R, et al. Comprehensive clinical plasma medicine: cold physical plasma for medical application. Cham: Springer; 2018.

Privat-Maldonado A, et al. ROS from physical plasmas: redox chemistry for biomedical therapy. Oxidative Med Cell Longev. 2019;2019:9062098.

Reuter S, et al. The kINPen-a review on physics and chemistry of the atmospheric pressure plasma jet and its applications. J Phys D Appl Phys. 2018;51(23):233001.

Winter J, et al. Atmospheric pressure plasma jets: an overview of devices and new directions. Plasma Sources Sci Technol. 2015;24(6):064001.

How Does Cold Plasma Work in Medicine?

Sander Bekeschus, Thomas von Woedtke, and Anke Schmidt

Contents

© Springer Nature Switzerland AG 2022
H.-R. Metelmann et al. (eds.), *Textbook of Good Clinical Practice in Cold Plasma Therapy*, https://doi.org/10.1007/978-3-030-87857-3_3

⊜ **Core Messages**

- Cold plasmas are a multi-component system consisting of electrons and ions, electric fields, UV and infrared radiation, and reactive oxygen and nitrogen species (ROS).
- Preclinical research points to ROS being the predominant effectors of cold plasma in medicine.
- Definite evidence of the specific roles of single plasma components is awaited as technical limitations hamper segregating their individual contribution to the biomedical effects observed.

3.1 Introduction

In simple terms, plasmas for medicine are energized (partially ionized), conductive, but electrically neutral gases (◘ Fig. 3.1) operated at body temperature (at or lower than 40 °C) at the target site for therapeutic purposes [1]. All devices are operated at room temperature and atmospheric pressure, and hence need no particular environment to be applied medically. This is mentioned because a major field in plasma physics is investigating plasma processes at low pressure. Due to temperature profile that does not cause thermal harm to tissues, cells, or proteins [2], it needs to be distinguished from another medical plasma concept, the argon plasma coagulation (APC) [3]. By definition from physics, APC is also a "cold" plasma and, technically speaking, belongs to cold plasma technology as well. However, and together with other instruments used in hemostasis and electrosurgery, these devices range from 60 °C to more than 100 °C [4], effectively necrotizing the treated tissue. The aim of these devices is not to regulate physiological processes in the tissue but rather to stop blood flow or to seal and cut more destructively. By contrast, the field of plasma medicine aims at utilizing plasma source

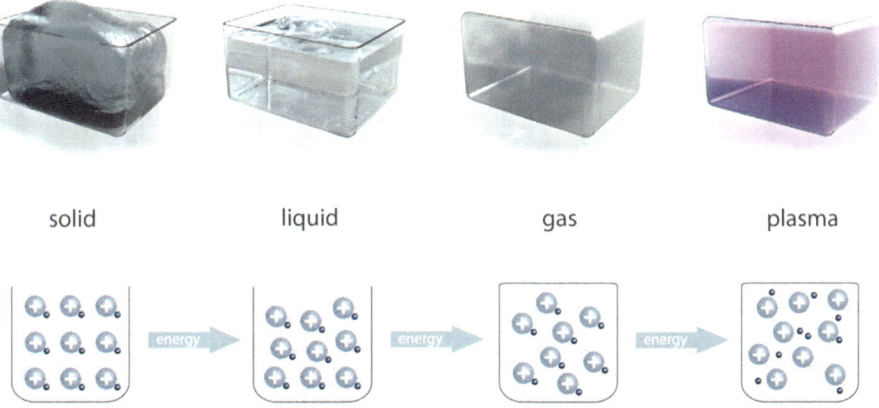

solid   liquid   gas   plasma

◘ **Fig. 3.1** Principle of the generation of physical plasma by adding energy to a gas. (Source: INP Greifswald)

concepts that do not change the tissue integrity by thermal means but rather to induce biological responses in a non-necrotizing fashion, virtually by being operated at body temperature. This is achieved by several components generated in "cold" physical plasmas. The main component, however, is the release of a variety of ROS that can be used therapeutically in a localized manner in the targeted tissue. In this book chapter, the different plasma components are discussed in terms of biomedical effects in vitro as well as in vivo in animal models as well as in human tissues. The chapter focusses on direct plasma applications, while taking into account results from studies using plasma-treated liquids (so-called "indirect" plasma treatment) as well as modeling studies without experimental evidence to a lesser extent. It, however, does not elaborate on specific contributions of plasma-derived components in disease resolution, since the many possible dermatological applications and diseases targeted in plasma medicine are too diverse and etiologically different to generate general conclusions with regard to individual effects of the plasma components.

3.2 Plasma Components and Source Concepts

The physicochemical characteristics of plasma are complex and depend on a multitude of parameters, including type and composition of the gas or gas mixture used for plasma generation, the energy being applied, the electrode configuration, and surroundings [5–7]. Since the 1990s, technologies for stable and reproducible plasma generation at body temperature under atmospheric conditions (cold atmospheric pressure plasma, CAP) are available on a larger scale, facilitating the generation of gas plasma devices also for medical applications [8, 9]. According to the current state of knowledge, free electrons, high-energy states of atoms and molecules along with ions and radicals in the plasma, and those generated in secondary reactions in the ambient air are the main components of plasmas [10, 11]. Over 500 chemical redox reactions occur in the plasma gas phase [12], with dozens of different types of ROS being generated simultaneously [13] that even show dynamic spatio-temporal concentrations [14]. In this chapter, the term ROS relates to both ROS and RNS simultaneously, as the latter also contains oxygen. Among the ROS identified in the best-investigated gas plasma device kINPen (see ▶ Chap. 16) in the fields of physics, biology, and medicine, are superoxide anion, hydroxyl radicals, peroxyl radicals, alkoxyl radicals, hydroperoxyl radicals, peroxynitrite, nitric oxide, singlet delta oxygen, and many others [15]. In addition to ROS, low electrical currents, electromagnetic radiation, mild ultraviolet (UV) light, and limited thermal radiation transferred to cells and tissue have the potential to elicit biological effects as well [16]. By definition, gas plasmas, therefore, are multi-component systems (◘ Fig. 3.2) with the amplitude and proportion of each of the components depending on the plasma device's geometry and operating conditions.

> ❯ Cold plasmas are multi-component systems consisting of electrons and ions, electric fields, UV and infrared radiation, and reactive oxygen and nitrogen species (ROS).

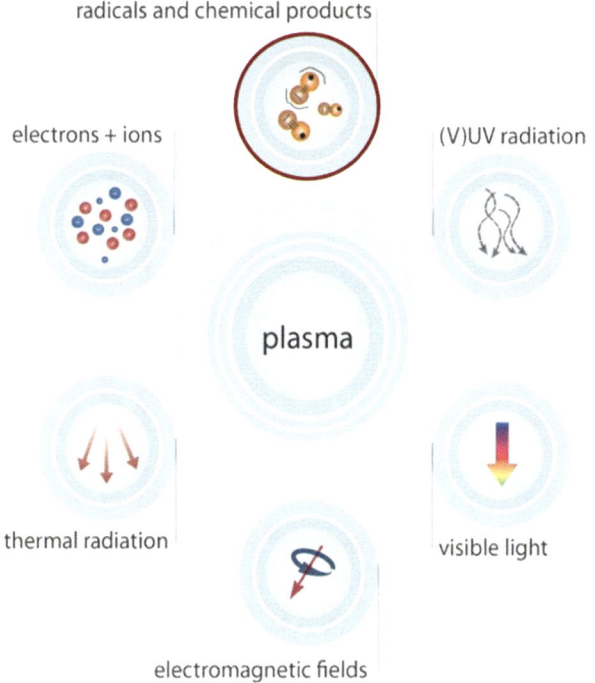

radicals and chemical products

electrons + ions

(V)UV radiation

plasma

thermal radiation

visible light

electromagnetic fields

■ **Fig. 3.2** The components of gas plasmas with ROS being the main biologically active compounds. (Source: INP Greifswald)

3.3 How Does Cold Plasma Work in Medicine: Conclusions Drawn from in Vitro Studies

Hundreds of studies have been conducted in the last twenty years based on observations made from plasma-treated cell cultures grown on plastic dishes in vitro. In general, it needs to be noted that plasma sources can differ considerably from each other in terms of geometry, electrical engineering, design, size, and mode of action. With an estimated three-digit number of plasma devices engineered for biomedical applications worldwide in the past two decades, with many of them being characterized to a sometimes-modest extent, this section is not intended to give a comprehensive overview of every single evidence presumably identified for the different types of devices. Instead, it will focus on the main findings made with commonly known plasma jets such as the kINPen and dielectric barrier discharges (DBD). The working principle of plasma jets and volume DBDs is shown below (■ Fig. 3.3), but also other well-studied DBD concepts with biomedical impact exist, such as surface DBDs [18–20]. For in vitro studies, an important factor to be considered is the presence of large amounts of liquids on top of and/or around the cultivated cells. This severely affects the biomass (cells) to liquid ratio in favor of the latter. Large amounts of liquids, in turn, attenuate several

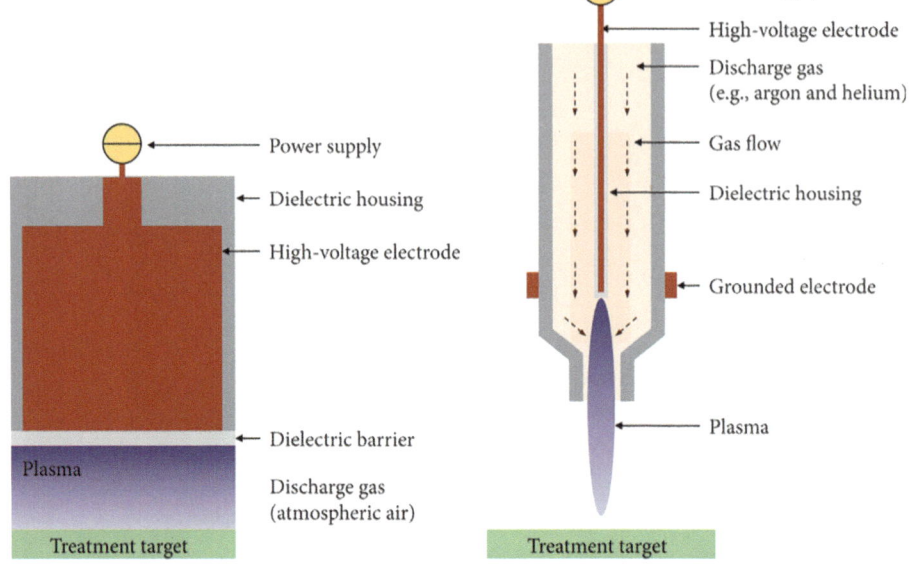

◘ Fig. 3.3   The two main principles of plasma sources, dielectric barrier discharges (left) and plasma jets (right). (Reproduced with permission from [17])

characteristics of plasma that otherwise might be possibly paramount in the direct treatment of tissue being rich in proteins and lipids. This is an essential factor to consider when concluding from in vitro studies for in vivo applications in plasma medicine. In vitro studies are nevertheless pivotal to explore the mechanistic basis of how plasma is perceived by cells and to make comparisons between different cell types, which is much more difficult to differentiate when treating tissues in vivo or ex vivo as these are composed of a multitude of different cell types and stromal compartments. Hence, it usually needs both to disentangle the basic mechanisms and the biomedical consequences of plasma treatment in medicine.

3.3.1   The Role of Plasma-Derived Electric Fields in Vitro

A putative role of electric fields as biomedical effectors of in vitro plasma treatment has been debated in several studies. As stated above, their role might depend on the type of device being investigated. For instance, it has been – although not comparatively – reported that helium plasma jets have strong electric fields that affect not only the plasma and plasma-treated droplets [21] but also the subsequent ROS generation [22]. Significant differences in gas phase-produced species (e.g., nitrogen metastables) were also observed in dependence of running the plasma in conductive mode (i.e., with the treated target directly "connecting" to the plasma) compared to the free-floating jet or DBD (with a gap distance of the plasma to the target) [23]. To treat a breast cancer cell line with a helium plasma jet, an increase of immediate (<30 min) cell permeabilization was reported and attributed to electric fields. Although appropriate controls were missing in this study to control for the simple drying effects of the feed gas flux that can lead to necrosis and immediate cell permeabilization [24]. For the kINPen argon plasma jet, it was found that its inherent electric fields are not strong enough to electroporate cells to facilitate the uptake of YO-PRO1 in a lymphocyte suspension, a dye commonly used in the field of bioelectrics to study membrane permeability [25]. By contrast, the application of pulsed electric fields, a method used in the clinic during electrochemotherapy [26], led to an instant uptake of YO-PRO1 at modest cytotoxicity rates, exemplifying the little strength of the electric field of the kINPen in this setting. For a well-known dielectric barrier discharge, the electric field can be studied by dipping the discharge into a liquid, disallowing plasma generation while generating an electric field. For the treatment of melanoma cells, an effect of this electric field alone was not observed, while the full plasma treatment exacerbated cell death in these tumor cells [27]. Yan and colleagues have recently claimed a new type of cell death induced via plasma-derived electric fields [28, 29]. However, several controls and molecular marker analysis, as required in cell death research [30], as well as the relevance in more complex tumor material such as 3D tumor spheroids lack, in order to determine a main role of plasma-derived electric fields unambiguously. Hence, electric fields persist during in vitro plasma treatment but are unlikely to play a major role during treatment of cells, a fact frequently observed in many in vitro studies that applied antioxidants to fully abolish plasma-induced effects (see below).

> ❯ Electrical fields are present during in vitro plasma treatment, but their role is limited for most plasma devices.

3.3.2 Role of Plasma-Derived Thermal Energy (Heat) in Vitro

The role of heat during in vitro treatment is negligible if the plasma sources' design acknowledges its biocompatibility, i.e., temperatures of less than 40 °C. For plasma jets, at moderate to high feed gas fluxes and sufficient distance to the target (usually a liquid containing cells), the gas flux even cools the treated target to a greater extent than heating it. Thermal cameras are available to measure the plasma device's dissipated thermal energy transfer to the target in vitro. This way, a lack of increasing the treated liquid temperatures to a supraphysiological level can be confirmed [31]. The kINPen has a temperature reported to be below 40 °C [2] and leads to an only modest increase in temperature within reasonable plasma treatment durations in vitro (■ Fig. 3.4).

> ❯ Appropriate biocompatible (<40 °C) plasma sources modestly elevate temperatures of a treated target suspension in vitro but are not doing so above physiological levels.

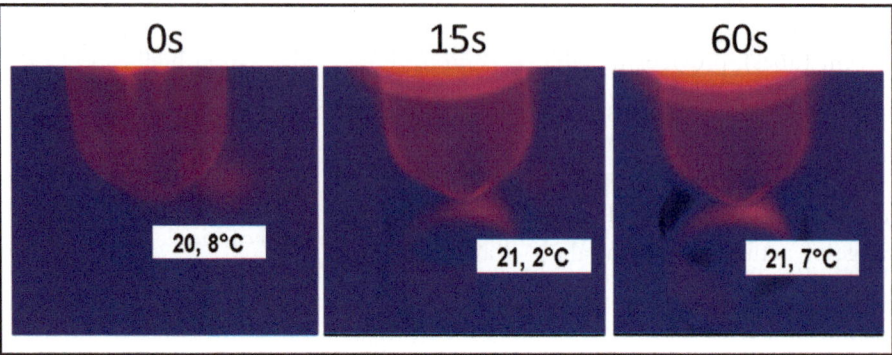

● **Fig. 3.4** Temperature of a saline solution at the beginning (left) and after 15 s (middle) and 60 s (right) of plasma treatment. (Source: INP Greifswald)

3.3.3 Role of Plasma-Derived Ultraviolet Radiation In Vitro

Ultraviolet (UV) radiation is segmented into UVA (315–400 nm), UVB (280–315 nm), and UVC (100–280 nm), and is produced during plasma generation [32]. Upon treatment of liquid, UV photolysis is capable of generating hydroxyl radicals in addition to those produced by the plasma [33]. Nevertheless, the lifetime of hydroxyl radicals is only about 100 ns, too short to appear at high concentrations in cells' direct vicinity. By contrast, hydroxyl radicals quickly deteriorate to more stable hydrogen peroxide, having significant biological effects in cells (see subsequent section). A similarly short range is known for vacuum and UVC radiation (<280 nm) that is quickly absorbed in air and at the gas-liquid interphase [34]. Accordingly, the hydrogen peroxide production of the vacuum UV portion of a plasma jet is about 100-fold less than that of the entire plasma, while the UV portion failed to generate noticeable amounts [35]. This is in line with a previous report showing a marked decline of antimicrobial activity of UV generated by an argon plasma jet (using a glass permitting only UV radiation but not ROS) when compared to the entire ROS generated by the plasma jet [36]. An analogous, despite less quantitative conclusion was reached by another study [37]. Nevertheless, another study concluded that UVC was more critical than ROS when it came to antimicrobial activity, although they reported at the same time that the antioxidant vitamin C abrogated most of the plasma-mediated antimicrobial activity [38]. This suggests one-time ROS exposure to not play a role in DNA damage since, in turn, UV radiation on intracellular DNA and subsequent DNA damage cannot be entirely counteracted by the addition of antioxidants. The failure of plasma treatment (that includes plasma-derived UV radiation known to have a minor intensity) has been recently demonstrated to directly and permanently damage DNA within intact cells to produce genotoxic events [39]. In-depth experimental characterizations of the plasma-derived UV portion on eukaryotic cells' viability and function are not available. Nevertheless, we would like to follow the conclusion drawn by Van Gils and colleagues up to this point. This states that the effects of heat, metastables (not discussed here, but investigated before [40]), ion- and UV-fluxes, electric fields, and gas flow (application of the pure and chemically inert noble gas argon or helium) do not have a prominent effect on the antimicrobial activity of plasma [34], which likely is also true to for the in vitro treatment of eukaryotic cells, at least for plasma jets. The low importance of UV is underlined by the frequent observation of radical scavengers abrogating plasma-effects, and by the effects seen with plasma-treated liquids [41].

❯ The impact of plasma-derived UV radiation during in vitro treatment of cells is low.

3.3.4 Role of Plasma-Derived ROS in Vitro

The current literature in plasma medicine states a myriad of reaction pathways, leading to the different ROS types in the plasma gas phase with different concentrations and compositions at different positions of the plasma streamers [15, 42–46]. An extensive review of the plasma chemistry and reaction products has been done before [43, 47] and is out of this chapter's scope. The intrinsic link between plasma medicine and redox biology, a field dealing with ROS's beneficial and detrimental effects in cells and tissues [48], has already been made by David Graves in 2012 [49]. Ever since, a plethora of studies have investigated and confirmed the causative relationship between plasma-derived ROS penetrating liquid and being the main effectors of the biomedical effects observed in vitro [50–53]. It delineates the different factors involved in cellular responses in vitro. These include the type of cell culture medium or liquid used in which the cells are immersed, any antioxidants included in these liquids, the type of plasma source, for plasma jets the feed gas composition, the intrinsic antioxidant defense and pro-survival signaling of the cell type(s) investigated, the time point of cellular investigation, stoichiometric considerations (i.e., the number of cells per volume unit of liquid in relation to plasma treatment energy or time), and – a recent field of investigation – the presence of organic molecules such as peptides and proteins that possibly attenuate or exacerbate the plasma effect on cells. A non-exhaustive list of studies is given in the following to exemplify these points.

The type of liquid in which the cells are immersed, as well as its composition, provides ROS-scavenging molecules to a different extent. For instance, the amount of hydrogen peroxide being deposited into (Roswell Park Memorial Institute [RPMI]) cell culture medium is twice as high as compared to, e.g., clinically relevant hydroxyethyl starch (HES) solution [54]. Moreover, the metabolic activity of cells exposed to plasma in Iscove's Modified Dulbecco's Medium (IMDM) compared to RPMI medium differs by a factor of 10 [55]. Hence, the choice of culture medium in an in vitro plasma medicine study is already a significant determinant of the outcome, and respective plasma treatment times are needed to achieve a biological effect. This is even more complicated considering cell culture medium additives, such as pyruvate, a major antioxidant shown to be decisive in protecting cells from plasma-induced oxidative stress [56]. Especially Dulbecco's Modified Eagle's Medium (DMEM) has variable amounts of pyruvate added, and care should be taken when choosing the specific type of DMEM for in vitro studies. Another additive sometimes found in culture medium is 2-mercaptoethanol, as this compound reduces the ROS being produced in heavily proliferating cells. We have found this additive to affect plasma in vitro effects as well (unpublished observation).

Another major factor influencing cellular responses is the type of ROS chemistry produced by the plasma. While this is an extensive field of (ongoing) research, it has been found for eukaryotic cells that at least two downstream reaction pathways exist. One leads to the accumulation of hydrogen peroxide, while the second yields vast amounts of hypochlorous acid, as outlined in detail in previous reports [57–59]. In principle, peroxynitrite has been observed to be formed, but a dominating biological effect over other species has been suggested rather than generally observed for many types of sources, at least at physiological pH [20, 50, 60, 61]. Depending on the target cells investigated, other species also come into play. For instance, superoxide was essential for antimicrobial inactivation [59] but not in the killing of lymphocytes (unpublished data). Especially for plasma jets, the ROS chemistry can be tuned to pronounce the production of some types of ROS, while attenuating the generation of other with subsequent biological consequences [62–64]. Nevertheless, after all, many studies report an abrogation of plasma effects in the presence of a scavenger being specific for the major classes of ROS being produced, such as catalase, N-acetylcysteine, glutathione, and mannitol. This once more exemplifies the pivotal role of ROS in plasma medicine research in vitro.

Moreover, the cell type being investigated has a significant effect on the biomedical response observed. Different cell types inherently differ by their capacity to cope with ROS-induced stress [65] and to succumb to cell death [66]. This phenomenon has also been observed in comparative studies in plasma medicine. For instance, non-malignant human keratinocytes are less sensitive to plasma-induced inactivation compared to human skin cancer cells [67], but more sensitive compared to human breast cancer cells [55]. Human leukemia cells of lymphocytic origin are more susceptible than those of myeloid origin [68]. While many similar observations have been made throughout the past years, the molecular basis accounting for these differences is less clear. We have recently suggested correlating the capability to import the antioxidant glutathione with the plasma-induced inactivation of cancer cells [69]. In contrast, others have proposed the expression of aquaporins (important for water and extracellular hydrogen peroxide transport into cells) to play a significant role [70, 71]. In the face of biology, it is natural that the findings often observed only reflect a cellular response's snapshot. For instance, apoptosis, a form of programmed cell death for many cell types, is a time-consuming process, not to be noted at significant levels before 12 h in, e.g., human lymphocytes, and peaking in about 24–48 h [72]. By contrast, rapidly proliferating cells such as B16F10 melanoma cells succumb very quickly to the plasma-induced cell death [73] and start to recover (and re-grow) already 12 h post-exposure, leading to a lower overall cytotoxic response at 24 h when compared to 12 h [74]. Bearing this in mind, it is needless to illustrate that the biological response to plasma treatment in vitro also is a function of the number of cells and the amount of liquid being treated. In simple terms, the more cells are present, the less ROS per cell are being effective, and the less intense (or cytotoxic) is the plasma treatment. By contrast, the more liquid is present during the treatment (with identical numbers of cells within it), the more the ROS are "diluted," and the less intense (or cytotoxic) is the response measured [55]. Hence, in vitro plasma treatment follows the pharmaceutical principles observed also with other agents.

Finally, a recent but exciting question on how plasma medicine works in vitro is investigating the contribution of oxidative modification of organic molecules. For instance, Tanaka and colleagues have identified lactate of *Ringer's* lactate solution to be oxidatively modified, and this modification confers the majority of the toxic effects observed with this plasma-treated liquid [75]. In our research, we have not only found plasma treatment to generate a highly diverse set of oxidative modifications in cysteine stemming from short-lived and not only long-lived (such as hydrogen peroxide) ROS [76] but also that plasma-treated cysteine by itself exerted distinct biological effect in cells in vitro [77]. This is exciting because this opens up a novel way of investigating the biomedical effects of plasma apart from the direct action of plasma-derived ROS or any other components on the cells. Current research lines are, therefore, exploring how those mechanisms could be further exploited therapeutically.

> The central role of plasma-derived ROS in exerting biomedical effects in vitro is undisputed. However, the type and amplitude of those responses depend on several factors, such as the cell culture medium used, the cell line being investigated, and the plasma source and specific ROS composition being generated.

3.4 How Does Cold Plasma Work in Medicine: Conclusions Drawn from in Vivo and Tissue-Based Studies

The in vivo role of plasma-derived electric fields, thermal energy, UV radiation, and ROS has been explored only to a limited extent yet. This is because of three limitations. The first is that it is nearly impossible to single out the individual component to disentangle their individual effects in vivo in the way of *exactly* matching the kinetics and intensity as derived from the plasma source. For instance, it was observed that plasma exposure of human skin ex vivo leads to a plasma treatment time-dependent increase in the proliferation of skin cells [78]. Whether this effect is a consequence of electric fields, thermal energy, UV radiation, ROS, or all or some of them is difficult to judge. This is further complicated because tissue as a "third electrode" impacts the plasma generation [17] so that studies of the plasma sources alone or in vitro studies with cell culture plastic do not accurately mimic treatment of a more complex tissue. The second limitation is that tissue comprises several types of cells. Observing a change in one cell type does not necessarily mean that these cells directly responded to the plasma treatment, but rather were affected by another cell type (e.g., via cytokines or cell-cell-communication) that responded to the plasma treatment. While this is a more hypothetical idea, it is known that, for instance, tissue-resident macrophages, despite being low in numbers, can dramatically affect nearby cells via inflammatory mediators [79]. The third limitation is the lack of methods to identify each of the plasma components' effect directly. There are currently no tools available in redox biology to differentiate the oxidation of cells or tissue components resulting from either hydroxyl radicals, atomic oxygen, or singlet delta oxygen.

Nevertheless, we here attempt to summarize the current knowledge of individual plasma-effectors on the tissue. The focus is predominantly on animal tissue, not mentioning some of the findings achieved in pseudo-tissue models such as alginate or collagen gels.

> It is difficult to disentangle the contribution of individual plasma components in tissues, mainly because of technical limitations of measuring their intensity in vivo.

3.4.1   The Role of Plasma-Derived Electric Fields in Vivo

An entire scientific community, bioelectrics, is devoted to the effects of pulsed electric fields in medicine, especially oncology. Hence, there is ample knowledge on how electric fields affect tissues. It is commonly assumed that electric fields in the microsecond range electroporate cells in tissues, but do not have any other effect except those stemming from the consequences of electroporation. By contrast, electric fields in the nanosecond range are thought to have distinct biological effects. The electric fields are commonly applied in patients or tissues using needle electrodes and field strengths [80]. As outlined above, direct evidence of plasma-derived electric field effects is lacking. However, one recent study found that a helium plasma jet had a decrease in voltage and current when in contact with a grounded human compared to an in vitro cell plastic culture dish [22]. This suggests that the electric field strength of in vivo plasma treatment is even smaller compared to those obtained from laboratory results. Such effect, however, may even be weaker in argon plasma jets as these are known to generate electric field strengths significantly below that of helium jets [81], with the latter having even higher values close to a target [82] that, moreover, depend on the excitation frequency of the jet [83].

> The in vivo effects of plasma-derived electric fields are unknown but likely stronger in helium than argon plasma jets.

3.4.2   The Role of Plasma-Derived Thermal Energy (Heat) in Vivo

The effect of elevated temperature on tissues, even at small scales, is undisputed [84]. Appropriate medical plasma devices are tissue compatible in terms of temperature, i.e., they do not exceed 40 °C and are thus void of generating thermal damage. Vice versa, some wounds display impaired healing below 28 °C [85], and a mild local increase of the temperature might even stimulate healing. It is known

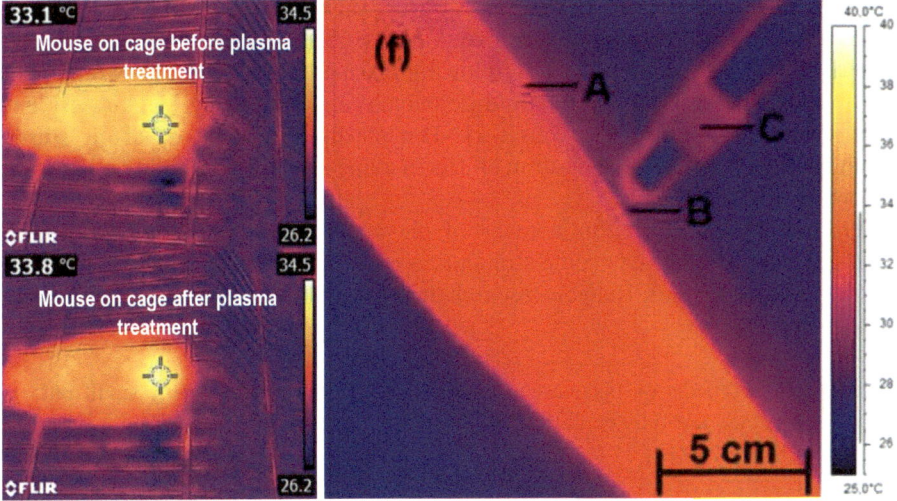

❏ Fig. 3.5 (left) A mouse sitting on a cage and imaged with a thermal camera to assess the temperature immediately before plasma treatment of the skin (upper image) and directly after (lower image) plasma treatment; a relevant increase was not observed. Reproduced with permission from [31]. (right) Temperature of a human forearm during plasma treatment with the argon plasma jet kINPen (C). The temperature at the plasma contact site (B) does not differ from the other part of the skin (A). (Source: INP Greifswald)

that mild temperature increase can elevate the expression of heat-shock proteins, which not only have protective and chaperone functions, but in turn, can also act as damage-associated molecular patterns to promote immune responses [86–89]. However, the exact contribution of plasma devices' temperature in terms of biomedical effects has not been studied sufficiently. Some studies have used thermal cameras to demonstrate the target tissue's temperature before and after plasma treatment. For instance (❏ Fig. 3.5), Saadati and colleagues measured the temperature of murine skin and did not find plasma treatment to cause any elevation [31]. The same is true for the medical plasma jet kINPen (unpublished data).

> ❯ The in vivo effect of plasma-mediated temperature is supposedly small as medical plasma sources operate at body temperature.

3.4.3   The Role of Plasma-Derived UV Radiation in Vivo

The role of UV radiation, especially in terms of safety, has been described in ▶ Chap. 5 of this book already. In general, UV radiation has substantial effects in tissues, motivating its medical use in dermatology across several types of diseases at modest intensities [90]. At the same time, chronically high levels of UV can damage the skin and support carcinogenesis. As outlined in ▶ Chap. 5, however, the

UV radiation of medical plasma devices during their recommended use is far less than even allowed for the most sensitive skin type. A good indication of this is the lack of skin erythema ("sunburn") following plasma treatment, which would otherwise appear if UV radiation would be perceived as damaging by skin-resident cells. From the clinical perspective, kINPen plasma treatment of acute, sterile wounds [91] did not show long-term effects in a one-year [92, 93] and five-year [94] follow-up study [94].

Despite the UV radiation intensity of plasma-devices being low, it cannot be excluded that UV still has some stimulating effects on the skin as observed with medical UV treatments. Reliable research data on this matter, however, are lacking in plasma medicine.

> The in vivo effects of plasma-generated UV radiation is supposedly small but experimentally not fully explored yet.

3.4.4 The Role of Plasma-Derived ROS in Vivo

Plasma-derived ROS are supposed to be the main effectors in biomedicine. While this fact is undisputed in vitro, supporting this claim in vivo is much more complicated. As outlined above, this mainly relates to the lack of specific redox biology tools to unambiguously track the ROS effects and, ideally, the type of ROS within tissues [95–99]. However, there is some direct and indirect evidence of plasma-derived ROS effects within tissues suggested so far. The by far most substantial evidence, in our hands, comes from our previous study in mice, where plasma treatment of wounds generated an intense increase in the expression of Nrf2 (nuclear factor erythroid 2-related factor 2), a redox-sensitive transcription factor that responds to altered ROS levels [100]. One of its transcriptional targets, heme oxygenase 1 (*HMOX1* / HO-1), was upregulated up to 300-fold in plasma-treated wounds compared to untreated control wounds, exemplifying massive redox regulation to be at work following plasma treatment.

One possibility to "catch" radicals where they appear is adding spin traps to an organism, such as a mouse, and measuring the tissue (post plasma treatment) using electron spin resonance (ESR/EPR) spectroscopy [101]. A recent study used spin-trap soaked tissue ex vivo following plasma treatment to estimate ROS penetration into that tissue [102]. Using different spin traps, the data evidenced the presence of hydroxyl and superoxide radicals being deposited by the plasma treatment into the tissue. This is the first and only study to measure radical formation inside plasma-treated tissues directly. However, it needs to be noted that the ESR/EPR is only a semi-quantitative method, as intra-tissue concentrations of the – usually expensive – spin trap compounds are usually lower than the amounts of ROS being generated. Nevertheless, more studies like this are needed to trace ROS trajectories into tissues to understand their biomedical consequences.

Another possibility to identify signatures of ROS in tissues is using mass spectrometry. For instance, this method can measure post-translational modifications such as 3-nitrotyrosine formation in proteins derived from tissues [103]. While we have successfully achieved this in tyrosine solutions following plasma treatment [50], studies investigating this product in vivo have not been performed yet. However, mass spectrometry can also identify oxidative post-translational modifications in lipids. To this end, we have recently treated the skin of human foreheads and found multiple oxidative modifications in subsequent lipidomics analysis, albeit to a lesser extent than expected [104]. This was confirmed in animal studies analyzing skin lipid oxidation (unpublished data). While mass spectrometry undoubtedly is among the most sensitive and precise methods to track oxidative modifications in tissue-derived material, it is at the same time also demanding on preparation time and accuracy as well as the scientific and data management and analysis infrastructure. Possibly due to these reasons, studies reporting ROS modifications in plasma-treated tissues are scarce.

Another option to assess the consequences of plasma-derived ROS in tissues is in vivo imaging. For instance, using hyperspectral-imaging technology, we have recently established a protocol measuring the immediate consequences of plasma treatment in mice, such as tissue oxygenation and water content [105]. Similar data were recorded in clinical reports with patients suffering from chronic wounds [106, 107]. With appropriate controls provided, such a method may also disentangle the different plasma components and their contributions to the immediate tissue reaction. Another option for imaging ROS in vivo is the use of fluorescent probes in animal models. For instance, fluorescent reporter proteins are available to monitor ROS explicitly generated in the cytosol or mitochondrial membrane in skin cells in vivo [108]. In botany research, many fluorescent redox-sensitive dyes have been developed in the past years and applied successfully [109, 110]. Reports on using fluorescent dyes for in vivo consequences and ROS tracing following plasma treatment are yet awaited. However, along those lines, we have recently used a luminescent probe injected in vivo to quantify the deposition of plasma-derived ROS into the skin in vivo (unpublished data) using bioluminescence imaging (☐ Fig. 3.6).

> Several technical possibilities exist to trace the in vivo trajectories of plasma-derived ROS into tissues. However, resolving those effects on a level of single reactive species currently is a technical challenge yet to be overcome.

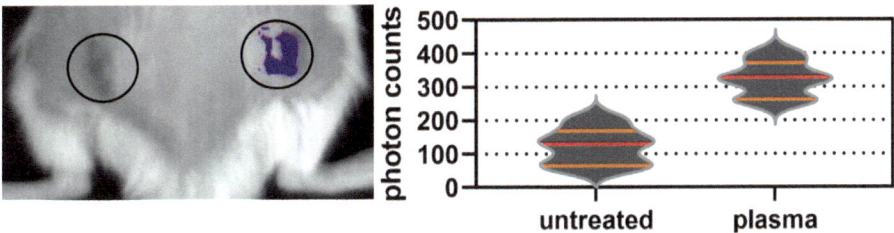

☐ **Fig. 3.6** (left) In vivo bioluminescence imaging of a non-treated (left circle) and plasma-treated area of a mouse with a dye indicating oxidation. (right) quantitative analysis of the signal of the left area (untreated) and right area (plasma-treated) of several mice. (Source: INP Greifswald)

Conclusion

The mechanistic investigations in plasma medicine face two challenges. The first is the nature of the plasma being a multi-component system, making it difficult – especially in complex samples such as tissues – to unambiguously identify the one or few main effectors responsible for the biomedical consequences of plasma treatment. The second is the lack of specific probes in science in general and redox biology specifically that – ideally even after fixation and cutting of tissues – would allow tracing the ROS inside of tissues. Nevertheless, from the studies published so far, it can be concluded that ROS are the main effectors driving plasma-medical effects, while mostly in vivo, the – presumably minor – contribution of other components such as low electric fields and mild UV radiation cannot be excluded as of now.

However, even though the specific role of different plasma components in vivo is not yet finally explored, some biological effects are proven to the extent that the application of cold atmospheric plasma in therapeutic settings has started. So far, the most critical medical plasma application is in wound healing. With a particular focus on chronic wounds, the primary objective of plasma application was to use its well-proven antimicrobial activity for wound antisepsis [111–113]. However, based on several in vitro experiments with cell cultures giving insight into cellular signal cascades that are relevant for cell proliferation, migration, and angiogenesis, in vivo studies on acute artificial wounds could demonstrate undoubtedly that cold atmospheric plasma is useful to accelerate the rate of wound closure at early stages after wounding, independent of any antiseptic effectivity [91, 114–117]. This was proven recently in a prospective, randomized, placebo-controlled, patient-blinded clinical trial in patients with diabetic foot ulcers, where a significant increase in wound healing was found independently from bacterial load reduction [118].

In cancer treatment, much more preclinical and clinical research is needed to allow cold plasma application in clinical settings. However, first applications are realized in palliative care to decontaminate infected head and neck cancer ulcerations [119]. As a secondary effect, in some cases, a partial and temporary remission of tumor growth was found [120]. These clinical observations are encouraging to follow the way to expand clinical plasma medicine to cancer treatment in the future.

The chapter offers a conceptual overview of the different plasma components and their presumable contribution to the biological effects observed in vitro and in vivo. Hence, this overview allows conclusions on how plasma works in biomedicine and outlines the principal routes of current research as well as technical and conceptual gaps needed for exploring the mechanisms of action in more detail in the future. Along those lines, it is out of the question that reactive oxygen and nitrogen species play a significant role in plasma medicine, but the exact extent remains to be investigated.

References

1. von Woedtke T, Reuter S, Masur K, Weltmann KD. Plasmas for medicine. Phys Rep. 2013;530:291–320. https://doi.org/10.1016/j.physrep.2013.05.005.
2. Weltmann KD, Kindel E, Brandenburg R, Meyer C, Bussiahn R, Wilke C, von Woedtke T. Atmospheric pressure plasma jet for medical therapy: plasma parameters and risk estimation. Contrib Plasma Physics. 2009;49:631–40. https://doi.org/10.1002/ctpp.200910067.
3. Grund KE, Straub T, Farin G. New haemostatic techniques: argon plasma coagulation. Baillieres Best Pract Res Clin Gastroenterol. 1999;13:67–84.
4. Zenker M. Argon plasma coagulation. GMS Krankenhhyg Interdiszip. 2008;3:Doc15.
5. Braithwaite NSJ. Introduction to gas discharges. Plasma Sources Sci Technol. 2000;9:517–27. https://doi.org/10.1088/0963-0252/9/4/307.
6. Conrads H, Schmidt M. Plasma generation and plasma sources. Plasma Sources Sci Technol. 2000;9:441–54. https://doi.org/10.1088/0963-0252/9/4/301.
7. Bogaerts A, Neyts E, Gijbels R, van der Mullen J. Gas discharge plasmas and their applications. Spectrochim Acta Part B At Spectrosc. 2002;57:609–58. https://doi.org/10.1016/S0584-8547(01)00406-2.
8. Park GY, Park SJ, Choi MY, Koo IG, Byun JH, Hong JW, Sim JY, Collins GJ, Lee JK. Atmospheric-pressure plasma sources for biomedical applications. Plasma Sources Sci Technol. 2012;21. https://doi.org/10.1088/0963-0252/21/4/043001.
9. Weltmann KD, von Woedtke T. Basic requirements for plasma sources in medicine. Eur Phys J Appl Phys. 2011;55:13807. https://doi.org/10.1051/epjap/2011100452.
10. Setsuhara Y. Low-temperature atmospheric-pressure plasma sources for plasma medicine. Arch Biochem Biophys. 2016;605:3–10. https://doi.org/10.1016/j.abb.2016.04.009.
11. Tanaka H, Ishikawa K, Mizuno M, Toyokuni S, Kajiyama H, Kikkawa F, Metelmann H-R, Hori M. State of the art in medical applications using non-thermal atmospheric pressure plasma. Rev Mod Plasma Phys. 2017;1:14–8. https://doi.org/10.1007/s41614-017-0004-3.
12. Schmidt-Bleker A, Winter J, Iseni S, Dunnbier M, Weltmann KD, Reuter S. Reactive species output of a plasma jet with a shielding gas device-combination of FTIR absorption spectroscopy and gas phase modelling. J Phys D Appl Phys. 2014;47:145201. https://doi.org/10.1088/0022-3727/47/14/145201.
13. Dunnbier M, Schmidt-Bleker A, Winter J, Wolfram M, Hippler R, Weltmann KD, Reuter S. Ambient air particle transport into the effluent of a cold atmospheric-pressure argon plasma jet investigated by molecular beam mass spectrometry. J Phys D Appl Phys. 2013;46:435203. https://doi.org/10.1088/0022-3727/46/43/435203.
14. Schmidt-Bleker A, Bansemer R, Reuter S, Weltmann K-D. How to produce an nox- instead of ox-based chemistry with a cold atmospheric plasma jet. Plasma Process Polym. 2016;13:1120–7. https://doi.org/10.1002/ppap.201600062.
15. Reuter S, von Woedtke T, Weltmann KD. The kINPen-a review on physics and chemistry of the atmospheric pressure plasma jet and its applications. J Phys D Appl Phys. 2018;51. https://doi.org/10.1088/1361-6463/aab3ad.
16. Weltmann KD, von Woedtke T. Plasma medicine-current state of research and medical application. Plasma Phys Control Fusion. 2017;59:014031. https://doi.org/10.1088/0741-3335/59/1/014031.
17. Privat-Maldonado A, Schmidt A, Lin A, Weltmann KD, Wende K, Bogaerts A, Bekeschus S. ROS from physical plasmas: redox chemistry for biomedical therapy. Oxidative Med Cell Longev. 2019;2019:9062098. https://doi.org/10.1155/2019/9062098.
18. Brandenburg R. Dielectric barrier discharges: progress on plasma sources and on the understanding of regimes and single filaments. Plasma Sources Sci Technol. 2017;26:053001. https://doi.org/10.1088/1361-6595/aa6426.
19. Lackmann JW, Baldus S, Steinborn E, Edengeiser E, Kogelheide F, Langklotz S, Schneider S, Leichert LIO, Benedikt J, Awakowicz P, Bandow JE. A dielectric barrier discharge terminally inactivates RNase a by oxidizing sulfur-containing amino acids and breaking structural disulfide bonds. J Phys D Appl Phys. 2015;48. https://doi.org/10.1088/0022-3727/48/49/494003.

3

20. Oehmigen K, Hahnel M, Brandenburg R, Wilke C, Weltmann KD, von Woedtke T. The role of acidification for antimicrobial activity of atmospheric pressure plasma in liquids. Plasma Process Polym. 2010;7:250–7. https://doi.org/10.1002/ppap.200900077.
21. Stancampiano A, Gallingani T, Gherardi M, Machala Z, Maguire P, Colombo V, Pouvesle J-M, Robert E. Plasma and aerosols: challenges, opportunities and perspectives. Appl Sci. 2019;9. https://doi.org/10.3390/app9183861.
22. Stancampiano A, Chung TH, Dozias S, Pouvesle JM, Mir LM, Robert E. Mimicking of human body electrical characteristic for easier translation of plasma biomedical studies to clinical applications. IEEE Trans Radiat Plasma Med Sci. 2020;4:335–42. https://doi.org/10.1109/trpms.2019.2936667.
23. Darny T, Pouvesle JM, Puech V, Douat C, Dozias S, Robert E. Analysis of conductive target influence in plasma jet experiments through helium metastable and electric field measurements. Plasma Sources Sci Technol. 2017;26:045008. https://doi.org/10.1088/1361-6595/aa5b15.
24. Sasaki S, Honda R, Hokari Y, Takashima K, Kanzaki M, Kaneko T. Characterization of plasma-induced cell membrane permeabilization: focus on oh radical distribution. J Phys D Appl Phys. 2016;49. https://doi.org/10.1088/0022-3727/49/33/334002.
25. Wolff CM, Kolb JF, Weltmann KD, von Woedtke T, Bekeschus S. Combination treatment with cold physical plasma and pulsed electric fields augments ROS production and cytotoxicity in lymphoma. Cancers (Basel). 2020;12:845. https://doi.org/10.3390/cancers12040845.
26. Wolff CM, Steuer A, Stoffels I, von Woedtke T, Weltmann K-D, Bekeschus S, Kolb JF. Combination of cold plasma and pulsed electric fields – a rationale for cancer patients in palliative care. Clin Plasma Med. 2019;16. https://doi.org/10.1016/j.cpme.2020.100096.
27. Lin A, Gorbanev Y, De Backer J, Van Loenhout J, Van Boxem W, Lemiere F, Cos P, Dewilde S, Smits E, Bogaerts A. Non-thermal plasma as a unique delivery system of short-lived reactive oxygen and nitrogen species for immunogenic cell death in melanoma cells. Adv Sci (Weinh). 2019;6:1802062. https://doi.org/10.1002/advs.201802062.
28. Yan D, Wang Q, Adhikari M, Malyavko A, Lin L, Zolotukhin DB, Yao X, Kirschner M, Sherman JH, Keidar M. A physically triggered cell death via transbarrier cold atmospheric plasma cancer treatment. ACS Appl Mater Interfaces. 2020;12:34548–63. https://doi.org/10.1021/acsami.0c06500.
29. Yan D, Wang Q, Malyavko A, Zolotukhin DB, Adhikari M, Sherman JH, Keidar M. The anti-glioblastoma effect of cold atmospheric plasma treatment: physical pathway v.s. chemical pathway. Sci Rep. 2020;10:11788. https://doi.org/10.1038/s41598-020-68585-z.
30. Galluzzi L, Vitale I, Warren S, Adjemian S, Agostinis P, Martinez AB, Chan TA, Coukos G, Demaria S, Deutsch E, et al. Consensus guidelines for the definition, detection and interpretation of immunogenic cell death. J Immunother Cancer. 2020;8. https://doi.org/10.1136/jitc-2019-000337.
31. Saadati F, Mahdikia H, Abbaszadeh HA, Abdollahifar MA, Khoramgah MS, Shokri B. Comparison of direct and indirect cold atmospheric-pressure plasma methods in the b16f10 melanoma cancer cells treatment. Sci Rep. 2018;8:7689. https://doi.org/10.1038/s41598-018-25990-9.
32. Weltmann KD, Kindel E, von Woedtke T, Hahnel M, Stieber M, Brandenburg R. Atmospheric-pressure plasma sources: prospective tools for plasma medicine. Pure Appl Chem. 2010;82:1223–37. https://doi.org/10.1351/Pac-Con-09-10-35.
33. Attri P, Kim YH, Park DH, Park JH, Hong YJ, Uhm HS, Kim KN, Fridman A, Choi EH. Generation mechanism of hydroxyl radical species and its lifetime prediction during the plasma-initiated ultraviolet (UV) photolysis. Sci Rep. 2015;5:9332. https://doi.org/10.1038/srep09332.
34. Van Gils C, Hofmann S, Boekema B, Brandenburg R, Bruggeman P. Mechanisms of bacterial inactivation in the liquid phase induced by a remote RF cold atmospheric pressure plasma jet. J Phys D Appl Phys. 2013;46:175203.
35. Jablonowski H, Bussiahn R, Hammer MU, Weltmann KD, von Woedtke T, Reuter S. Impact of plasma jet vacuum ultraviolet radiation on reactive oxygen species generation in bio-relevant liquids. Phys Plasmas. 2015;22:122008. https://doi.org/10.1063/1.4934989.

36. Brandenburg R, Lange H, von Woedtke T, Stieber M, Kindel E, Ehlbeck J, Weltmann KD. Antimicrobial effects of UV and VUV radiation of nonthermal plasma jets. IEEE Trans Plasma Sci. 2009;37:877–83. https://doi.org/10.1109/Tps.2009.2019657.

37. Schneider S, Lackmann J-W, Ellerweg D, Denis B, Narberhaus F, Bandow JE, Benedikt J. The role of VUV radiation in the inactivation of bacteria with an atmospheric pressure plasma jet. Plasma Process Polym. 2012;9:561–8. https://doi.org/10.1002/ppap.201100102.

38. Judee F, Wattieaux G, Merbahi N, Mansour M, Castanie-Cornet MP. The antibacterial activity of a microwave argon plasma jet at atmospheric pressure relies mainly on UV-C radiations. J Phys D Appl Phys. 2014;47. https://doi.org/10.1088/0022-3727/47/40/405201.

39. Bekeschus S, Schutz CS, Niessner F, Wende K, Weltmann KD, Gelbrich N, von Woedtke T, Schmidt A, Stope MB. Elevated H2AX phosphorylation observed with kINPen plasma treatment is not caused by ROS-mediated DNA damage but is the consequence of apoptosis. Oxidative Med Cell Longev. 2019;2019:8535163. https://doi.org/10.1155/2019/8535163.

40. Bekeschus S, Iseni S, Reuter S, Masur K, Weltmann KD. Nitrogen shielding of an argon plasma jet and its effects on human immune cells. IEEE Trans Plasma Sci. 2015;43:776–81. https://doi.org/10.1109/Tps.2015.2393379.

41. Yan D, Sherman JH, Keidar M. The application of the cold atmospheric plasma-activated solutions in cancer treatment. Anti Cancer Agents Med Chem. 2018;18:769–75. https://doi.org/10.2174/1871520617666170731115233.

42. Adamovich I, Baalrud SD, Bogaerts A, Bruggeman PJ, Cappelli M, Colombo V, Czarnetzki U, Ebert U, Eden JG, Favia P, et al. The 2017 plasma roadmap: low temperature plasma science and technology. J Phys D Appl Phys. 2017;50:323001. https://doi.org/10.1088/1361-6463/aa76f5.

43. Bruggeman PJ, Kushner MJ, Locke BR, Gardeniers JGE, Graham WG, Graves DB, Hofman-Caris RCHM, Maric D, Reid JP, Ceriani E, et al. Plasma-liquid interactions: a review and roadmap. Plasma Sources Sci Technol. 2016;25:053002. https://doi.org/10.1088/0963-0252/25/5/053002.

44. Norberg SA, Johnsen E, Kushner MJ. Formation of reactive oxygen and nitrogen species by repetitive negatively pulsed helium atmospheric pressure plasma jets propagating into humid air. Plasma Sources Sci Technol. 2015;24. https://doi.org/10.1088/0963-0252/24/3/035026.

45. Schmidt-Bleker A, Norberg SA, Winter J, Johnsen E, Reuter S, Weltmann KD, Kushner MJ. Propagation mechanisms of guided streamers in plasma jets: the influence of electronegativity of the surrounding gas. Plasma Sources Sci Technol. 2015;24. https://doi.org/10.1088/0963-0252/24/3/035022.

46. Lietz AM, Kushner MJ. Air plasma treatment of liquid covered tissue: long timescale chemistry. J Phys D Appl Phys. 2016;49. https://doi.org/10.1088/0022-3727/49/42/425204.

47. Jablonowski H, von Woedtke T. Research on plasma medicine-relevant plasma–liquid interaction: what happened in the past five years? Clin Plasma Med. 2015;3:42–52. https://doi.org/10.1016/j.cpme.2015.11.003.

48. Sies H. Oxidative stress: a concept in redox biology and medicine. Redox Biol. 2015;4:180–3. https://doi.org/10.1016/j.redox.2015.01.002.

49. Graves DB. The emerging role of reactive oxygen and nitrogen species in redox biology and some implications for plasma applications to medicine and biology. J Phys D Appl Phys. 2012;45:263001. https://doi.org/10.1088/0022-3727/45/26/263001.

50. Bekeschus S, Kolata J, Winterbourn C, Kramer A, Turner R, Weltmann KD, Broker B, Masur K. Hydrogen peroxide: a central player in physical plasma-induced oxidative stress in human blood cells. Free Radic Res. 2014;48:542–9. https://doi.org/10.3109/10715762.2014.892937.

51. Judee F, Fongia C, Ducommun B, Yousfi M, Lobjois V, Merbahi N. Short and long time effects of low temperature Plasma Activated Media on 3D multicellular tumor spheroids. Sci Rep. 2016;6:21421. https://doi.org/10.1038/srep21421.

52. Kaushik N, Uddin N, Sim GB, Hong YJ, Baik KY, Kim CH, Lee SJ, Kaushik NK, Choi EH. Responses of solid tumor cells in DMEM to reactive oxygen species generated by nonthermal plasma and chemically induced ROS systems. Sci Rep. 2015;5:8587. https://doi.org/10.1038/srep08587.

53. Zhao S, Xiong Z, Mao X, Meng D, Lei Q, Li Y, Deng P, Chen M, Tu M, Lu X, Yang G, He G. Atmospheric pressure room temperature plasma jets facilitate oxidative and nitrative stress and lead to endoplasmic reticulum stress dependent apoptosis in HepG2 cells. PLoS One. 2013;8:e73665. https://doi.org/10.1371/journal.pone.0073665.

54. Freund E, Liedtke KR, Gebbe R, Heidecke AK, Partecke L-I, Bekeschus S. In vitro anticancer efficacy of six different clinically approved types of liquids exposed to physical plasma. IEEE Trans Radiat Plasma Med Sci. 2019;3:588–96. https://doi.org/10.1109/trpms.2019.2902015.

55. Wende K, Reuter S, von Woedtke T, Weltmann KD, Masur K. Redox-based assay for assessment of biological impact of plasma treatment. Plasma Process Polym. 2014;11:655–63. https://doi.org/10.1002/ppap.201300172.

56. Tornin J, Mateu-Sanz M, Rodriguez A, Labay C, Rodriguez R, Canal C. Pyruvate plays a main role in the antitumoral selectivity of cold atmospheric plasma in osteosarcoma. Sci Rep. 2019;9:10681. https://doi.org/10.1038/s41598-019-47128-1.

57. Wende K, Williams P, Dalluge J, Gaens WV, Aboubakr H, Bischof J, von Woedtke T, Goyal SM, Weltmann KD, Bogaerts A, Masur K, Bruggeman PJ. Identification of the biologically active liquid chemistry induced by a nonthermal atmospheric pressure plasma jet. Biointerphases. 2015;10:029518. https://doi.org/10.1116/1.4919710.

58. Bekeschus S, Wende K, Hefny MM, Rodder K, Jablonowski H, Schmidt A, Woedtke TV, Weltmann KD, Benedikt J. Oxygen atoms are critical in rendering thp-1 leukaemia cells susceptible to cold physical plasma-induced apoptosis. Sci Rep. 2017;7:2791. https://doi.org/10.1038/s41598-017-03131-y.

59. Kondeti V, Phan CQ, Wende K, Jablonowski H, Gangal U, Granick JL, Hunter RC, Bruggeman PJ. Long-lived and short-lived reactive species produced by a cold atmospheric pressure plasma jet for the inactivation of pseudomonas aeruginosa and staphylococcus aureus. Free Radic Biol Med. 2018;124:275–87. https://doi.org/10.1016/j.freeradbiomed.2018.05.083.

60. Lukes P, Dolezalova E, Sisrova I, Clupek M. Aqueous-phase chemistry and bactericidal effects from an air discharge plasma in contact with water: evidence for the formation of peroxynitrite through a pseudo-second-order post-discharge reaction of H_2O_2 and HNO_2. Plasma Sources Sci Technol. 2014;23:015019.

61. Xu DH, Cui QJ, Xu YJ, Liu ZJ, Chen ZY, Xia WJ, Zhang H, Liu DX, Chen HL, Kong MG. NO_2^- and NO_3^- enhance cold atmospheric plasma induced cancer cell death by generation of $ONOO^-$. AIP Adv. 2018;8 https://doi.org/10.1063/1.5046353.

62. Winter J, Sousa JS, Sadeghi N, Schmidt-Bleker A, Reuter S, Puech V. The spatio-temporal distribution of He (2^3S_1) metastable atoms in a MHZ-driven helium plasma jet is influenced by the oxygen/nitrogen ratio of the surrounding atmosphere. Plasma Sources Sci Technol. 2015;24:25015–25.

63. Winter J, Wende K, Masur K, Iseni S, Dunnbier M, Hammer MU, Tresp H, Weltmann KD, Reuter S. Feed gas humidity: a vital parameter affecting a cold atmospheric-pressure plasma jet and plasma-treated human skin cells. J Phys D Appl Phys. 2013;46:295401. https://doi.org/10.1088/0022-3727/46/29/295401.

64. Winter T, Bernhardt J, Winter J, Mader U, Schluter R, Weltmann KD, Hecker M, Kusch H. Common versus noble bacillus subtilis differentially responds to air and argon gas plasma. Proteomics. 2013;13:2608–21. https://doi.org/10.1002/pmic.201200343.

65. Chandel NS, Budinger GR. The cellular basis for diverse responses to oxygen. Free Radic Biol Med. 2007;42:165–74. https://doi.org/10.1016/j.freeradbiomed.2006.10.048.

66. Galluzzi L, Vitale I, Aaronson SA, Abrams JM, Adam D, Agostinis P, Alnemri ES, Altucci L, Amelio I, Andrews DW, et al. Molecular mechanisms of cell death: recommendations of the nomenclature committee on cell death 2018. Cell Death Differ. 2018;25:486–541. https://doi.org/10.1038/s41418-017-0012-4.

67. Pasqual-Melo G, Nascimento T, Sanches LJ, Blegniski FP, Bianchi JK, Sagwal SK, Berner J, Schmidt A, Emmert S, Weltmann KD, von Woedtke T, Gandhirajan RK, Cecchini AL, Bekeschus S. Plasma treatment limits cutaneous squamous cell carcinoma development in vitro and in vivo. Cancers (Basel). 1993;2020:12. https://doi.org/10.3390/cancers12071993.

68. Schmidt A, Rodder K, Hasse S, Masur K, Toups L, Lillig CH, von Woedtke T, Wende K, Bekeschus S. Redox-regulation of activator protein 1 family members in blood cancer cell lines

exposed to cold physical plasma-treated medium. Plasma Process Polym. 2016;13:1179–88. https://doi.org/10.1002/ppap.201600090.

69. Bekeschus S, Eisenmann S, Sagwal SK, Bodnar Y, Moritz J, Poschkamp B, Stoffels I, Emmert S, Madesh M, Weltmann KD, von Woedtke T, Gandhirajan RK. xCT (SLC7A11) expression confers intrinsic resistance to physical plasma treatment in tumor cells. Redox Biol. 2020;30:101423. https://doi.org/10.1016/j.redox.2019.101423.

70. Yan D, Talbot A, Nourmohammadi N, Sherman JH, Cheng X, Keidar M. Toward understanding the selective anticancer capacity of cold atmospheric plasma--a model based on aquaporins (review). Biointerphases. 2015;10:040801. https://doi.org/10.1116/1.4938020.

71. Yan DY, Xiao HJ, Zhu W, Nourmohammadi N, Zhang LG, Bian K, Keidar M. The role of aquaporins in the anti-glioblastoma capacity of the cold plasma-stimulated medium. J Phys D Appl Phys. 2017;50. https://doi.org/10.1088/1361-6463/aa53d6.

72. Bekeschus S, von Woedtke T, Kramer A, Weltmann K-D, Masur K. Cold physical plasma treatment alters redox balance in human immune cells. Plasma Med. 2013;3:267–78. https://doi.org/10.1615/PlasmaMed.2014011972.

73. Sagwal SK, Pasqual-Melo G, Bodnar Y, Gandhirajan RK, Bekeschus S. Combination of chemotherapy and physical plasma elicits melanoma cell death via upregulation of SLC22A16. Cell Death Dis. 2018;9:1179. https://doi.org/10.1038/s41419-018-1221-6.

74. Bekeschus S, Rodder K, Fregin B, Otto O, Lippert M, Weltmann KD, Wende K, Schmidt A, Gandhirajan RK. Toxicity and immunogenicity in murine melanoma following exposure to physical plasma-derived oxidants. Oxidative Med Cell Longev. 2017;2017:4396467. https://doi.org/10.1155/2017/4396467.

75. Tanaka H, Nakamura K, Mizuno M, Ishikawa K, Takeda K, Kajiyama H, Utsumi F, Kikkawa F, Hori M. Non-thermal atmospheric pressure plasma activates lactate in ringer's solution for anti-tumor effects. Sci Rep. 2016;6:36282. https://doi.org/10.1038/srep36282.

76. Lackmann JW, Wende K, Verlackt C, Golda J, Volzke J, Kogelheide F, Held J, Bekeschus S, Bogaerts A, Schulz-von der Gathen V, Stapelmann K. Chemical fingerprints of cold physical plasmas - an experimental and computational study using cysteine as tracer compound. Sci Rep. 2018;8:7736. https://doi.org/10.1038/s41598-018-25937-0.

77. Heusler T, Bruno G, Bekeschus S, Lackmann J-W, von Woedtke T, Wende K. Can the effect of cold physical plasma-derived oxidants be transported via thiol group oxidation? Clin Plasma Med. 2019;14. https://doi.org/10.1016/j.cpme.2019.100086.

78. Hasse S, Duong Tran T, Hahn O, Kindler S, Metelmann HR, von Woedtke T, Masur K. Induction of proliferation of basal epidermal keratinocytes by cold atmospheric-pressure plasma. Clin Exp Dermatol. 2016;41:202–9. https://doi.org/10.1111/ced.12735.

79. Adamson R. Role of macrophages in normal wound healing: an overview. J Wound Care. 2009;18:349–51. https://doi.org/10.12968/jowc.2009.18.8.43636.

80. Akiyama H, Heller R. Bioelectrics. Chiyoda-ku: Springer; 2017.

81. Passaras D, Amanatides E, Kokkoris G. Predicting the flow of cold plasma jets in kINPen: a critical evaluation of turbulent models. J Phys D Appl Phys. 2020;53. https://doi.org/10.1088/1361-6463/ab7d6d.

82. Orr K, Tang Y, Simeni Simeni M, van den Bekerom D, Adamovich IV. Measurements of electric field in an atmospheric pressure helium plasma jet by the e-fish method. Plasma Sources Sci Technol. 2020;29. https://doi.org/10.1088/1361-6595/ab6e5b.

83. Slikboer E, Acharya K, Sobota A, Garcia-Caurel E, Guaitella O. Revealing plasma-surface interaction at atmospheric pressure: imaging of electric field and temperature inside the targeted material. Sci Rep. 2020;10:2712. https://doi.org/10.1038/s41598-020-59345-0.

84. Yarmolenko PS, Moon EJ, Landon C, Manzoor A, Hochman DW, Viglianti BL, Dewhirst MW. Thresholds for thermal damage to normal tissues: an update. Int J Hyperth. 2011;27:320–43. https://doi.org/10.3109/02656736.2010.534527.

85. Kramer A, Lademann J, Bender C, Sckell A, Hartmann B, Münch S, Hinz P, Ekkernkamp A, Matthes R, Koban I, et al. Suitability of tissue tolerable plasmas (TTP) for the management of chronic wounds. Clin Plasma Med. 2013;1:11–8. https://doi.org/10.1016/j.cpme.2013.03.002.

86.   Akerfelt M, Trouillet D, Mezger V, Sistonen L. Heat shock factors at a crossroad between stress and development. Ann N Y Acad Sci. 2007;1113:15–27. https://doi.org/10.1196/annals.1391.005.

87.   Bellaye PS, Burgy O, Causse S, Garrido C, Bonniaud P. Heat shock proteins in fibrosis and wound healing: good or evil? Pharmacol Ther. 2014;143:119–32. https://doi.org/10.1016/j.pharmthera.2014.02.009.

88.   Li Z, Menoret A, Srivastava P. Roles of heat-shock proteins in antigen presentation and cross-presentation. Curr Opin Immunol. 2002;14:45–51. https://doi.org/10.1016/s0952-7915(01)00297-7.

89.   Rodriguez ME, Cogno IS, Milla Sanabria LS, Moran YS, Rivarola VA. Heat shock proteins in the context of photodynamic therapy: autophagy, apoptosis and immunogenic cell death. Photochem Photobiol Sci. 2016;15:1090–102. https://doi.org/10.1039/c6pp00097e.

90.   Chen H, Weng QY, Fisher DE. Uv signaling pathways within the skin. J Invest Dermatol. 2014;134:2080–5. https://doi.org/10.1038/jid.2014.161.

91.   Metelmann H-R, von Woedtke T, Bussiahn R, Weltmann K-D, Rieck M, Khalili R, Podmelle F, Waite PD. Experimental recovery of CO_2-laser skin lesions by plasma stimulation. Am J Cosmet Surg. 2012;29:52–6. https://doi.org/10.5992/ajcs-d-11-00042.1.

92.   Metelmann H-R, Vu TT, Do HT, Le TNB, Hoang THA, Phi TTT, Luong TML, Doan VT, Nguyen TTH, Nguyen THM, et al. Scar formation of laser skin lesions after cold atmospheric pressure plasma (CAP) treatment: a clinical long term observation. Clin Plasma Med. 2013;1:30–5. https://doi.org/10.1016/j.cpme.2012.12.001.

93.   Jablonowski L, Kocher T, Schindler A, Muller K, Dombrowski F, von Woedtke T, Arnold T, Lehmann A, Rupf S, Evert M, Evert K. Side effects by oral application of atmospheric pressure plasma on the mucosa in mice. PLoS One. 2019;14:e0215099. https://doi.org/10.1371/journal.pone.0215099.

94.   Rutkowski R, Daeschlein G, von Woedtke T, Smeets R, Gosau M, Metelmann HR. Long-term risk assessment for medical application of cold atmospheric pressure plasma. Diagnostics (Basel). 2020;10. https://doi.org/10.3390/diagnostics10040210.

95.   Wu L, Sedgwick AC, Sun X, Bull SD, He XP, James TD. Reaction-based fluorescent probes for the detection and imaging of reactive oxygen, nitrogen, and sulfur species. Acc Chem Res. 2019;52:2582–97. https://doi.org/10.1021/acs.accounts.9b00302.

96.   Paulsen CE, Carroll KS. Cysteine-mediated redox signaling: chemistry, biology, and tools for discovery. Chem Rev. 2013;113:4633–79. https://doi.org/10.1021/cr300163e.

97.   Jiang X, Wang L, Carroll SL, Chen J, Wang MC, Wang J. Challenges and opportunities for small-molecule fluorescent probes in redox biology applications. Antioxid Redox Signal. 2018;29:518–40. https://doi.org/10.1089/ars.2017.7491.

98.   Chen X, Tian X, Shin I, Yoon J. Fluorescent and luminescent probes for detection of reactive oxygen and nitrogen species. Chem Soc Rev. 2011;40:4783–804. https://doi.org/10.1039/c1cs15037e.

99.   Hou J-T, Yu K-K, Sunwoo K, Kim WY, Koo S, Wang J, Ren WX, Wang S, Yu X-Q, Kim JS. Fluorescent imaging of reactive oxygen and nitrogen species associated with pathophysiological processes. Chem. 2020;6:832–66. https://doi.org/10.1016/j.chempr.2019.12.005.

100. Schmidt A, von Woedtke T, Vollmar B, Hasse S, Bekeschus S. Nrf2 signaling and inflammation are key events in physical plasma-spurred wound healing. Theranostics. 2019;9:1066–84. https://doi.org/10.7150/thno.29754.

101. Villamena FA, Zweier JL. Detection of reactive oxygen and nitrogen species by EPR spin trapping. Antioxid Redox Signal. 2004;6:619–29. https://doi.org/10.1089/152308604773934387.

102. Weiss M, Barz J, Ackermann M, Utz R, Ghoul A, Weltmann KD, Stope MB, Wallwiener D, Schenke-Layland K, Oehr C, Brucker S, Loskill P. Dose-dependent tissue-level characterization of a medical atmospheric pressure argon plasma jet. ACS Appl Mater Interfaces. 2019;11:19841–53. https://doi.org/10.1021/acsami.9b04803.

103. Carballal S, Bartesaghi S, Radi R. Kinetic and mechanistic considerations to assess the biological fate of peroxynitrite. Biochim Biophys Acta. 1840;2014:768–80. https://doi.org/10.1016/j.bbagen.2013.07.005.

104. Striesow J, Lackmann JW, Ni Z, Wenske S, Weltmann KD, Fedorova M, von Woedtke T, Wende K. Oxidative modification of skin lipids by cold atmospheric plasma (CAP): a standardizable approach using RP-LC/MS^2 and DI-ESI/MS^2. Chem Phys Lipids. 2020;226:104786. https://doi.org/10.1016/j.chemphyslip.2019.104786.
105. Schmidt A, Niessner F, von Woedtke T, Bekeschus S. Hyperspectral imaging of wounds reveals augmented tissue oxygenation following cold physical plasma treatment in vivo. IEEE Trans Radiat Plasma Med Sci. 2020:1–1. https://doi.org/10.1109/trpms.2020.3009913.
106. Kulcke A, Holmer A, Wahl P, Siemers F, Wild T, Daeschlein G. A compact hyperspectral camera for measurement of perfusion parameters in medicine. Biomed Tech (Berl). 2018. https://doi.org/10.1515/bmt-2017-0145.
107. Daeschlein G, Rutkowski R, Lutze S, von Podewils S, Sicher C, Wild T, Metelmann HR, von Woedkte T, Junger M. Hyperspectral imaging: innovative diagnostics to visualize hemodynamic effects of cold plasma in wound therapy. Biomed Tech (Berl). 2018. https://doi.org/10.1515/bmt-2017-0085.
108. Wolf AM, Nishimaki K, Kamimura N, Ohta S. Real-time monitoring of oxidative stress in live mouse skin. J Invest Dermatol. 2014;134:1701–9. https://doi.org/10.1038/jid.2013.428.
109. Schwarzlander M, Dick TP, Meyer AJ, Morgan B. Dissecting redox biology using fluorescent protein sensors. Antioxid Redox Signal. 2016;24:680–712. https://doi.org/10.1089/ars.2015.6266.
110. Schwarzlander M, Finkemeier I. Mitochondrial energy and redox signaling in plants. Antioxid Redox Signal. 2013;18:2122–44. https://doi.org/10.1089/ars.2012.5104.
111. Isbary G, Morfill G, Schmidt HU, Georgi M, Ramrath K, Heinlin J, Karrer S, Landthaler M, Shimizu T, Steffes B, et al. A first prospective randomized controlled trial to decrease bacterial load using cold atmospheric argon plasma on chronic wounds in patients. Br J Dermatol. 2010;163:78–82. https://doi.org/10.1111/j.1365-2133.2010.09744.x.
112. Isbary G, Heinlin J, Shimizu T, Zimmermann JL, Morfill G, Schmidt HU, Monetti R, Steffes B, Bunk W, Li Y, Klaempfl T, Karrer S, Landthaler M, Stolz W. Successful and safe use of 2 min cold atmospheric argon plasma in chronic wounds: results of a randomized controlled trial. Br J Dermatol. 2012;167:404–10. https://doi.org/10.1111/j.1365-2133.2012.10923.x.
113. Brehmer F, Haenssle HA, Daeschlein G, Ahmed R, Pfeiffer S, Gorlitz A, Simon D, Schon MP, Wandke D, Emmert S. Alleviation of chronic venous leg ulcers with a hand-held dielectric barrier discharge plasma generator (PlasmaDerm® VU-2010): results of a monocentric, two-armed, open, prospective, randomized and controlled trial (NCT01415622). J Eur Acad Dermatol Venereol. 2015;29:148–55. https://doi.org/10.1111/jdv.12490.
114. Arndt S, Unger P, Wacker E, Shimizu T, Heinlin J, Li YF, Thomas HM, Morfill GE, Zimmermann JL, Bosserhoff AK, Karrer S. Cold atmospheric plasma (CAP) changes gene expression of key molecules of the wound healing machinery and improves wound healing in vitro and in vivo. PLoS One. 2013;8:e79325. https://doi.org/10.1371/journal.pone.0079325.
115. Heinlin J, Zimmermann JL, Zeman F, Bunk W, Isbary G, Landthaler M, Maisch T, Monetti R, Morfill G, Shimizu T, Steinbauer J, Stolz W, Karrer S. Randomized placebo-controlled human pilot study of cold atmospheric argon plasma on skin graft donor sites. Wound Repair Regen. 2013;21:800–7. https://doi.org/10.1111/wrr.12078.
116. Vandersee S, Richter H, Lademann J, Beyer M, Kramer A, Knorr F, Lange-Asschenfeldt B. Laser scanning microscopy as a means to assess the augmentation of tissue repair by exposition of wounds to tissue tolerable plasma. Laser Phys Lett. 2014;11:115701. https://doi.org/10.1088/1612-2011/11/11/115701.
117. Schmidt A, Bekeschus S, Wende K, Vollmar B, von Woedtke T. A cold plasma jet accelerates wound healing in a murine model of full-thickness skin wounds. Exp Dermatol. 2017;26:156–62. https://doi.org/10.1111/exd.13156.
118. Stratmann B, Costea TC, Nolte C, Hiller J, Schmidt J, Reindel J, Masur K, Motz W, Timm J, Kerner W, Tschoepe D. Effect of cold atmospheric plasma therapy vs standard therapy placebo on wound healing in patients with diabetic foot ulcers: a randomized clinical trial. JAMA Netw Open. 2020;3:e2010411. https://doi.org/10.1001/jamanetworkopen.2020.10411.
119. Metelmann H-R, Nedrelow DS, Seebauer C, Schuster M, von Woedtke T, Weltmann K-D, Kindler S, Metelmann PH, Finkelstein SE, Von Hoff DD, Podmelle F. Head and neck cancer

treatment and physical plasma. Clin Plas Med. 2015;3:17–23. https://doi.org/10.1016/j.cpme.2015.02.001.

120. Metelmann H-R, Seebauer C, Miller V, Fridman A, Bauer G, Graves DB, Pouvesle J-M, Rutkowski R, Schuster M, Bekeschus S, et al. Clinical experience with cold plasma in the treatment of locally advanced head and neck cancer. Clin Plasma Med. 2018;9:6–13. https://doi.org/10.1016/j.cpme.2017.09.001.

3

Suggested Reading

Mechanisms of Physico-Chemical and Biomedical Mechanisms of Plasmas

Privat-Maldonado A, Schmidt A, Lin A, Weltmann KD, Wende K, Bogaerts A, Bekeschus S. ROS from physical plasmas: redox chemistry for biomedical therapy. Oxidative Med Cell Longev. 2019;9062098 https://doi.org/10.1155/2019/9062098. eCollection 2019

von Woedtke T, Schmidt A, Bekeschus S, Wende K, Weltmann KD. Plasma medicine: a field of applied redox biology. In Vivo. 2019;33:1011–26. https://doi.org/10.21873/invivo.11570.

Principles of the Best-Characterized Medical Plasma Jet

Reuter S, von Woedtke T, Weltmann KD. The kINPen-a review on physics and chemistry of the atmospheric pressure plasma jet and its applications. J Phys D Appl Phys. 2018;51(23):233001. https://doi.org/10.1088/1361-6463/aab3ad.

Preclinical and Clinical Effects of a Plasma Jet in Dermatology

Bekeschus S, Schmidt A, Weltmann KD, von Woedtke T. The plasma jet kINPen – a powerful tool for wound healing. Clin Plasma Med. 2016;4(1):19–28. https://doi.org/10.1016/j.cpme.2016.01.001.

Bernhardt T, Semmler ML, Schäfer M, Bekeschus S, Emmert S, Boeckmann L. Plasma medicine: applications of cold atmospheric pressure plasma in dermatology. Oxid Med Cell Longev. 2019;2019(3873928) https://doi.org/10.1155/2019/3873928.

Landmarks to Differentiate Between Reliable and Questionable Devices for Application in Plasma Medicine

Thomas von Woedtke,
Klaus-Dieter Weltmann, Steffen Emmert,
and Hans-Robert Metelmann

Contents

© Springer Nature Switzerland AG 2022
H.-R. Metelmann et al. (eds.), *Textbook of Good Clinical Practice in
Cold Plasma Therapy*, https://doi.org/10.1007/978-3-030-87857-3_4

4

☎ **Core Messages**

- Plasma medicine focuses on the use of cold atmospheric plasma (CAP) in direct treatment of the living body in therapeutic settings.
- It is necessary to differentiate carefully between reliable and rather dubious offers and devices for plasma medical application.
- CE certification as a medical device is not a guarantee for the reliability of a plasma device concerning its offered purpose in medical application.
- Minimum technical information to estimate basic performance characteristics of a plasma device for reliable medical application includes feed gas, power and frequency for plasma generation, plasma temperature, and radiation emission spectrum of the plasma. Additionally, basic biological and clinical performance data have to be available.
- CAP devices that mainly fulfil these preconditions are kINPen® MED (neoplas tools GmbH, Greifswald, Germany), SteriPlas (ADTEC, Hounslow, UK), PlasmaDerm® (CINOGY GmbH, Duderstadt, Germany), and plasma care® (terraplasma medical GmbH, Garching, Germany); see ▶ Chaps. 16, 17, 18 and 19.
- Devices using glassy vacuum electrodes (also labelled as HF electrodes) are based on historic devices from the end of the nineteenth century and need much more characterization before a reliable medical application is responsible.

4.1 Introduction

Plasma medicine is a growing field that opens up promising applications in medicine. Currently, clinical success is reported mostly in wound healing, but plasma application in cancer treatment is the next very attractive and promising field. The great progress in basic research in recent years provides the basis for promising clinical applications. In the end, such transfer from bench to bedside depends on manufacturers and distributors who provide safe and reliable plasma devices. Only based on a triumvirate of basic research, clinics, and industry, plasma medicine will be able to become an integral and successful part of modern medicine in the twenty-first century.

The beginning success of plasma medicine is attracting several companies yet, but also freeloaders who want to profit from this success story and use for their own benefit the huge scientific background that was necessary to bring plasma medicine into the clinics. Therefore, it is unfortunately necessary to differentiate carefully between reliable and rather dubious offers and devices for plasma medical application. This is not always simple. As a matter of course, plasma devices for medical application have to be medical devices. However, CE certification as a medical device alone is not a guarantee for the reliability of such plasma device concerning its offered purpose in plasma-specific medical application.

There are different plasma devices on the market offered for medical applications, like wound healing, skin treatment, and much more, including cosmetic applications. In most cases, the manufacturer or distributor, respectively, gives a list of more or less precise application fields. However, this information is very often not accompanied by meaningful information allowing an independent estimation on the plasma device itself and its performance in biological or clinical settings. In many cases, offered medical applications are based on claims made by the manufacturer or distributor, only, without robust scientific references.

Because of the relative novelty of plasma medicine, basic knowledge about specific features of this group of medical devices is not that common as it is with regard to other comparable devices such as medical lasers or electrosurgical equipment. Therefore, some basic information is necessary to assess a plasma device and to estimate its usability for reliable medical application.

This chapter will give some basic guidelines that might be followed to estimate the reliability of a plasma device for medical application. It will start with a basic device classification followed by some characteristics that should be disclosed by a manufacturer or supplier of such a device. Afterwards, some examples of approved plasma devices for application in the field of plasma medicine will be given followed by some final remarks on plasma device and marketing concepts that are not really reliable.

The aim of this chapter is neither to distinguish nor to criticize or condemn individual devices but to give the potential user some kind of guideline to form an independent opinion regarding the reliability and applicability of a plasma device for application in the field of plasma medicine.

Plasma medicine is a new and promising field with growing and successful applications in several field of clinical practice. Therefore, all players in this new field, including researchers, manufacturers, and clinicians have a high responsibility to establish plasma medicine as part of modern medicine on a sound scientific basis and to anticipate any dubious applications without substance.

4.2 General Classification of Devices for Plasma Medicine

Basics on plasma medicine and on plasma devices used in this field are given in the preceding ▶ Chaps. 2 and 3, as well as in ▶ Chap. 15. As it is explained there, plasma medicine in its proper sense is focused on the therapeutic application of cold atmospheric plasma (CAP).

> ❯ **Important to Know**
> Plasma medicine to our current understanding focuses on the use of cold atmospheric plasma (CAP) in direct treatment of parts of the living body in therapeutic settings. Biological effects of CAP are not based on thermal impact, but on specific interactions of reactive oxygen and nitrogen species (ROS, RNS) with cell and tissue components partially supported by electrical fields and ultraviolet radiation.

Consequently, any medical plasma application should be related to these basic characteristics with regard to their claimed or proven effects.

However, medical application of physical plasma in general comprises other applications beyond non-thermal, cold plasma, which are well established for decades. Therefore, it should be useful to differentiate physical plasma devices for medical applications into at least **three basic categories**:

- **Cold atmospheric-pressure plasma (CAP) devices** generate plasma in direct contact or in close vicinity to the target to be treated (wound, skin, etc.) with a temperature below 40 °C at the target site of treatment. These devices are meant when speaking of plasma medicine, and these devices and applications are the subject of this book.

- **Electrosurgical plasma devices** are well-established tools for blood coagulation, cauterization, tissue ablation, and cutting, respectively. The effects of these plasma devices are mainl y based on thermal impact resulting in tissue shrinking and/or carbonization [1–3]. This is of course also application of physical plasma in medicine, but is not in the main focus of the new field of plasma medicine.

- Some **devices** use plasma **to generate gases or gas mixtures** for therapeutic use, e.g., nitric oxide [4, 5] or ozone [6–8]. This is kind of "indirect" plasma application with no direct plasma contact to the target that will be treated.

Even if in some cases a strong separation between these three categories is not that easy, a careful differentiation is very important. The vast majority of recent publications in plasma medicine on biological plasma effects and, above all, on the safety of plasma devices refers to cold atmospheric plasma (CAP) and its intervention in redox-controlled cellular processes [9], but not to thermal plasma or plasma-generated gases. For some non-CAP devices or applications offered sometimes in public media or by companies, this is not always apparent, above all if they refer to actual research and clinical success of plasma medicine. Therefore, this differentiation and careful identification of the technical basis of a plasma device needs special attention because it will define the nature of biological effects caused by such a device.

❶ Caution

It has to be pointed out that all investigations on safety of plasma application in the field of plasma medicine were done using cold atmospheric pressure plasmas with distinct biological activity based on redox-controlled processes. Any reference to these results on safety of plasma use in medicine has to ensure that the respective devices are really based on this working principle.

4.3 Basic Characterization of CAP Devices

To be able to make a sound differentiation, for any plasma device for medical application, scientifically based characteristics of both basic physical parameters and basic biological and clinical performance data have to be available.

First, basic technical features of a plasma device like mode of plasma excitation (high voltage, microwave, or others), power and frequency, and operating gas used for plasma generation are essential.

One of the most important performance parameters is the **temperature** of the plasma. It is common knowledge that at temperatures higher than 40 °C, hyperthermia and time-dependent cell death and devitalization of living tissue starts. These effects are not only dependent on the plasma temperature itself but also on the technique of plasma application. For instance, in the case of higher plasma temperature, thermal impact on treated tissue can be reduced by internal cooling of the plasma or by simple moving of the plasma above the target to reduce the local contact time. Independent of details that might be very specific for different plasma devices, for a reliable CAP device, information on plasma temperature should be available to decide about the plasma application mode as well as to estimate if any effects of the plasma are caused by thermal impact or not.

A second meaningful parameter is the **radiation emission** of the plasma. As explained in ▶ Chaps. 2, 3, and 15, respectively, plasma is generated by supplying energy to a gas resulting in excitation and ionization of atoms or molecules of the gas. This is the main precondition for the generation of biologically active ROS and RNS and the resulting biological reactivity of cold atmospheric plasma. An additional result of these ionization and excitation processes is the emission of radiation by the plasma, which can be measured by optical emission spectroscopy (OES). Emission spectra of CAP may range from ultraviolet to visible range, i.e., from 200 to 1000 nm. For biomedical CAP applications, ultraviolet C (UV-C, 200–280 nm), ultraviolet B (UV-B, 280–315 nm) and ultraviolet A (UV-A, 315–400 nm) are of particular interest. ◻ Figure 4.1 presents an example OES spectrum of a plasma jet operated with argon.

Primarily, such an emission spectrum contains information about the wavelength and, in the case of a calibrated spectrometer, the intensity of UV radiation of the plasma. With a more detailed and informed evaluation, the spectrum gives information about excited species composition of the plasma. Looking at the spectrum presented in ◻ Fig. 4.1, there is a distinct UV-B emission around 309 nm

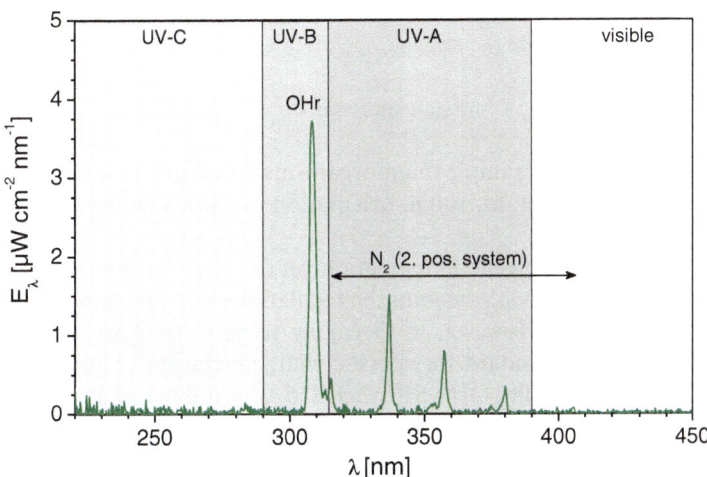

◻ **Fig. 4.1** Typical ultraviolet emission spectrum including intensity of irradiance of an argon-driven cold atmospheric-pressure plasma jet [10, 11]

caused by hydroxyl radical (OHr), some UV-A emission of excited nitrogen (N_2), but nearly no emission in the UV-C range.

Generally, together with specifications on plasma temperature, an annotated OES spectrum provides basic information on plasma characteristics that allows a first estimation of possible biologic effects of a given plasma device. Therefore, the presentation of a representative emission spectrum should be mandatory for any plasma device.

Even if a plethora of further parameters are measurable that are useful for detailed plasma diagnostics and are absolutely valuable for research purposes, this basic set of physical and technical parameters is sufficient to get a basic picture of the plasma device itself.

Additionally, some data related to the biological performance of the plasma device should be available. These data may be dependent on the intended use of the plasma device. However, the effectivity to kill microorganisms is a useful and meaningful parameter. Simple basic microbiological test procedures like inhibition zone assay or quantitative suspension test are customary. In all cases, specification of microorganisms, cultivation conditions, and experimental setup of the test should be disclosed. In a very simple view, the ability of a cold plasma to kill microorganisms is the first and basic test to prove if there is any biological effect.

Furthermore, testing of the plasma impact on the viability of mammalian cells is an additional very meaningful characterization parameter. Here, because of the current most promising CAP application in wound healing and dermatology, skin cells (keratinocytes, fibroblasts) are very often used. Again, cell line, cultivation conditions, and experimental setup have to be recorded and some specifications of the test method that has been used to evaluate cell viability after plasma treatment.

> **Important to Know**
>
> For a meaningful basic characterization, allowing a general classification of plasma devices for intended medical use, the following data should be available:
> - Technical features: mode of plasma excitation (high voltage, microwave, or others), power and frequency, and operating gas
> - Plasma temperature
> - Representative plasma emission spectrum

Data on inactivation of example microorganisms and impact on mammalian cells can give basic information for rough orientation purposes on biological effects of the plasma device.

Up to now, there is no general regulation yet on what parameters are necessary specifically for plasma devices beyond the regulations that are mandatory for medical devices in general. However, in Germany some years ago, an initiative was started to establish a standard for specific characterization of plasma devices in medicine. As a first result, DIN SPEC 91315 was published in 2014 as a pre-standard defining "General requirements for plasma sources in medicine" [11, 12]. This DIN SPEC defines both physical, but also biological, performance parameters that should become mandatory to characterize basic operating features for medical plasma devices. Activities are still ongoing to develop this pre-standard to a regular national and subsequently international standard. The most important intention of such a standard is to force, above all, manufacturers or suppliers to present a basic set of research data before any medical application of their plasma devices should be recommended.

Of course, basic information on clinical performance of a plasma device related to its intended use is desirable naturally. Even if, in general, randomized controlled trials (RCTs) are the gold standard to prove the effectiveness of medical treatments, it has to be kept in mind that RCTs for medical devices so far are not obligatory to the same extent as in the field of pharmaceutical drugs. This is caused by several practical and regulatory reasons. However, because plasma medicine is a new field whose effectivity and applicability in medicine have yet to be proven, any recommendation of a plasma device for specific therapeutic purposes should be based on valid data from clinical trials or at least systematic case reports. It is not sufficient to present before-after pictures from single plasma treatments only to prove any success in specific indications. In addition, documentation of enthusiastic statements of individual medical doctors is not sufficient as a reliable proof of clinical performance and reliability of a plasma device or a specific plasma treatment.

4.4 Approved CAP Devices

With these basic considerations, the first and most important criterion to estimate if a plasma device is reliable for medical application is the availability of some basic information on its physical characterization and biological performance as it was executed above. Such information has to be provided by the manufacturer or supplier and should be requested by any user. There are different possibilities to present such information, ranging from manufacturer's own test reports up to research studies published in scientific journals, in several cases, by research institutions that cooperate with the plasma device manufacturer. In every case, exact references for these data must be given. This is also true for any clinical data and reports.

Based on these premises, currently at least four CAP devices are on the market which mainly fulfil these preconditions:

- The argon-driven high-frequency (HF) plasma jet kINPen® MED (neoplas tools GmbH, Greifswald, Germany)
- The argon-driven microwave plasma torch SteriPlas (ADTEC, Hounslow, UK)
- PlasmaDerm® (CINOGY GmbH, Duderstadt, Germany), a device based on a dielectric barrier discharge (DBD) that uses atmospheric air as working gas
- The DBD-based plasma care® (terraplasma medical GmbH, Garching, Germany), also driven in atmospheric air

These devices are comprehensively presented in ► Chaps. 16, 17, 18 and 19.

Development of these plasma devices up to clinically applicable as well as certifiable medical devices has been preceded by more or less long-term scientific research of scientific institutions, as Leibniz Institute for Plasma Science and Technology (INP) Greifswald, Germany (kINPen® MED), Max Planck Institute for Extraterrestrial Physics (MPE) Garching, Germany (SteriPlas, plasma care®), or University of Applied Sciences and Arts together with the Fraunhofer Institute for Surface Engineering and Thin Films IST Göttingen, Germany (PlasmaDerm®).

These research institutions compiled the physical, technological, and biological basics for the plasma devices, transferred this knowledge to the companies and further support their clinical proving and application. Consequently, a lot of scientific studies and results are available for these plasma devices covering the complete spectrum from plasma physics to clinical data. References are available in this book but also in the comprehensive textbooks "Plasmamedizin" (in German) and "Comprehensive Clinical Plasma Medicine" (see suggestions for further reading).

Of course, it is possible and will become usual practice in future, that new plasma devices from other manufacturers will be referred to these first and pioneering devices. This is quite acceptable and welcome as long as appropriate references are given and basic data are disclosed that allow estimating similarities or differences to other approved devices. In the case of new developments, e.g., based on innovative techniques of plasma generation, scientifically sound studies to characterize these devices as medically applicable tools are demanded.

All these demands sound very challenging and restrictive. However, to point it out again, plasma medicine is a new field that is on its way to clinical practice to become a successful part of modern medicine based on a sound scientific fundament. Therefore, we have to be careful that this course is not stopped or delayed by unwanted side effects that are caused by inappropriately prepared and tested devices.

4.5 Questionable Plasma Devices

Finally, some remarks will be given on more or less problematic plasma devices on the market. Of course, it is impossible to assess the complete range of plasma devices on offer. Above all, the World Wide Web is a platform for a huge number of uncontrollable activities also with respect to plasma applications in the field of healthcare. This is not the place to give any extended statements on detailed pros and cons of plasma devices that would have to be categorized as "questionable" based on the landmarks given in this chapter. However, the readers should get some feeling on possible twilight zones on the market and should be encouraged to form their own opinion based on the available information.

One specific group of devices seems to be relatively widespread on the market and, therefore, should be addressed particularly in this chapter. These devices are based on so-called vacuum electrodes. In a glass vessel with different possible geometries, a glow discharge is created under low-pressure conditions by an inserted electrode using a high-voltage high-frequency discharge. The plasma inside the vessel often emits violet light, even if the colour of this light may change dependent on the gas used inside the vessel. This kind of device was invented at the turn of the nineteenth to the twentieth century. Known as "violet ray" or "violet wand" or also as high frequency (HF) therapy, it was widely used in the first decades of the twentieth century. Announced indications were more or less exactly defined, ranging from promotion of blood circulation, increasing of oxidizing power of the blood, increasing cellular chemical processes or vaso-motor activities, to mention some examples only. Germicidal activity via ozone generation was also announced. According to the state of knowledge of the time, these applications finally should lead to a restoration of the general harmony of a body's physiology. There are reports on therapeutic success in the field of dermatology, but also in the case of diseases of the digestive system, the blood and heart, the respiratory tract, metabolic, infectious, and malignant diseases, or diseases of the nervous system (see [13] for a historical review). ◘ Figure 4.2 gives an example of a historical violet ray apparatus.

Even if there is some more or less serious historical literature on various biological and physiological effects of these devices, also with respect to the state of knowledge at this time, there is no real proof of their therapeutic efficacy available. With our present perspective at the beginning of the twenty-first century, all these indications are very vague. From the middle of the twentieth century, these kinds of therapies were no longer part of regular medicine.

However, the increasing success of scientifically based plasma medicine also supports the resurgence of this kind of vacuum or HF electrode applications. There are several devices available via the World Wide Web and by other distributors that look identical to the historic devices as given in ◘ Fig. 4.2. In several cases, the marketing of these devices is promoted by more or less dramatic stories about saving this technology through World War II and East-European dictatorships and its re-invention against the resistance of the modern and dominating healthcare industry. Nowadays, the indications for these devices range from more or less specific applications in dentistry to a general promotion as "oxy miracle medicine" with a broad spectrum of applications in healthcare, beauty, and wellness (see for example [14]).

Bringing this vacuum electrode closely to an external conductive surface like skin, a plasma is generated under atmospheric air conditions between the glass electrode

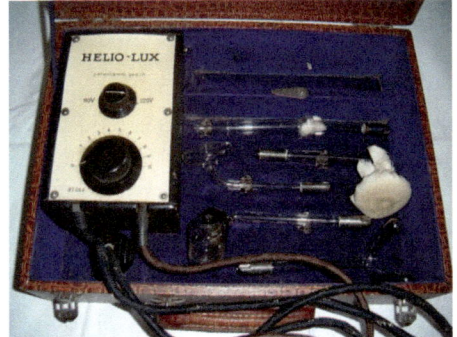 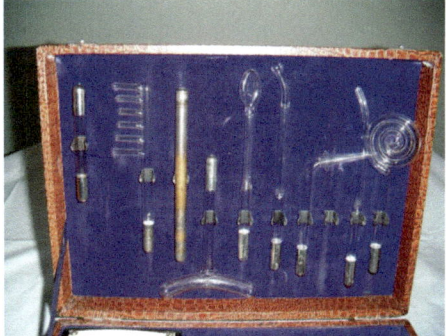

◘ **Fig. 4.2** Suitcase containing control unit as well as set of glassy vacuum electrodes of the antique HELIO-LUX high frequency (HF) apparatus. (Picture source: Ramona Meißner-Kellotat, Medical Historic Collection of the Institute of Ethics and History of Medicine, University Medicine Greifswald, Germany)

and the skin as a kind of dielectric barrier discharge (see ▶ Chap. 15). The reported germicidal activity via ozone generation of the historic devices was based most probably on this externally generated atmospheric pressure plasma. However, systematic investigations on biological effects of these specific vacuum or HF electrodes are missed now as before. Recently, there were some sporadic reports on antimicrobial activity of historic as well as current vacuum electrode devices tested in vitro demonstrating some antimicrobial activity [15, 16]. Its applicability for disinfection purposes in the oral cavity was estimated in comparison to other local antimicrobial therapies using liquid antiseptics [16]. In an in vitro study on periodontal wound healing, it was stated that cold atmospheric plasma generated by a vacuum electrode has regulatable effects on markers of periodontal wound healing [17].

Summarizing these few exact knowledge on biological effects of vacuum or HF electrodes, there is some evidence of a mild antimicrobial effect that may be used in wound healing or treatment of dermatological diseases or in dentistry. However, to establish these devices in medical practice, much more systematic pre-clinical and clinical research is needed that should lead to exact indications of its use in medicine. All other "esoteric" indications have to be rejected quite distinctly. This is all the more true if the marketing of such devices and indications is referring to plasma medicine as an innovative field of cold plasma application for medical therapy!

> **Important to Know**
> Plasma devices based on glassy vacuum electrodes (also named HF electrodes) are based on historic devices from the end of the nineteenth century and are re-launched for several years. Its announced performance in health care, beauty, and wellness is mainly based on historic reports, but not sufficiently documented by scientific investigations. Therefore, any reference of these devices to the results of plasma medicine has to be considered with caution.

Conclusion
Plasma medicine is an innovative field of application of physical devices in medicine comparable to the inauguration of laser medicine in the middle of the twentieth century. A lot of basic and applied research has been done during the last years to recognize the potential of cold atmospheric plasma (CAP) for medical applications and to explain its biological action mechanisms. Meanwhile, both the scientific basis and the successful application of CAP in wound healing or cancer treatment in future is no longer questionable. One of the most important preconditions to establish plasma medicine in daily healthcare practice is the availability of reliable CAP devices. Consequently, it is highly welcome that more and more medical device manufacturers are becoming active in the field of plasma medicine. However, to further guarantee the respectability and safety of plasma medicine, a close cooperation between basic research, clinics, and industry is essential. CAP devices for medical application have not only to fulfil the basic requirements of the medical device regulations but should be characterized specifically concerning its technical and biological performance. There are some devices on the market yet that fulfil these preconditions. The use of these devices in medical practice will foster the development of plasma medicine.

Other devices like the vacuum or HF electrodes might have also potential for specific medical applications. Here, much more systematic preclinical and clinical research is needed. It is not sufficient to refer to its supposed success in the historical past and to accompany its re-launch with conspiracy theories as well as the promise of miraculous success in healthcare, beauty, and wellness. Especially the reference of such "esoteric" fields of plasma application to the scientific basis of plasma medicine must be rejected vigorously.

References

1. Raiser J, Zenker M. Argon plasma coagulation for open surgical and endoscopic applications: state of the art. J Phys D Appl Phys. 2006;39:3520–3.
2. Canady J, Wile K, Ravo B. Argon plasma coagulation and the future applications for dual-mode endoscopic probes. Rev Gastroenterol Disord. 2006;6:1–12.
3. Weiss M, Utz R, Ackermann M, Taran F-A, Krämer B, Hahn M, Wallwiener D, Brucker S, Haupt M, Barz J, Oehr C. Characterization of a non-thermally operated electrosurgical argon plasma source by electron spin resonance spectroscopy. Plasma Process Polym. 2019;16:e1800150.
4. Vasilets VN, Shekhter AB, Guller AE, Pekshev AV. Air plasma-generated nitric oxide in treatment of skin scars and articular musculoskeletal disorders: preliminary review of observations. Clin Plasma Med. 2015;3:32–9.
5. Shekhter AB, Pekshev AV, Vagapov AB, Telpukhov VI, Panyushkin PV, Rudenko TG, Fayzullin AL, Sharapov NA, Vanin AF. Physicochemical parameters of NO-containing gas flow affect wound healing therapy. An experimental study. Eur J Pharm Sci. 2019;128:193–201.
6. Martínez-Sánchez G, Al-Dalain SM, Menéndez S, Re L, Giuliani A, Candelario-Jalil E, Álvarez H, Fernández-Montequín JI, León OS. Therapeutic efficacy of ozone in patients with diabetic foot. Eur J Pharmacol. 2005;523:151–61.
7. Gupta S, Deepa D. Applications of ozone therapy in dentistry. J Oral Res Rev. 2016;8:86–91.
8. Tiwari S, Avinash A, Katiyar S, Iyer AA, Jain S. Dental applications of ozone therapy: a review of literature. Saudi J Dent Res. 2017;8:105–11.
9. von Woedtke T, Schmidt A, Bekeschus S, Wende K, Weltmann K-D. Plasma medicine: a field of applied redox biology. In Vivo. 2019;33:1011–26.
10. Bussiahn R, Lembke N, Gesche R, von Woedtke T, Weltmann K-D. Plasma sources for biomedical applications. Hyg Med. 2013;38(5):212–6. (in German)
11. Mann MS, Tiede R, Gavenis K, Daeschlein G, Bussiahn R, Weltmann K-D, Emmert S, von Woedtke T, Ahmed R. Introduction to DIN-specification 91315 based on the characterization of the plasma jet kINPen MED. Clin Plasma Med. 2016;4:35–45.
12. DIN SPEC 91315:2014-6. General requirements for plasma sources in medicine. DIN Deutsches Institut für Normung e.V./ Beuth Verlag, Berlin 2014 (in German).
13. Graves DB. Lessons from tesla for plasma medicine. IEEE Trans Radiat Plasma Med Sci. 2018;2(6):594–607.
14. Halen V. Die Oxy Wunder Medizin. Norderstedt: BoD – Books on Demand; 2014. (in German)
15. Daeschlein G, Napp M, von Podewils S, Scholz S, Arnold A, Emmert S, Haase H, Napp J, Spitzmueller R, Gümbel D, Jünger M. Antimicrobial efficacy of a historical high-frequency plasma apparatus in comparison with 2 modern, cold atmospheric pressure plasma devices. Surg Innov. 2015;22(4):394–400.
16. Hafner S, Ehrenfeld M, Neumann A-C, Wieser A. Comparison of the bactericidal effect of cold atmospheric pressure plasma (CAPP), antimicrobial photodynamic therapy (aPDT), and polihexanide (PHX) in a novel wet surface model to mimic oral cavity application. J Craniomaxillofac Surg. 2018;46:2197–202.
17. Kleineidam B, Nokhbehsaim M, Deschner J, Wahl G. Effect of cold plasma on periodontal wound healing—an in vitro study. Clin Oral Investig. 2019;23:1941–50.

4

Further Reading

Arndt S, Schmidt A, Karrer S, von Woedtke T. Comparing two different plasma devices kINPen and Adtec SteriPlas regarding their molecular and cellular effects on wound healing. Clin Plasma Med. 2018;9:24–33.

Bernhardt T, Semmler ML, Schäfer M, Bekeschus S, Emmert S, Boeckmann L. Plasma medicine: applications of cold atmospheric pressure plasma in dermatology. Oxidative Med Cell Longev. 2019;2019:3873928.

Boeckmann L, Bernhardt T, Schäfer M, Semmler ML, Kordt M, Waldner A-C, Wendt F, Sagwal S, Bekeschus S, Berner J, Kwiatek E, Frey A, Fischer T, Emmert S. Aktuelle Indikationen der Plasmatherapie in der Dermatologie. Hautarzt. 2020;71:109–13. (in German)

Metelmann H-R, von Woedtke TH, Weltmann K-D, editors. Plasmamedizin. Kaltplasma in der medizinischen Anwendung. Berlin Heidelberg: Springer-Verlag; 2016. (in German)

Metelmann H-R, von Woedtke TH, Weltmann K-D, editors. Comprehensive clinical plasma medicine. Cold physical plasma for medical application. Cham: Springer International Publishing AG, part of Springer Nature; 2018.

Privat-Maldonado A, Schmidt A, Lin A, Weltmann K-D, Wende K, Bogaerts A, Bekeschus S. ROS from physical plasmas: redox chemistry for biomedical therapy. Oxidative Med Cell Longev. 2019;2019:9062098.

How Safe is Plasma Treatment in Clinical Applications?

Anke Schmidt and Sander Bekeschus

Contents

© Springer Nature Switzerland AG 2022
H.-R. Metelmann et al. (eds.), *Textbook of Good Clinical Practice in
Cold Plasma Therapy*, https://doi.org/10.1007/978-3-030-87857-3_5

Core Messages

— Evaluation strategies for risk assessment and determination of the patient's safety are essential prerequisites for a clinical application of cold physical plasma.

— Cold physical plasma potentially poses chemical, biochemical, and/or physical risks in humans, which must be evaluated in preclinical and long-term studies and clinical trials.

— Risk management of plasma applications in the clinics includes the identification and evaluation of risk factors, a description of potential consequences for human health, and qualitative and quantitative analysis of any potential risk of the application in humans.

5.1 Introduction

Cold physical plasmas are a valuable tool in biomedical research and a promising option for multi-ROS (reactive oxygen and nitrogen species) therapy in several types of diseases [1, 2]. Application areas of cold physical plasma therapy cover its use in dermatology (e.g., treatment of skin diseases, chronic wound healing), dermato-oncology, and dentistry [3–5], and very recently, selective killing of cancer cells by the extensive triggering of intracellular apoptotic pathways (reviewed in [6]). However, for a clinical application of cold physical plasma, evaluation strategies for risk assessment are essential prerequisites. A comprehensive risk assessment is defined as any self-contained systematic procedure to answer, for example, the following questions:

— How much of each hazard or suspected component is contained per plasma treatment culminating in the question of plasma treatment intensity or time, respectively?

— Are microorganisms becoming resistant to plasma treatment?

— Which general and disease-specific short- or long-term adverse side effects might appear during plasma treatment?

The general aim of this chapter is to summarize the knowledge of potential plasma risks connected with a comprehensive risk assessment and to evaluate the safety of plasma treatment in the clinics in the light of the current literature available.

5.2 Fundamentals in Risk Management and Mitigation Strategies

Cold physical plasma, from here on referred to as plasma, potentially poses chemical, biochemical, and/or physical threats to humans. There exists a multiplicity of plasma sources differing in their principle of plasma generation and technology, configuration, gas composition, application field with a specific operation and treatment strategy, and efficacy [7, 8]. To ensure the safety of patients and clinical staff, each plasma source and exposure process has to be carefully described and validated by a comprehensive physical, chemical, and biological characterization to assess its potential risks. Consequently, evaluation strategies for risk management and a safety assessment of any plasma source are essential prerequisites in a clinical plasma application.

Comprehensive risk management, including risk mitigation strategies, contains a systematic process for describing and quantifying risks associated with plasma treatment. Briefly, the risk assessment depicts, specifies, and evaluates the potential of the plasma device to release or introduce hazardous agents into the human body. During plasma source development, the relevant conditions and characteristics of plasma-generated components should be identified and quantified. This requires a detailed analysis of plasma constituents (e.g., radicals, electromagnetic and UV radiation), and types, amounts, timing and the release of toxic components, and energy as well as other potential risk agents of plasma treatment. Appropriate methods and model systems as well as clinical trials are then needed to evaluate any adverse side effects. This also includes a description of intensity, frequency, and duration of plasma exposure at biologically active plasma treatment intensities or times, respectively.

Judging the significance of risk factors along with qualitative and quantitative analysis of observed risk and their potential consequences for human health is a critical step in this process. This includes the analysis of adverse side effects, ranging from minor to severe or life-threatening in humans. Therefore, the relationship between specified exposure to plasma and the health consequences of this exposure in humans has to be depicted, including delayed and/or sustained effects (illness, injury, etc.). As such, beneficial or detrimental effects of plasma use must be investigated in long-term preclinical studies and clinical trials for the determination of the patient's safety. Finally, the risk acceptance should be monitored by developing and applying quality standards for estimating health consequences in humans. Other information should be further included in the risk-evaluation process to produce quantitative measures of health risks, including measurements of the estimated amount of humans with a potential health impact related to the treatment, any adverse effects observed, and uncertainties in these estimates (◻ Fig. 5.1). Finally, all points have to be integrated into standard protocols for developing guidelines estimating the health consequences of plasma use in clinical plasma medicine.

> At higher concentrations or intensities, respectively, the physico-chemical components of cold physical plasma potentially pose harm in humans. Therefore, risk estimations always played an essential role in developing the field of plasma medicine. Risk assessment and management to develop standard protocols of plasma health risks include the identification of potentially hazardous components and evaluation of risk factors, a description of potential consequences for human health, and qualitative and quantitative analysis of resulting risks.

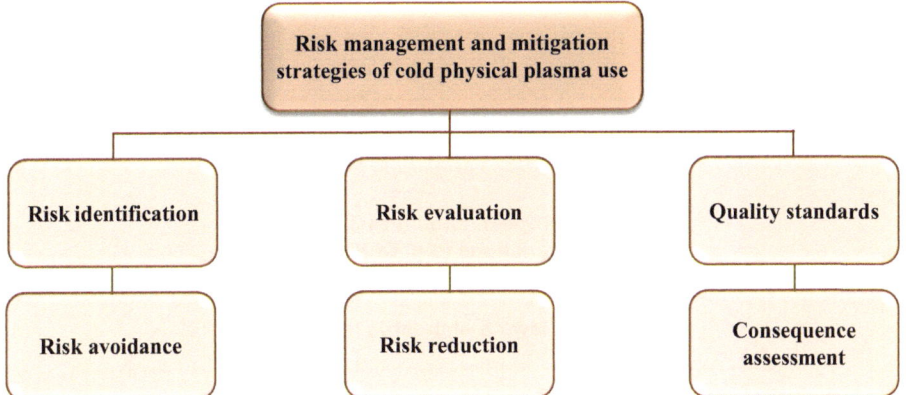

☐ Fig. 5.1 Risk classification and scope for clinical use of cold physical plasma. Risk management and mitigation strategies include a systematic process for describing and quantifying any potential risk associated with cold physical plasma treatment. Risk identification of hazard components, conditions, and/or events, as well as their avoidance and reduction strategies, are parts of the risk assessment. A reliable risk assessment reduces any adverse side effects ranging from minor over severe to life-threatening in humans. The risk acceptance should be monitored by developing and applying quality standards for estimating health consequences in humans

5.3 National and International Consensus Statements on Safety Standards in Clinical Plasma Medicine

Global standardization in plasma medicine has the mission to identify plasma sources, which are useful for biomedical investigations and their therapeutic applications. Standards in plasma medicine, including basic requirements, should improve the design and construction of medical plasma devices, which are useful to both therapeutic efficacy and safety for investigators, patients, and therapists. Standards should be established for simple and generally applicable physical methods (e.g., temperature, thermal capacity, optical emission spectrometry, leakage current, ultraviolet radiation and gas emission, etc.), and biological test methods (inactivation of microorganisms, cytotoxicity assays, detection of chemical species in liquids, genotoxicity testing, etc.) [9]. National and international standardization protocols and guidelines help consolidate application-oriented aspects of research resulting in an intensive and interdisciplinary scientific exchange within the field of plasma medicine worldwide. In the near future, it is also necessary to support the industry and authorities by developing European and international standards to enhance the acceptance and reputation of plasma medicine for patients and health insurances alike (☐ Fig. 5.2).

A multiplicity of plasma devices have been developed for a plethora of therapeutic applications. Clinical translation, however, is considerably low. Plasma can be generated by a variety of technologies (jet vs. DBD differing in, e.g., electrode design and size) using different gases (summarized in [10, 11]). Comparability between different plasma devices should not only be based on physical and technical parameters but mostly on their biophysical and biochemical as well as medical

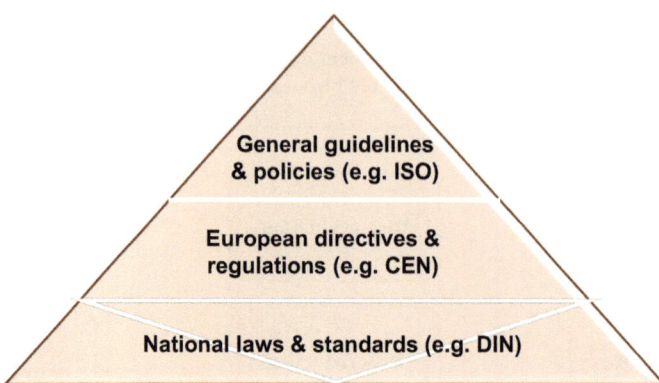

■ **Fig. 5.2** Safety standards in clinical plasma medicine. Guidelines on risk assessment and hazard prevention accumulate in specifications and standards to assure that plasma devices are safe and effective for their intended use. National laws and acts (e.g., medical devices act and operator ordinance), European directives and regulations concerning marketing, operation, and clinical studies (e.g., AIMDD, IVDD, and EWGMDD), general guidelines and policies at the international level (e.g., good clinical practice, Declaration of Helsinki) are essential to human safety and health to a maximal extent during any type of therapy

performance. While the latter is crucial for clinical applications, previous studies demonstrated the general performance of plasma sources with similar biological effects in mammalian cells or microorganisms [12]. To promote clinical translation, there is a growing interest among physicians, biologists, and physicists in analyzing the adverse effects of non-standard plasma devices in terms of any potential risks and how to mitigate such effects. However, the literature only provides little advice regarding the application of such non-standard devices in clinics. Due to the lack of international standardization, the proof of the efficacy of the plasma sources worldwide is difficult. To address this issue, the plasma community should launch a series of studies, particularly clinical trials, to provide a broad international perspective on the current state of research.

On the national level, the first German DIN specification entitled "General requirements for medical plasma sources" was published together with the German Institute for Standardization (DIN e.V., Berlin, Germany) in June 2014. This specification, DIN-SPEC 91315, describes simple and generally applicable biological and physical test methods to estimate the beneficial and potential side effects of plasma sources in therapeutic applications. The standards and specifications were described and characterized using the kINPen®Med (neoplas med GmbH, Greifswald, Germany) plasma jet [13]. Subsequently, it was demonstrated that several other plasma sources such as PlasmaDerm (Cinogy GmbH, Duderstadt, Germany), MicroPlaSter®/SteriPlas (Adtec, Hounslow, UK) and the plasma care® (terraplasma medical GmbH, Garching, Germany) are safe and effective concerning physical, chemical, and biological requirements (summarized in [9]). Manufacturers, e.g., Adtec, did a full risk assessment under ISO 14961 to ensure that their plasma device is safe for all participants [14]. With the declaration of conformity based on EU Council Directive 93/42/EEC, manufacturers guarantee the highest safety standards for patients and users by the implementation of a complete quality management system based on DIN EN ISO 13485 [15]. However, the Regulation (EU) 2017/745 on Medical Devices (MDR) changed the European legal framework for medical devices. New responsibilities for the European Medicines Agency (EMA) and the respective national authorities were introduced in 2017 and will fully apply in 2020. The guideline clarifies expectations and addresses new requirements of medical devices. Medical devices have to undergo a conformity assessment to demonstrate that they meet legal requirements to ensure they are safe and perform as intended (e.g., proof of effectiveness).

> International standards (ISO) should be established for simple and generally applicable biological test procedures and physical test methods to obtain first and basic information about performance characteristics as well as the effectiveness and safety of medical plasma sources. Medical devices in the European Union (EU) have to undergo a conformity assessment to ensure they are safe and perform as intended. National standards, such as the DIN-SPEC 91315 ("General requirements for medical plasma sources"), describe obligatory and essential criteria for the characterization of plasma sources for medical use in Germany.

5.4 Technical Demands on Plasma Devices and Their Multi-Component Signatures as Potential Hazards

The multi-component signature of plasma is unique, with a different but specific shape for each device. It needs to be analyzed as precise as possible, as each component may interplay with biological tissues, subsequently triggering well-known, unknown, and potential adverse effects in humans. The plasma components include neutral particles, free moving charged carriers (ions, electrons), radiation from the ultraviolet (UV) over visible light (VIS) to near-infrared range (NIR) and heat, electromagnetic and electric fields, and a sophisticated cocktail of chemical compounds such as reactive oxygen and nitrogen species (here summarized as ROS) and radicals (◻ Fig. 5.3) [16].

At supra-physiological concentrations or amounts, all plasma components (e.g., UV radiation, electric fields, radicals) have a specific risk profile that needs to be determined, quantified, and characterized for each plasma device. The presence of reactive molecules such as ROS is crucial for antimicrobial and biological effects (e.g., oxidative stress and tissue damage) [17]. At high amounts, UV radiation poses a mutagenic and cytotoxic potential due to interaction with biomolecules and especially DNA. Direct contact of patients with high voltage (e.g., electric spark, joule heating) is dangerous for human health and should be avoided by using dielectric materials and grounded components. A supra-physiological thermal impact on tissues (via, e.g., direct plasma application on the skin, electromagnetic energy transfer, etc.) may induce potential damage of tissue, including necrosis, damage of lipid bilayers, and proteins denaturation. Gas particles may trigger further physico-chemical reactions. Other potential side effects of plasma must be investigated in

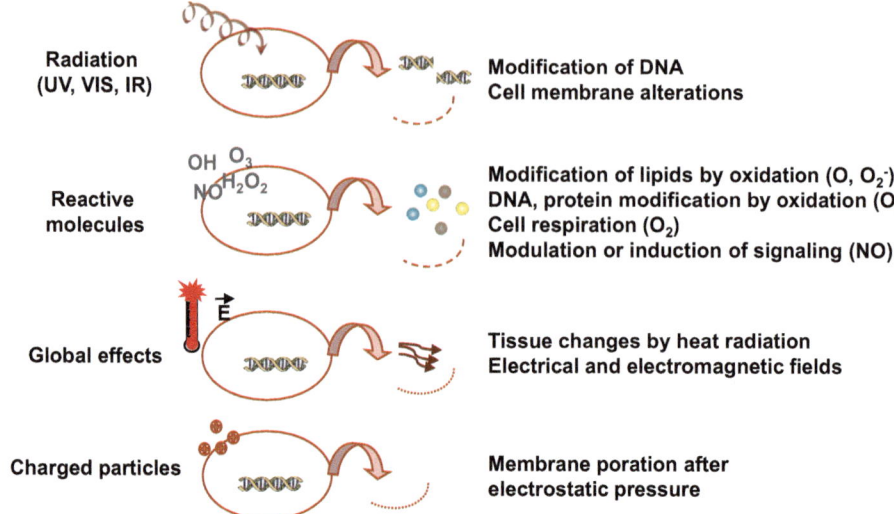

Fig. 5.3 Plasma-generated biological active components and consequences of plasma effectors in cells. The presence of plasma-generated reactive molecules such as ROS is crucial for antimicrobial and biological effects. Ultraviolet radiation has mutagenic and cytotoxic potential. Direct contact of patients with high voltage is dangerous for human health and should be avoided by dielectric materials and grounded components. Thermal impact on tissues may induce potential damage of lipid bilayers and proteins by denaturation

long-term studies in preclinical models and clinical trials for the determination of patient safety (■ Fig. 5.4).

The potential risk factors of plasma applications in humans are as diverse as plasma-generated biological active components and existing plasma devices. For this reason, all relevant parameters for safety are described in more detail in the following.

5.4.1 Electric Fields

Electric currents and fields must be considered for each plasma device type separately (e.g., jet, dielectric barrier discharge). Plasma ignition includes charging transporters such as ions and electrons carrying electric currents. High electric currents are often used in technical applications of plasma [18, 19]. Biomedical plasma devices possess lower electric currents, which, however, cannot be circumvented. Notably, volume dielectric barrier discharges (DBDs) use the skin as a counter electrode [3]. For all plasma devices with an internal electrode configuration (e.g., central electrode), there is no or low current flowing through the biological target (e.g., kINPen) – in contrast to a volume-DBD. According to international guidelines and national rules (IEC and DIN EN 60601-1-6:2010 + A1:2013), devices should be constructed using appropriate materials to avoid risks with high voltage components in plasma (e.g., electromagnetic interference, physical damage) [20].

Medical plasma devices

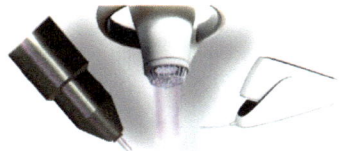

**No severe adverse
effects observed**

Potential risky components

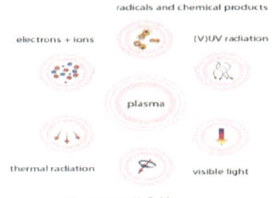

**Separation of the contribution of
individual components challenging**

**How safe is clinical
plasma medicine?**

**No tumor promotion of plasma
treatment observed so far**

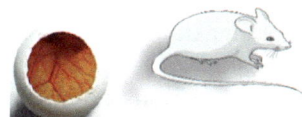

**Long-term studies in
pre-clinical models**

**Documented risk assessment in proband
performed for accredited plasma devices**

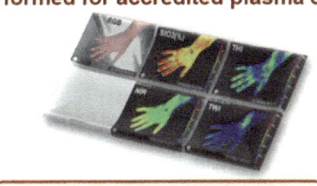

Clinical trials

◘ Fig. 5.4 How safe is clinical plasma medicine? There exists a multiplicity of plasma sources differing in their configuration, principle of plasma generation, and technology, with specific types of treatment and efficacy. The output of plasma-generated components is of great medical importance as they have essential roles as regulatory molecules in a range of biological processes. Potentially risky plasma components have to be identified, quantified, and characterized. Beneficial or adverse side effects of plasma use must be proven in long-term studies in preclinical models and clinical trials for the determination of patient safety

Moreover, plasma devices can be specifically developed to change or tune parameters, for example, by pulsing [21, 22].

Electric fields are mediators of biological plasma effects and interact with biological targets like cell membranes [23, 24]. Accordingly, the electric field of plasma could, in principle, lead to a change of transmembrane potential, oxidation of lipids of the plasma membrane, and fluidity changes. A subsequent pore formation in cell membranes, generated through electric fields, might enable the entry and penetration of reactive (plasma) species into the cell core [25], facilitating cell growth and respiratory changes [26, 27]. Pores may also promote the therapeutic transfer of drugs or creams in medical plasma applications. In sum, adverse side effects evoked by electric fields are not known so far but should be further investigated for any plasma source.

> Electric fields may penetrate treated tissue and may contribute to the clinical plasma effects. If the recommendation for design and use are respected, no adverse side effects are expected.

5.4.2 Thermal Energy

To avoid hyperthermia of biological targets (tissues, organs, cells), medical plasma sources should be working at a temperature of not more than 40 °C at the target site of treatment. Consequences of higher temperatures through electromagnetic energy transfer [28] are thermal damage of cellular components of the membrane lipid bilayer and molecular structures by denaturation of proteins and collagens, eventually culminating in cell death (e.g., apoptosis, necrosis) [29]. To prevent non-physiological temperatures, cold plasma devices were developed for biomedical applications operated at body temperature and under atmospheric pressure. Non-invasive optical emission spectroscopy, pyrometry, or fiber optic temperature sensors are available for the determination of specific thermal properties of plasma sources [20].

Several studies investigated the thermal profile of a plasma device in relation to its axial distance. For most technical concepts (e.g., DBD, torch, jet), gas temperatures below 40 °C are present [30, 31]. An optimal treatment distance between 9 and 12 mm and a treatment velocity between 6–10 mm/s was determined for the kINPen [32]. Preclinical studies in murine wound models found no skin damage, an intact epithelial layer, and an unchanged dermal skin layer morphology after repetitive plasma treatment [33, 34]. Studies on mammalian skin tissues confirmed a lack of thermal damage for up to 5 min of plasma treatment [35]. Moreover, previous case studies in humans using different plasma sources excluded any adverse effects due to thermal impact [36–42]. Spacers can be used for avoiding tissue treatment outside the recommended plasma-to-target-distance.

> Thermal impact on tissues via direct plasma application on skin may induce potential damage of lipid bilayers and proteins by denaturation. Using low-temperature plasma devices, thermal damage can be excluded if the recommendation for use is respected.

5.4.3 Ultraviolet Radiation

The plasma device geometry, electrode configuration, and working gas composition dictate the specific spectral characteristics being hallmarks of plasma-emitted components [43]. Such components may be hazardous at higher levels and should be determined for any plasma device. Depending on the emitted light intensity and the wavelength, photochemical events can be present in large biomolecules such as proteins and DNA. Particularly, ultraviolet (UV) radiation is the most important risk factor for the promotion of skin cancer (e.g., basal or squamous cell carcinoma, malignant melanoma), and many other skin disorders (e.g., pigmentation disorders, atrophy, degenerative aging). UV radiation as a component of the electromagnetic spectrum ranges between visible light and radiation, and its energy can be classified into UVA (315–400 nm), UVB (280–315 nm), and UVC (100–280 nm) [44].

UV radiation must be considered in plasma applications (e.g., wound or cancer treatment) with regard to its penetration depth. The penetration depth of radiation into intact biological systems like the skin is variable and correlates inversely with the total energy and wavelength. UV light can penetrate deeper skin layers, evoking adverse effects like cell aging and skin tumor formation. Each UV component affects biological targets by breaking chemical bonds in biomolecules [45]. Such processes allow oxidation and/or dimerization of nucleotides resulting in DNA damage and induction of DNA double-strand breaks (DSBs), UVA-related senescence, and a cancer-related transformation of skin cells [45]. Moreover, plasma treatment of damaged targets of the skin (e.g., wound) must be taken into account due to the loss of the top skin layers such as the *stratum corneum*, which serves as a protective barrier to the environment [46]. Nonetheless, UV also has beneficial effects by mediating the natural synthesis of vitamin D in the skin, demonstrating the dual and complex roles of UV in human health. Several studies have shown the gainful effects of UV radiation in cancer [47, 48], psoriasis [49], and vitiligo [50, 51].

Plasma jets like the k*IN*Pen or DBDs were investigated for UV radiation, showing that its exposure is lower than the recommended limits of the International Commission on Non-Ionizing Radiation Protection (ICNIRP) guidelines (30 J/m^2 per day) [52, 53]. Plasma-emitted UV radiation was an order of magnitude lower than the minimal erythema dose, which is necessary to produce sunburn in the human skin [38]. Health risk evaluation was also done using a microwave-driven jet (APJ) [54]. The limiting UV exposure duration for the APJ with a calculated maximum effective irradiance of 2.6 µW/cm^2 is around 19 min, based on the exposure limits of ICNIRP.

> ❯ Plasma treatment emits UV radiation. It should be ensured that the doses released into the treated tissue do not extend beyond that defined in the ICNIRP guidelines.

5.4.4 Chemical Energy

Chemical energy can be found in molecules and atoms and is released during chemical reactions in the gas phase and liquid environments, and subsequently onto cells and tissues [55].

Plasma devices are designed with a variety of different materials (metals, ceramics, quartz, glass, polymers, etc.), which can react with another. For clinical applications, mainly inert materials are used for the dielectric barrier and the housing to minimize corrosion and etching. However, polymeric organic material with a chain of carbon atoms may be attacked by plasma components evoking a break of bonds, etching, and loss of polymeric material. Finally, arising products can be potentially toxic (e.g., polytetrafluoroethylene, PTFE; polyvinylidene fluoride, PVDF; polyvinyl fluoride, PVF) by a plasma-induced release of fluorine in the case of fluor-containing polymers [43]. The generation and release of such toxic components must be avoided.

Typically, plasma sources work with non-toxic, ambient air (e.g., several types of DBDs) or inert gases like helium, argon, or neon as bulk gas with small admixtures of reactive working gases (nitrogen, oxygen) or liquids (water) [56, 57]. Gases are usually used in the highest purity of medical-grade [58]. No toxic effects are expected in the external use of noble gases on skin surfaces due to a lack of generating stable chemical products under the ambient conditions [43]. During use in the human body (e.g., endoscopic plasma devices), noble gases are a potential health risk because of their weak solubility in water and should be avoided.

Diverse short- and long-lived ROS are the primary mediators of biological plasma effects. These ROS cause hundreds of chemical reactions in the liquid environment, leading to primary and secondary plasma effects in biological targets [59]. Using kINPen plasma jets, acute health risks are not to be expected due to the low temperature, the local and only short-term application of plasma, and the lack of potentially toxic nitrogen dioxide formation [32]. Other plasma-generated gases such as ozone (O_3) are in the range of MAK (maximum working concentration) value of 0.1 ppm in close vicinity (<10 cm) to the plasma effluent of the kINPen jet [52]. The ozone generation depends on the working gas used, e.g., the admixture of oxygen into the working gas leads to increased ozone formation in contrast to the use of noble gas alone. Moreover, the plasma temperature is important. Ozone is produced to a greater extent at lower temperatures. The plasma devices like DBDs produce more ozone, which is relatively stable and poorly soluble in water [60, 61]. The unpleasant odor of ozone might be removed using filters or by working under appropriate hoods or in rooms with extensive air-conditioning. Nonetheless, ROS, including ozone, are crucial for antimicrobial plasma effects [62]. NO is an important signaling molecule in a variety of biological processes and serves as a vasodilator [63]. NO concentrations >2500 ppm are toxic in mice [38]. Generally, clinical plasma sources do not generate a large amount of NO so that the maximum MAK value of 0.5 ppm is not exceeded. Concentrations of approximately 40 ppm NO were determined after treatment with radiofrequency jets, but at longer distances, the NO concentration exponentially decreases [64].

Plasma-induced biological effects are mainly attributed to ROS and its downstream products, as shown in numerous in vitro and in vivo studies, as reviewed recently [1]. In close proximity to the treated biological surfaces, plasma-generated types of ROS include, for instance, superoxide anion ($O_2^{-\bullet}$), singlet delta oxygen (Δ^1O_2), atomic oxygen (O), peroxide (O_2^{-2}), hydrogen peroxide (H_2O_2), and the hydroxyl ion (OH-) and radical ($^\bullet$OH). Each of the ROS have individual life-times and reactivity with other components in the range from nanoseconds ($^\bullet$OH) over microseconds (Δ^1O_2) to seconds (O_2^-) [65, 66]. The range of chemical reactions, reaction products (e.g., organic radicals, hydrogen peroxide, dimeric, and hydroxylated molecules), and rates constants differ over several orders of magnitude [59, 67]. They are also determined by the diffusion rate and chemical environment [68, 69]. At excessive concentrations, each of the species may have harmful effects. As of now, it is technically impossible to investigate the amount of each of the many types of ROS being deposited into the tissue via plasma treatment.

> Reactive gases but not the non-excited noble gases formed by plasma devices can be potentially harmful. For polymers within the plasma-generating device being in direct contact to the plasma, the possible release of polymeric and putatively toxic compounds should be investigated to ascertain their safe use in medical plasma systems. A variety of components of cold physical plasma is known: reactive oxygen and nitrogen species (ROS), electric and electromagnetic fields, UV and heat emission, visible and near-infrared radiation, electrons, and ions. Components created by the plasma sources can be potentially harmful during use. However, all plasma components contribute to the desired plasma effects.

5.5 Genotoxic and Mutagenic Risk Assessment of Plasma Utilization

Plasma is not only useful for the treatment of wounds, including bacterial killing and stimulation of tissue regeneration, therapy of skin diseases, or induction of programmed cell death in cancer cells [3, 6, 22, 70, 71], but may also be harmful to human tissue. Through direct biological/clinical effects of plasma-generated ROS, oxidative stress may be increased, resulting in cytotoxic effects in the liquid environment of target cells [72]. At very high treatment intensities or times, respectively, the potential for the development of bacterial resistance and delayed effects such as induction of malignancies, mutagenic, and/or genetic effects are given. Resulting consequences include changes in secondary and tertiary protein structure and oxidation of lipids, proteins, or nucleic acids (e.g., pore formation, changes of cell proliferation and cycle, repair processes) [73]. Therefore, studies investigating all potential toxic effects following plasma treatment are of essential importance to evaluate fundamental risks and the safety of plasma technology.

5.5.1 Studies on the Potential Cytotoxicity, Genotoxicity, and Mutagenicity in Biomedical Plasma Applications in Vitro and in Ovo

Plasma-generated ROS directly or indirectly interact with a plethora of cellular molecules (e.g., nucleotides, fatty acids, sugar, amino acids) and its larger components (proteins, lipids of cell bilayer, carbohydrates, etc.), evoking potential harmful products [74–76]. Lipid peroxidation occurs by oxygen derivatives; however, products are often signaling molecules evoking an activation of cellular responses

[77]. Several studies have demonstrated a strong antioxidative Nrf2-mediated response [78, 79], which seems to be a direct effect of lipid peroxidation or formation of pores in the cell membranes [77]. Although a small amount of nuclear-localized Nrf2 maintains cellular redox homeostasis by regulation of basal expression of antioxidant genes, an oncogenic characteristic was suggested after constitutive Nrf2 activation in skin tumorigenesis [80], leading to a transition of a cancer-associated fibroblast phenotype [81] and resistance to chemotherapy [82]. However, after repeated plasma treatments over 3 months, the global transcriptomic profile of keratinocytes identifies genes, reflecting adaptions to frequent redox stress [83]. The exposure to plasma evokes acute oxidative stress but is not cytotoxic. Most cytotoxic effects are counterbalanced by the complex and finely tuned antioxidative defense system. Such transient activation of Nrf2 after plasma treatment does not increase the cytoplasmic-to-nuclear translocation and thereby prevents cancer formation [84]. Moreover, such molecules are promising clinical targets to reduce oxidative stress [85, 86].

Still, ROS, generated by plasma and following secondary cellular reactions, react persistent with chemical structures in DNAs and RNAs. Oxidative DNA damage and resulting mutagenic processes are tightly linked to aging, inflammation, and the development of cancer [87]. Consequently, one focus on the assessment of plasma risks lies in investigations of genetic stability after plasma utilization. Structural damage and decay of naked plasma-treated DNA (e.g., plasmid DNA) [88] were obtained in several cell lines (e.g., HeLa, HaCaT, mucosal cells) using a helium plasma needle [89] and air DBD [90, 91], which is, however, in biological context irrelevant. Within the cell, the nuclear DNA in the cellular environment is highly protected and stable (e.g., supercoiled in histone proteins), and the diffusion distance of reactive species is limited due to the thiol-group rich cytosol and short-lived ROS [92]. Moreover, primary oxidative DNA damage is mediated by extensive DNA repair mechanisms. The wild-type tumor suppressor p53 protein coordinates these responses and is a key determinant of antioxidant and cytoprotective functions at different stress levels [93]. Plasma-induced phosphorylation and activation of up-stream inducers of p53 signaling emphasized the assumption that a protein kinase-dependent branch of cellular redox homeostasis exists. Specifically, a serine/threonine-protein kinase (e.g., ATM/ATR kinases) might act as a redox sensor controlling levels of reactive species and initiates protective signaling subsequently. H2AX, a marker for double-strand breaks (DSBs), facilitates the recruitment of DNA repair proteins [94] and becomes phosphorylated (γ-H2AX) as a downstream effect of the apoptosis cascade and in response to DNA replication stress [95]. The finding that only a minor increase in histone 2AX phosphorylation was detected substantiated this [92]. However, after long-lasting plasma treatment over 3 months, an increased presence of γ-H2AX suggests that genomic stress was perceived throughout the treatment. No significant modulation of ATR expression was found [83], which corroborates the results of a previous study investigating the transcriptome in cold plasma-treated corneas [96]. Contrary, DNA damages were postulated in genotoxic studies through detection of γ-H2AX in cancer cells (e.g., MCF10A, B16F10, HCT116 spheroids [62, 97, 98]) or ex vivo in porcine [99] and human skin [100]. Very recently, it was pointed out that elevated

H2AX phosphorylation observed with plasma treatment is not caused by ROS-mediated DNA damage, but is the consequence of apoptosis. Despite γH2AX induction, UV, but not plasma treatment, led to significantly increased micronucleus formation, which is a functional read-out of genotoxic DNA DSBs [101]. For intact cells, the utilized plasma treatment intensities for clinical use are not sufficient to trigger DSBs.

According to OECD- (Organization for Economic Cooperation and Development) based protocols, several studies with different plasma devices demonstrated mainly no evidence of genotoxicity and mutagenicity in human cells in vitro and in ovo. To prove genetic safety, the estimation of micronuclei in cells was applied according to the OECD 487/2010 "Guidelines for testing of chemicals: in vitro mammalian cell micronucleus (MN) assay", and for mammalian erythrocytes to the OECD 474/1997 "Guidelines for testing of chemicals". In accordance with ISO norms, a plasma jet treatment with the k*INP*en did not display a mutagenic potential in multiple cell lines, MN, and colony formation assay [102]. The absence of newly formed MN in any feed gas condition added to a plasma jet was also demonstrated using a high-throughput MN assay in a lymphocyte cell line k*INP*en [103]. In two other studies, an increased mutation rate and cell death were detected in long-term DBD treatment of the brain cancer cell line T98G [104] and an argon plasma jet treatment of lymphoblastoid cells [105]. Plasma treatment on chicken embryos also demonstrated a plasma-induced lethality after 4 min using a DBD device [106]. Such differences in the identification of DNA damage and toxicity have many reasons, e.g., treatment parameters and methodology, cell targets, and exposure time. However, in ovo, genotoxic investigation using hen's egg test (HET) for MN induction showed no genotoxicity in fertilized eggs [107]. Moreover, safety in terms of promotion of metastasis after plasma treatment was tested in 3D tumor spheroids and tumor tissue grown on chicken embryos. As an important result, the authors found a lack of plasma-spurred metastatic behavior of 3D tumor spheroid outgrowth and the absence of an increase of metabolically active cells physically or chemically detached with plasma treatment [108].

Plasma treatment options in oncology are based on the induction of programmed cell death (apoptosis) or necrosis, cell cycle arrest, and changes in mitochondrial membrane potential [6, 22]. Furthermore, the recognition of damage-associated molecular patterns (DAMPs) and higher sensitivity of plasma in tumor cells was shown [109–114]. However, the limitation of plasma-induced killing effects on tumor cells and the identification of harmful side effects need to be considered. An important field of plasma use is, therefore, the ability to induce immunogenic cell death in tumors, which allows the explanation of plasma effects in deeper layers [68, 113, 115, 116]. For screening of plasma-induced inflammation, a modified hens'' egg test (HET)-CAM can be applied [117]. Plasma-induced apoptosis in pancreatic tumor cells identified decreased cell viability of cancer cells in a chorioallantoic membrane (CAM) assay [118]. Another study demonstrated little to no side effects after the plasma treatment of the pancreatic cancer cell tumor model [119].

To analyze the mutagenicity induced in V79 Chinese hamster cells, longer plasma treatment times were applied and analyzed using the hypoxanthine-guanine phosphoribosyltransferase (HPRT) mutation assay. Generally, a MiniFlatPlaSter-

DBD, a microwave-driven argon jet MicroPlaSter®, and an argon plasma jet kIN-Pen was applied for HRPT assay. To define a safe application window, the results show that a DBD plasma treatment of up to 240 s and repeated treatments of 30 s every 12 h did not induce mutagenicity at the Hprt locus beyond naturally occurring spontaneous mutations [120]. No mutagenicity was also detected in the HPRT assay even after repetitive plasma treatments up to 10 min every day over 5 days using the MicroPlaSter® [121]. Moderate plasma treatment up to 180 s with kIN-Pen plasma jet did not increase genotoxicity in HRPT assay in all cell types investigated [102]. Otherwise, the presence of epithelial cell mutants was reported after plasma exposure using high-voltage volume DBD [72], requiring further studies with any plasma device to exclude such effects.

5.5.2 Plasma-Derived ROS Therapies in Preclinical Studies

The absence of local inflammation as a sign of skin sensitization was shown in a murine wound model [122]. Other risk estimation studies in animals permitted a clinical application of plasma due to the absence of toxicity and good plasma tolerability [37]. A one-year follow-up wound healing study in mice that had received 14 repetitive plasma treatment sessions validated the finding of a lack of excessive inflammation. Additionally, no cells' metastatic behavior and tumor formation were found, as shown by non-invasive methods such as anatomical magnetic-resonance imaging and positron emission tomography-computed tomography [34]. Side effects by oral application of cold plasma on the mucosa were investigated in 180 mice showing no cytological atypia, loss of weight, and ongoing inflammation [123]. Consistent with mouse studies of Schmidt and co-workers [33, 79], MicroPlaSter® treatment of skin wounds showed similar effects regarding wound epithelialization and cytokine expression with an absence of toxic side effects in a rodent wound model [124–126]. Short-term plasma treatment accelerates wound healing without vital organ toxicity in rats [127] and pigs without microscopic skin damage due to the blood clotting [99]. Synergistic effects of plasma and polihexanide were shown to promote the healing of chronic wounds without adverse side effects in vivo [128]. Nevertheless, some other studies found early skin damage after long-term plasma treatment using a helium plasma jet [129], suggesting for these specific plasma sources detailed monitoring and control of plasma parameters like temperature – to exclude thermal damage – and oxidative stress generation.

5.5.3 Clinical Plasma Devices, Their Risk Assessments, and Application in Clinical Trials

Plasma-derived ROS therapy was applied with the aid of numerous sources in clinical approaches [1]. A plethora of plasma sources is available such as plasma jets and torches, floating electrode (FE-) [130] and dielectric barrier discharge (DBD), surface micro barrier discharge (SMD), microwave, and corona discharge [73]. For biomedical research, different conformations (needle, jet, torch, DBD, etc.) and gas compositions (e.g., air, argon, helium, etc.) are used [21, 70, 131, 132]. The majority of plasma sources with validation and/or use in clinical trials and patient pilot studies were developed mainly for alternative solutions of wound healing and microbial reduction as well as for the treatment of chronic and pathogen-based skin diseases [9]. A predominant number of studies were based on the use of PlasmaDerm, MicroPlaSter, and k*INP*en and stated no evidence for detrimental side effects.

> Several plasma sources received medical device accreditation for the treatment of infective skin diseases and wound healing. On the European market, for all medical plasma devices with a CE-certification as a medical IIa product, a sophisticated characterization of biological and physical effects is present, including the risk assessment for the use of plasma for the treatment of diseases in humans.

An important finding of studies was that the plasma application remains without risk for humans. Neither the plasma-induced UV radiation, temperature increase, nor the formation of radicals poses a potential risk to the treated patients [40]. Ex vivo treated skin biopsies revealed stimulating effects in deeper layers without harming cells on the skin surface [35, 133]. Improved wound healing along with the reduction of the bacterial load was reported for all medical plasma products such as kINPen®Med [134, 135], MicroPlaSter (trial ID: ISRCTN17491903) [136], PlasmaDerm (NCT01415622) [15, 41, 137, 138], PlasmaCare (trial ID: ISRCTN98384076) in clinical trials and pilot studies with and without randomizations. Despite wound healing, the broad antimicrobial benefit and the safe plasma use has been demonstrated in randomized controlled clinical trials in patients with chronic wounds [139, 140]. Such effects were successfully validated using k*INP*en [141, 142], using PlasmaDerm in 14 patients [41], using MicroPlaSter in 24 patients [36, 136] as well as 40 patients [143], in 46 patients for reduction of pruritus [144], and using surface micro barrier discharge [145]. All studies stated no side effects such as pain, and dermal damage, inflammation, or infections, which was also reported after k*INP*en treatment of wound healing disorders [42, 146], and in microcirculatory investigations using single or repetitive PlasmaDerm treatments [147, 148]. An interventional, non-blinded phase I clinical trial with the *plasoma* device investigating the efficiency of antimicrobial killing and safety aspects, including thermal damages of human skin, was finalized in the Netherlands (Association of Dutch Burn Centres, NCT03007264). Additionally, a clinical trial evaluating wound healing was recently finished in the USA using the *RenewalNail* device (NCT03072550, NCT03216200). At the State Scientific Centre of Coloproctology in Moscow, a plasma treatment after hemorrhoidectomy is currently ongoing in Russia (NCT03907306). In Germany, the investigator-initiated "Kaltplasma-Wund-Trial" was performed to prove beneficial effects of cold plasma in wound healing of diabetic foot independent of the reduction of bacterial load in a randomized bi-center study at the Ruhr University Bochum (NCT04205942) [142]. Cervical intraepithelial neoplasia will be treated with cold plasma at the University Women's Hospital Tübingen (NCT03218436). At *The Skin Center Dermatology Group* association in the United States of America, a study for efficacy and adverse effects using imaging techniques treats skin diseases such as actinic keratosis, acne, verruca plana, tinea, and alopecia (NCT02759900). An argon DBD-based source called *P-Jet* without accreditation as a medical device reduces the microbial burden and increases the healing of pressure ulcers [149]. This non-exhaustive list of clinical trials is complemented by recent review papers on this topic [3, 150]. From this perspective, plasma treatment may be regarded as safe for use in biomedical applications.

> ❯ The success of plasma therapeutic strategies is demonstrated in multiple in vitro, in ovo, ex vivo, in vivo, preclinical, and clinical studies. Clinical results with plasma sources developed for biomedical applications contain studies showing an improvement of chronic wound healing by reducing the bacterial burden and local pain. Despite the effectivity of plasma therapies varying between patients, consequences of plasma-therapeutic applications in clinical trials should be beneficial with no or negligible side effects regarding genotoxicity and mutagenicity.

5.6 Perspectives, Challenges, Limitations, and Concluding Remarks

The treatment with plasma-derived ROS is a novel tool in redox biology. However, the evidence level for many indications and their success is limited at the moment. This is related to the absence of large-scale multicenter studies and their subsequent meta-analysis. Beside tissue regeneration and skin disinfection in infective skin diseases and dentistry (e.g., implantology, caries, orthodontics), research fields of immunology, general surgery, aesthetic medicine, and pigmentation disorders are promising areas for plasma treatments. Moreover, treatment of malignancies, such as adjuvant cancer therapy, is promising but has been used only to a minimal extent in plasma research. These new fields of plasma medicine are potentially linked to the development of specialized plasma sources with increased safety requirements. A particular challenge for plasma medicine arises from a (work in progress) definition of generally applicable basic criteria and test procedures. These would be required to characterize such plasma devices in a standardized fashion and to compare their potential for specific experimental applications and/or prospective therapeutic uses.

Generally, the risks coming with plasma treatment are minimal and not severe. The remaining risks associated with plasma exposure can be reduced, though not entirely eliminated. Experimental data and preclinical studies conclude that plasma treatment is devoid of toxic side effects such as abnormal morphological changes, tumor formation or promotion of metastasis, mutagenicity, and genotoxicity. Plasma sources are safe if recommendations, guidelines, and standards (e.g., DIN-specification) for clinical use are followed. However, the lack of global standardization protocols of risk factor evaluation and the limited number of clinical trials exemplifies the large workload ahead as a prerequisite to a global and fully accepted clinical plasma medicine.

> This chapter offers a conceptual overview of risk assessment and management to define safety standards and potential health risks in plasma-treated humans, and to eliminate some of the confusion associated with cold plasma treatment. Testing the safety of plasma treatment in multiple studies, data demonstrate beneficial healing effects in chronic wounds and antibacterial effects in the decontamination of biological surfaces. Moreover, plasma treatment, as an add-on adjuvant strategy, may maximize the effectiveness of the therapeutic intervention in oncology. Generally, currently available data lead to the conclusion that plasma treatment is devoid of toxic side effects such as abnormal morphological changes, tumor formation, and promotion of metastasis as well as mutagenicity and genotoxicity. Future research may aid in further deciphering the consequences of plasma treatment, taking into account the safety aspects and risk factor assessment.

References

1. Privat-Maldonado A, Schmidt A, Lin A, Weltmann KD, Wende K, Bogaerts A, et al. ROS from physical plasmas: redox chemistry for biomedical therapy. Oxidative Med Cell Longev. 2019;2019:9062098. https://doi.org/10.1155/2019/9062098.

2. Graves DB. The emerging role of reactive oxygen and nitrogen species in redox biology and some implications for plasma applications to medicine and biology. J Phys D Appl Phys [Internet]. 2012;45:263001 p.

3. Bernhardt T, Semmler ML, Schafer M, Bekeschus S, Emmert S, Boeckmann L. Plasma medicine: applications of cold atmospheric pressure plasma in dermatology. Oxidative Med Cell Longev. 2019;2019:3873928. https://doi.org/10.1155/2019/3873928.

4. Izadjoo M, Zack S, Kim H, Skiba J. Medical applications of cold atmospheric plasma: state of the science. J Wound Care. 2018;27(Sup9):S4–S10. https://doi.org/10.12968/jowc.2018.27.Sup9.S4.

5. Metelmann H-R, Von Woedtke T, Weltmann K-D. Comprehensive clinical plasma medicine: cold physical plasma for medical application. Berlin: Springer; 2018.

6. Semmler ML, Bekeschus S, Schafer M, Bernhardt T, Fischer T, Witzke K, et al. Molecular mechanisms of the efficacy of cold atmospheric pressure plasma (CAP) in cancer treatment. Cancers (Basel). 2020;12(2). https://doi.org/10.3390/cancers12020269.

7. Weltmann KD, von Woedtke T. Plasma medicine-current state of research and medical application. Plasma Phys Control Fusion. 2017;59(1):014031. https://doi.org/10.1088/0741-3335/59/1/014031.

8. Helmke A, Gerling T, Weltmann K-D. Plasma sources for biomedical applications. In: Metelmann H-R, von Woedtke T, Weltmann K-D, editors. Comprehensive clinical plasma medicine. Cham: Springer International Publishing; 2018. p. 23–41.

9. Metelmann H-R, von Woedtke T, Weltmann K-D. Comprehensive clinical plasma medicine. Cham: Springer International Publishing; 2018.

10. Adamovich I, Baalrud SD, Bogaerts A, Bruggeman PJ, Cappelli M, Colombo V, et al. The 2017 plasma roadmap: low temperature plasma science and technology. J Phys D Appl Phys. 2017;50(32):323001. https://doi.org/10.1088/1361-6463/aa76f5.

11. Reuter S, von Woedtke T, Weltmann KD. The kINPen-a review on physics and chemistry of the atmospheric pressure plasma jet and its applications. J Phys D Appl Phys. 2018;51(23). https://doi.org/10.1088/1361-6463/aab3ad.

12. von Woedtke T, Schmidt A, Bekeschus S, Wende K, Weltmann KD. Plasma medicine: A field of applied redox biology. In Vivo. 2019;33(4):1011–26. https://doi.org/10.21873/invivo.11570.

13. Mann MS, Tiede R, Gavenis K, Daeschlein G, Bussiahn R, Weltmann K-D, et al. Introduction to DIN-specification 91315 based on the characterization of the plasma jet kINPen® MED. Clin Plasma Med. 2016;4(2):35–45. https://doi.org/10.1016/j.cpme.2016.06.001.

14. Herbst F, van Schalkwyk J, McGovern M. MicroPlaSter and SteriPlas. In: Metelmann H-R, von Woedtke T, Weltmann K-D, editors. Comprehensive Clinical Plasma Medicine. Cham: Springer International Publishing; 2018. p. 503–9.
15. Wandke D. PlasmaDerm® - based on di_CAP technology. In: Metelmann H-R, von Woedtke T, Weltmann K-D, editors. Comprehensive clinical plasma medicine. Cham: Springer International Publishing; 2018. p. 495–502.
16. von Woedtke T, Reuter S, Masur K, Weltmann KD. Plasmas for medicine. Phys Rep. 2013;530(4):291–320. https://doi.org/10.1016/j.physrep.2013.05.005.
17. Memar MY, Ghotaslou R, Samiei M, Adibkia K. Antimicrobial use of reactive oxygen therapy: current insights. Infect Drug Resist. 2018;11:567–76. https://doi.org/10.2147/Idr.S142397.
18. Fan HG, Kovacevic R. A unified model of transport phenomena in gas metal arc welding including electrode, arc plasma and molten pool. J Phys D Appl Phys. 2004;37(18):2531–44. https://doi.org/10.1088/0022-3727/37/18/009.
19. Khakpour A, Franke S, Uhrlandt D, Gorchakov S, Methling R-P. Electrical arc model based on physical parameters and power calculation. IEEE Transactions on Plasma Science. 2015;43(8):2721–9. https://doi.org/10.1109/tps.2015.2450359.
20. Gerling T, Helmke A, Weltmann K-D. Relevant plasma parameters for certification. In: Comprehensive Clinical Plasma Medicine; 2018. p. 43–70. https://doi.org/10.1007/978-3-319-67627-2_3.
21. Brandenburg R. Dielectric barrier discharges: progress on plasma sources and on the understanding of regimes and single filaments. Plasma Sources Sci Technol. 2017;26(5):053001. https://doi.org/10.1088/1361-6595/aa6426.
22. Bekeschus S, Lin A, Fridman A, Wende K, Weltmann KD, Miller V. A comparison of floating-electrode DBD and kINPen jet: plasma parameters to achieve similar growth reduction in colon cancer cells under standardized conditions. Plasma Chem Plasma Process. 2018;38(1):1–12. https://doi.org/10.1007/s11090-017-9845-3.
23. Wolff CM, Steuer A, Stoffels I, von Woedtke T, Weltmann K-D, Bekeschus S, et al. Combination of cold plasma and pulsed electric fields – A rationale for cancer patients in palliative care. Clin Plasma Med 2020. https://doi.org/10.1016/j.cpme.2020.100096.
24. Steuer A, Schmidt A, Laboha P, Babica P, Kolb JF. Transient suppression of gap junctional intercellular communication after exposure to 100-nanosecond pulsed electric fields. Bioelectrochemistry. 2016;112:33–46. https://doi.org/10.1016/j.bioelechem.2016.07.003.
25. Yusupov M, Van der Paal J, Neyts EC, Bogaerts A. Synergistic effect of electric field and lipid oxidation on the permeability of cell membranes. Biochim Biophys Acta Gen Subj. 2017;1861(4):839–47. https://doi.org/10.1016/j.bbagen.2017.01.030.
26. Steuer A, Wolff CM, von Woedtke T, Weltmann KD, Kolb JF. Cell stimulation versus cell death induced by sequential treatments with pulsed electric fields and cold atmospheric pressure plasma. PLoS One. 2018;13(10):e0204916. https://doi.org/10.1371/journal.pone.0204916.
27. Babaeva NY, Tian W, Kushner MJ. The interaction between plasma filaments in dielectric barrier discharges and liquid covered wounds: electric fields delivered to model platelets and cells. J Phys D Appl Phys. 2014;47(23). https://doi.org/10.1088/0022-3727/47/23/235201.
28. Koch R. The coupling of electromagnetic power to plasmas. Fusion Sci Technol. 2017;45(2T):193–202. https://doi.org/10.13182/fst04-a483.
29. Yarmolenko PS, Moon EJ, Landon C, Manzoor A, Hochman DW, Viglianti BL, et al. Thresholds for thermal damage to normal tissues: an update. Int J Hyperth. 2011;27(4):320–43. https://doi.org/10.3109/02656736.2010.534527.
30. Kuchenbecker M, Bibinov N, Kaemlimg A, Wandke D, Awakowicz P, Viol W. Characterization of DBD plasma source for biomedical applications. J Phys D Appl Phys. 2009;42(4):045212. https://doi.org/10.1088/0022-3727/42/4/045212.
31. Bussiahn R, Lembke N, Gesche R, von Woedtke T, Weltmann K-D. Plasma sources for biomedical applications. Hyg Med. 2013;38:212–6.
32. Weltmann KD, Kindel E, Brandenburg R, Meyer C, Bussiahn R, Wilke C, et al. Atmospheric pressure plasma jet for medical therapy: plasma parameters and risk estimation. Contrib Plasma Phys. 2009;49(9):631–40. https://doi.org/10.1002/ctpp.200910067.

33. Schmidt A, Bekeschus S, Wende K, Vollmar B, von Woedtke T. A cold plasma jet accelerates wound healing in a murine model of full-thickness skin wounds. Exp Dermatol. 2017;26(2):156–62. https://doi.org/10.1111/exd.13156.

34. Schmidt A, Woedtke TV, Stenzel J, Lindner T, Polei S, Vollmar B, et al. One year follow-up risk assessment in SKH-1 mice and wounds treated with an argon plasma jet. Int J Mol Sci. 2017;18(4). https://doi.org/10.3390/ijms18040868.

35. Hasse S, Duong Tran T, Hahn O, Kindler S, Metelmann HR, von Woedtke T, et al. Induction of proliferation of basal epidermal keratinocytes by cold atmospheric-pressure plasma. Clin Exp Dermatol. 2016;41(2):202–9. https://doi.org/10.1111/ced.12735.

36. Isbary G, Heinlin J, Shimizu T, Zimmermann JL, Morfill G, Schmidt HU, et al. Successful and safe use of 2 min cold atmospheric argon plasma in chronic wounds: results of a randomized controlled trial. Br J Dermatol. 2012;167(2):404–10. https://doi.org/10.1111/j.1365-2133.2012.10923.x.

37. von Woedtke T, Metelmann HR, Weltmann KD. Clinical plasma medicine: state and perspectives of in VivoApplication of cold atmospheric plasma. Contrib Plasma Physics. 2014;54(2):104–17. https://doi.org/10.1002/ctpp.201310068.

38. Lademann J, Richter H, Alborova A, Humme D, Patzelt A, Kramer A, et al. Risk assessment of the application of a plasma jet in dermatology. J Biomed Opt. 2009;14(5):054025. https://doi.org/10.1117/1.3247156.

39. Lademann J, Richter H, Patzelt A, Meinke MC, Fluhr JW, Kramer A, et al. Antisepsis of the skin by treatment with tissue-tolerable plasma (TTP): risk assessment and perspectives. In: Plasma for bio-decontamination, medicine and food security. Dordrecht: Springer; 2012. p. 281–91.

40. Lademann J, Ulrich C, Patzelt A, Richter H, Kluschke F, Klebes M, et al. Risk assessment of the application of tissue-tolerable plasma on human skin. Clin Plasma Med. 2013;1(1):5–10. https://doi.org/10.1016/j.cpme.2013.01.001.

41. Brehmer F, Haenssle HA, Daeschlein G, Ahmed R, Pfeiffer S, Gorlitz A, et al. Alleviation of chronic venous leg ulcers with a hand-held dielectric barrier discharge plasma generator (PlasmaDerm((R)) VU-2010): results of a monocentric, two-armed, open, prospective, randomized and controlled trial (NCT01415622). J Eur Acad Dermatol Venereol. 2015;29(1):148–55. https://doi.org/10.1111/jdv.12490.

42. Rutkowski R, Daeschlein G, von Woedtke T, Smeets R, Gosau M, Metelmann HR. Long-term risk assessment for medical application of cold atmospheric pressure plasma. Diagnostics (Basel). 2020;10:4. https://doi.org/10.3390/diagnostics10040210.

43. Wende K, Schmidt A, Bekeschus S. Safety aspects of non-thermal plasmas. In: Metelmann H-R, von Woedtke T, Weltmann K-D, editors. Comprehensive clinical plasma medicine. Cham: Springer International Publishing; 2018. p. 83–109.

44. Bekeschus S, Schmidt A, Weltmann K-D, von Woedtke T. The plasma jet kINPen – A powerful tool for wound healing. Clin Plasma Med. 2016;4(1):19–28. https://doi.org/10.1016/j.cpme.2016.01.001.

45. Sinha RP, Hader DP. UV-induced DNA damage and repair: a review. Photochem Photobiol Sci. 2002;1(4):225–36.

46. Proksch E, Brandner JM, Jensen JM. The skin: an indispensable barrier. Exp Dermatol. 2008;17(12):1063–72. https://doi.org/10.1111/j.1600-0625.2008.00786.x.

47. Dolmans DE, Fukumura D, Jain RK. Photodynamic therapy for cancer. Nat Rev Cancer. 2003;3(5):380–7. https://doi.org/10.1038/nrc1071.

48. Dos Santos AF, De Almeida DRQ, Terra LF, Baptista MS, Labriola L. Photodynamic therapy in cancer treatment - an update review. J Cancer Metastasis Treat. 2019;2019. https://doi.org/10.20517/2394-4722.2018.83.

49. Weischer M, Blum A, Eberhard F, Rocken M, Berneburg M. No evidence for increased skin cancer risk in psoriasis patients treated with broadband or narrowband UVB phototherapy: a first retrospective study. Acta Derm Venereol. 2004;84(5):370–4. https://doi.org/10.1080/00015550410026948.

50. Schallreuter KU, Wood JM, Lemke KR, Levenig C. Treatment of vitiligo with a topical application of pseudocatalase and calcium in combination with short-term UVB exposure: a case study on 33 patients. Dermatology. 1995;190(3):223–9. https://doi.org/10.1159/000246690.

51. Scherschun L, Kim JJ, Lim HW. Narrow-band ultraviolet B is a useful and well-tolerated treatment for vitiligo. J Am Acad Dermatol. 2001;44(6):999–1003. https://doi.org/10.1067/mjd.2001.114752.

52. Bussiahn R, Lembke N, Gesche R, von Woedtke T, Weltmann K-D. Plasmaquellen für biomedizinische Applikationen. Hyg Med. 2013;38:212–6.

53. European Union. Directive 2006/25/EC on the minimum health and safety requirements regarding the exposure of workers to risks arising from physical agents (artificial optical radiation) (19th individual Directive within the meaning of Article 16(1) of Directive 89/391/EEC). 2006(L 114):0038–59.

54. Lehmann A, Pietag F, Arnold T. Human health risk evaluation of a microwave-driven atmospheric plasma jet as medical device. Clin Plasma Med. 2017;7-8:16–23. https://doi.org/10.1016/j.cpme.2017.06.001.

55. Wende K, von Woedtke T, Weltmann KD, Bekeschus S. Chemistry and biochemistry of cold physical plasma derived reactive species in liquids. Biol Chem. 2018;400(1):19–38. https://doi.org/10.1515/hsz-2018-0242.

56. Winter J, Wende K, Masur K, Iseni S, Dunnbier M, Hammer MU, et al. Feed gas humidity: a vital parameter affecting a cold atmospheric-pressure plasma jet and plasma-treated human skin cells. J Phys D Appl Phys. 2013;46(29):295401. https://doi.org/10.1088/0022-3727/46/29/295401.

57. Frenking G, Koch W, Reichel F, Cremer D. Light noble gas chemistry: structures, stabilities, and bonding of helium, neon, and argon compounds. J Am Chem Soc. 1990;112:4240–56.

58. Ohorodnik SD, DeGendt S, Tong SL, Harrison WW. Consideration of the chemical reactivity of trace impurities glow discharge. J Anal At Spectrom. 1993;8:859–65.

59. Schmidt-Bleker A, Winter J, Iseni S, Dunnbier M, Weltmann KD, Reuter S. Reactive species output of a plasma jet with a shielding gas device-combination of FTIR absorption spectroscopy and gas phase modelling. J Phys D Appl Phys. 2014;47(14):145201. https://doi.org/10.1088/0022-3727/47/14/145201.

60. Kogoma M, Okazaki S. Raising of ozone formation efficiency in a homogeneous glow discharge plasma at atmospheric pressure. J Phys D Appl Phys. 1994;27(9):1985–7. https://doi.org/10.1088/0022-3727/27/9/026.

61. Zhang S, van Gaens W, van Gessel B, Hofmann S, van Veldhuizen E, Bogaerts A, et al. Spatially resolved ozone densities and gas temperatures in a time modulated RF driven atmospheric pressure plasma jet: an analysis of the production and destruction mechanisms. J Phys D Appl Phys. 2013;46(20). https://doi.org/10.1088/0022-3727/46/20/205202.

62. Kalghatgi S, Azizkhan-Clifford J. DNA damage in mammalian cells by atmospheric pressure microsecond-pulsed dielectric barrier discharge plasma is not mediated via lipid peroxidation. Plasma Med. 2011;1(2):167–77. https://doi.org/10.1615/PlasmaMed.2011003798.

63. Victor VM, Rocha M, De la Fuente M. Immune cells: free radicals and antioxidants in sepsis. Int Immunopharmacol. 2004;4(3):327–47. https://doi.org/10.1016/j.intimp.2004.01.020.

64. van Gessel A, Alards K, Bruggeman P. NO production in an RF plasma jet at atmospheric pressure. J Phys D Appl Phys. 2013;46(26):265202.

65. Hanschmann EM, Godoy JR, Berndt C, Hudemann C, Lillig CH. Thioredoxins, glutaredoxins, and peroxiredoxins--molecular mechanisms and health significance: from cofactors to antioxidants to redox signaling. Antioxid Redox Signal. 2013;19(13):1539–605. https://doi.org/10.1089/ars.2012.4599.

66. Bielski BHJ, Cabelli DE, Arudi RL, Ross AB. Reactivity of HO_2/O_2^- radicals in aqueous solution. J Phys Chem Ref Data. 1985;14(4):1041–100. https://doi.org/10.1063/1.555739.

67. Schmidt-Bleker A, Bansemer R, Reuter S, Weltmann K-D. How to produce an NO_x- instead of O_x-based chemistry with a cold atmospheric plasma jet. Plasma Process Polym. 2016;13(11):1120–7. https://doi.org/10.1002/ppap.201600062.

68. Bekeschus S, Brautigam L, Wende K, Hanschmann EM. Oxidants and redox Signaling: perspectives in cancer therapy, inflammation, and plasma medicine. Oxidative Med Cell Longev. 2017;2017:4020253. https://doi.org/10.1155/2017/4020253.

69. Winterbourn CC. Reconciling the chemistry and biology of reactive oxygen species. Nat Chem Biol. 2008;4(5):278–86. https://doi.org/10.1038/nchembio.85.

70. Winter J, Brandenburg R, Weltmann KD. Atmospheric pressure plasma jets: an overview of devices and new directions. Plasma Sources Sci Technol. 2015;24(6):064001. https://doi.org/10.1088/0963-0252/24/6/064001.

71. Daeschlein G, Napp M, von Podewils S, Lutze S, Emmert S, Lange A, et al. In vitro susceptibility of multidrug resistant skin and wound pathogens against low temperature atmospheric pressure plasma jet (APPJ) and dielectric barrier discharge plasma (DBD). Plasma Process Polym. 2014;11(2):175–83. https://doi.org/10.1002/ppap.201300070.

72. Boehm D, Heslin C, Cullen PJ, Bourke P. Cytotoxic and mutagenic potential of solutions exposed to cold atmospheric plasma. Sci Rep. 2016;6:21464. https://doi.org/10.1038/srep21464.

73. Boehm D, Bourke P. Safety implications of plasma-induced effects in living cells - a review of in vitro and in vivo findings. Biol Chem. 2018;400(1):3–17. https://doi.org/10.1515/hsz-2018-0222.

74. Fahy E, Cotter D, Sud M, Subramaniam S. Lipid classification, structures and tools. Biochim Biophys Acta. 2011;1811(11):637–47. https://doi.org/10.1016/j.bbalip.2011.06.009.

75. Maheux S, Frache G, Thomann JS, Clément F, Penny C, Belmonte T, et al. Small unilamellar liposomes as a membrane model for cell inactivation by cold atmospheric plasma treatment. J Phys D Appl Phys. 2016;49(34). https://doi.org/10.1088/0022-3727/49/34/344001.

76. Choe E, Min DB. Chemistry and reactions of reactive oxygen species in foods. J Food Sci. 2006;70(9):R142–R59. https://doi.org/10.1111/j.1365-2621.2005.tb08329.x.

77. Gueraud F, Atalay M, Bresgen N, Cipak A, Eckl PM, Huc L, et al. Chemistry and biochemistry of lipid peroxidation products. Free Radic Res. 2010;44(10):1098–124. https://doi.org/10.3109/10715762.2010.498477.

78. Schmidt A, Bekeschus S. Redox for repair: cold physical plasmas and Nrf2 Signaling promoting wound healing. Antioxidants (Basel). 2018;7(10):146. https://doi.org/10.3390/antiox7100146.

79. Schmidt A, von Woedtke T, Vollmar B, Hasse S, Bekeschus S. Nrf2 signaling and inflammation are key events in physical plasma-spurred wound healing. Theranostics. 2019;9(4):1066–84. https://doi.org/10.7150/thno.29754.

80. Rolfs F, Huber M, Kuehne A, Kramer S, Haertel E, Muzumdar S, et al. Nrf2 activation promotes keratinocyte survival during early skin carcinogenesis via metabolic alterations. Cancer Res. 2015;75(22):4817–29. https://doi.org/10.1158/0008-5472.CAN-15-0614.

81. Hiebert P, Wietecha MS, Cangkrama M, Haertel E, Mavrogonatou E, Stumpe M, et al. Nrf2-mediated fibroblast reprogramming drives cellular senescence by targeting the matrisome. Dev Cell. 2018;46(2):145–61. e10. https://doi.org/10.1016/j.devcel.2018.06.012.

82. Shibata T, Kokubu A, Gotoh M, Ojima H, Ohta T, Yamamoto M, et al. Genetic alteration of Keap1 confers constitutive Nrf2 activation and resistance to chemotherapy in gallbladder cancer. Gastroenterology. 2008;135(4):1358–68, 68 e1-4. https://doi.org/10.1053/j.gastro.2008.06.082.

83. Schmidt A, von Woedtke T, Bekeschus S. Periodic exposure of keratinocytes to cold physical plasma: an in vitro model for redox-related diseases of the skin. Oxidative Med Cell Longev. 2016;2016(Harmful and Beneficial Role of ROS (HBR)):9816072. https://doi.org/10.1155/2016/9816072.

84. Schmidt A, Dietrich S, Steuer A, Weltmann KD, von Woedtke T, Masur K, et al. Non-thermal plasma activates human keratinocytes by stimulation of antioxidant and phase II pathways. J Biol Chem. 2015;290(11):6731–50. https://doi.org/10.1074/jbc.M114.603555.

85. Tukaj S, Gruner D, Zillikens D, Kasperkiewicz M. Hsp90 blockade modulates bullous pemphigoid IgG-induced IL-8 production by keratinocytes. Cell Stress Chaperones. 2014;19(6):887–94. https://doi.org/10.1007/s12192-014-0513-8.

86. Voll EA, Ogden IM, Pavese JM, Huang X, Xu L, Jovanovic BD, et al. Heat shock protein 27 regulates human prostate cancer cell motility and metastatic progression. Oncotarget. 2014;5(9):2648–63. https://doi.org/10.18632/oncotarget.1917.

87. Poetsch AR. The genomics of oxidative DNA damage, repair, and resulting mutagenesis. Comput Struct Biotechnol J. 2020;18:207–19. https://doi.org/10.1016/j.csbj.2019.12.013.

88. Arjunan KP, Sharma VK, Ptasinska S. Effects of atmospheric pressure plasmas on isolated and cellular DNA-a review. Int J Mol Sci. 2015;16(2):2971–3016. https://doi.org/10.3390/ijms16022971.

89. García-Alcantara E, Lopez-Callejas R, Serment-Guerrero J, Peña-Eguiluz R, Muñoz-Castro A, Rodriguez-Mendez B, et al. Toxicity and Genotoxicity in HeLa and E. coli cells caused by a helium plasma needle. Appl Phys Res. 2013;5(5):21.

90. Blackert S, Haertel B, Wende K, von Woedtke T, Lindequist U. Influence of non-thermal atmospheric pressure plasma on cellular structures and processes in human keratinocytes (HaCaT). J Dermatol Sci. 2013;70(3):173–81. https://doi.org/10.1016/j.jdermsci.2013.01.012.

91. Tiede R, Hirschberg J, Viöl W, Emmert S. A μs-pulsed dielectric barrier discharge source: physical characterization and biological effects on human skin fibroblasts. Plasma Process Polym. 2016;13(8):775–87. https://doi.org/10.1002/ppap.201500190.

92. Schmidt A, Bekeschus S, Jarick K, Hasse S, von Woedtke T, Wende K. Cold physical plasma modulates p53 and mitogen-activated protein kinase signaling in keratinocytes. Oxidative Med Cell Longev. 2019;2019:1–16. https://doi.org/10.1155/2019/7017363.

93. Murray D, Mirzayans R. Non-linearities in the cellular response to ionizing radiation and the role of p53 therein. Int J Radiat Biol. 2020:1–42. https://doi.org/10.1080/09553002.2020.1721602.

94. Rogakou EP, Pilch DR, Orr AH, Ivanova VS, Bonner WM. DNA double-stranded breaks induce histone H2AX phosphorylation on serine 139. J Biol Chem. 1998;273(10):5858–68.

95. Ward IM, Chen JJ. Histone H2AX is phosphorylated in an ATR-dependent manner in response to replicational stress. J Biol Chem. 2001;276(51):47759–62. https://doi.org/10.1074/bjc.C100569200.

96. Rosani U, Tarricone E, Venier P, Brun P, Deligianni V, Zuin M, et al. Atmospheric-pressure cold plasma induces transcriptional changes in ex vivo human corneas. PLoS One. 2015;10(7):e0133173. https://doi.org/10.1371/journal.pone.0133173.

97. Kim CH, Bahn JH, Lee SH, Kim GY, Jun SI, Lee K, et al. Induction of cell growth arrest by atmospheric non-thermal plasma in colorectal cancer cells. J Biotechnol. 2010;150(4):530–8. https://doi.org/10.1016/j.jbiotec.2010.10.003.

98. Judee F, Fongia C, Ducommun B, Yousfi M, Lobjois V, Merbahi N. Short and long time effects of low temperature plasma activated media on 3D multicellular tumor spheroids. Sci Rep. 2016;6:21421. https://doi.org/10.1038/srep21421.

99. Wu AS, Kalghatgi S, Dobrynin D, Sensenig R, Cerchar E, Podolsky E, et al. Porcine intact and wounded skin responses to atmospheric nonthermal plasma. J Surg Res. 2013;179(1):e1–e12. https://doi.org/10.1016/j.jss.2012.02.039.

100. Isbary G, Köritzer J, Mitra A, Li YF, Shimizu T, Schroeder J, et al. Ex vivo human skin experiments for the evaluation of safety of new cold atmospheric plasma devices. Clin Plasma Med. 2013;1(1):36–44. https://doi.org/10.1016/j.cpme.2012.10.001.

101. Bekeschus S, Schütz CS, Niessner F, Wende K, Weltmann K-D, Gelbrich N, et al. Elevated H2AX phosphorylation observed with kINPen plasma treatment is not caused by ROS-mediated DNA damage but is the consequence of apoptosis. Oxidative Med Cell Longev. 2019;2019:8535163. https://doi.org/10.1155/2019/8535163.

102. Wende K, Bekeschus S, Schmidt A, Jatsch L, Hasse S, Weltmann KD, et al. Risk assessment of a cold argon plasma jet in respect to its mutagenicity. Mutat Res Genet Toxicol Environ Mutagen. 2016;798-799:48–54. https://doi.org/10.1016/j.mrgentox.2016.02.003.

103. Bekeschus S, Schmidt A, Kramer A, Metelmann HR, Adler F, von Woedtke T, et al. High throughput image cytometry micronucleus assay to investigate the presence or absence of mutagenic effects of cold physical plasma. Environ Mol Mutagen. 2018;59(4):268–77. https://doi.org/10.1002/em.22172.

104. Kaushik NK, Uhm H, Choi EH. Micronucleus formation induced by dielectric barrier discharge plasma exposure in brain cancer cells. Appl Phys Lett. 2012;100(8):084102 Artn 08410210. https://doi.org/10.1063/1.3687172.

105. Hong SH, Szili EJ, Fenech M, Gaur N, Short RD. Genotoxicity and cytotoxicity of the plasma jet-treated medium on lymphoblastoid WIL2-NS cell line using the cytokinesis block micronucleus cytome assay. Sci Rep. 2017;7(1):3854. https://doi.org/10.1038/s41598-017-03754-1.

106. Zhang JJ, Jo JO, Huynh DL, Ghosh M, Kim N, Lee SB, et al. Lethality of inappropriate plasma exposure on chicken embryonic development. Oncotarget. 2017;8(49):85642–54. https://doi.org/10.18632/oncotarget.21105.

107. Kluge S, Bekeschus S, Bender C, Benkhai H, Sckell A, Below H, et al. Investigating the mutagenicity of a cold argon-plasma jet in an HET-MN model. PLoS One. 2016;11(9):e0160667. https://doi.org/10.1371/journal.pone.0160667.

108. Bekeschus S, Freund E, Spadola C, Privat-Maldonado A, Hackbarth C, Bogaerts A, et al. Risk assessment of kINPen plasma treatment of four human pancreatic cancer cell lines with respect to metastasis. Cancers (Basel). 2019;11(9):1237. https://doi.org/10.3390/cancers11091237.

109. Schlegel J, Köritzer J, Boxhammer V. Plasma in cancer treatment. Clin Plasma Med. 2013;1(2):2–7. https://doi.org/10.1016/j.cpme.2013.08.001.

110. Gjika E, Pal-Ghosh S, Tang A, Kirschner M, Tadvalkar G, Canady J, et al. Adaptation of operational parameters of cold atmospheric plasma for in vitro treatment of cancer cells. ACS Appl Mater Interfaces. 2018;10(11):9269–79. https://doi.org/10.1021/acsami.7b18653.

111. Bauer G. Increasing the endogenous NO level causes catalase inactivation and reactivation of intercellular apoptosis signaling specifically in tumor cells. Redox Biol. 2015;6:353–71. https://doi.org/10.1016/j.redox.2015.07.017.

112. Bauer G. The antitumor effect of singlet oxygen. Anticancer Res. 2016;36(11):5649–63. https://doi.org/10.21873/anticanres.11148.

113. Bauer G, Sersenova D, Graves DB, Machala Z. Dynamics of singlet oxygen-triggered, RONS-based apoptosis induction after treatment of tumor cells with cold atmospheric plasma or plasma-activated medium. Sci Rep. 2019;9(1):13931. https://doi.org/10.1038/s41598-019-50329-3.

114. Khlyustova A, Labay C, Machala Z, Ginebra MP, Canal C. Important parameters in plasma jets for the production of RONS in liquids for plasma medicine: a brief review. Front Chem Sci Eng. 2019;13(2):238–52. https://doi.org/10.1007/s11705-019-1801-8.

115. Bekeschus S, Clemen R, Metelmann H-R. Potentiating anti-tumor immunity with physical plasma. Clin Plasma Med. 2018;12:17–22. https://doi.org/10.1016/j.cpme.2018.10.001.

116. Bekeschus S, Mueller A, Miller V, Gaipl U, Weltmann K-D. Physical plasma elicits immunogenic cancer cell death and mitochondrial singlet oxygen. IEEE Trans Radiat Plasma Med Sci. 2018;2(2):138–46. https://doi.org/10.1109/trpms.2017.2766027.

117. Bender C, Partecke LI, Kindel E, Doring F, Lademann J, Heidecke CD, et al. The modified HET-CAM as a model for the assessment of the inflammatory response to tissue tolerable plasma. Toxicol In Vitro. 2011;25(2):530–7. https://doi.org/10.1016/j.tiv.2010.11.012.

118. Partecke LI, Evert K, Haugk J, Doering F, Normann L, Diedrich S, et al. Tissue tolerable plasma (TTP) induces apoptosis in pancreatic cancer cells in vitro and in vivo. BMC Cancer. 2012;12(1):473. https://doi.org/10.1186/1471-2407-12-473.

119. Liedtke KR, Bekeschus S, Kaeding A, Hackbarth C, Kuehn JP, Heidecke CD, et al. Non-thermal plasma-treated solution demonstrates antitumor activity against pancreatic cancer cells in vitro and in vivo. Sci Rep. 2017;7(1):8319. https://doi.org/10.1038/s41598-017-08560-3.

120. Boxhammer V, Li YF, Koritzer J, Shimizu T, Maisch T, Thomas HM, et al. Investigation of the mutagenic potential of cold atmospheric plasma at bactericidal dosages. Mutat Res. 2013;753(1):23–8. https://doi.org/10.1016/j.mrgentox.2012.12.015.

121. Maisch T, Bosserhoff AK, Unger P, Heider J, Shimizu T, Zimmermann JL, et al. Investigation of toxicity and mutagenicity of cold atmospheric argon plasma. Environ Mol Mutagen. 2017;58(3):172–7. https://doi.org/10.1002/em.22086.

122. van der Linde J, Liedtke KR, Matthes R, Kramer A, Heidecke C-D, Partecke LI. Repeated cold atmospheric plasma application to intact skin does not cause sensitization in a standardized murine model. Plasma Med. 2017;7(4):383–93. https://doi.org/10.1615/PlasmaMed.2017019167.

123. Jablonowski L, Kocher T, Schindler A, Muller K, Dombrowski F, von Woedtke T, et al. Side effects by oral application of atmospheric pressure plasma on the mucosa in mice. PLoS One. 2019;14(4):e0215099. https://doi.org/10.1371/journal.pone.0215099.

124. Arndt S, Schmidt A, Karrer S, von Woedtke T. Comparing two different plasma devices kINPen and Adtec SteriPlas regarding their molecular and cellular effects on wound healing. Clin Plasma Med. 2018;9:24–33. https://doi.org/10.1016/j.cpme.2018.01.002.

125. Arndt S, Unger P, Berneburg M, Bosserhoff AK, Karrer S. Cold atmospheric plasma (CAP) activates angiogenesis-related molecules in skin keratinocytes, fibroblasts and endothelial cells and improves wound angiogenesis in an autocrine and paracrine mode. J Dermatol Sci. 2018;89(2):181–90. https://doi.org/10.1016/j.jdermsci.2017.11.008.

126. Arndt S, Unger P, Wacker E, Shimizu T, Heinlin J, Li YF, et al. Cold atmospheric plasma (CAP) changes gene expression of key molecules of the wound healing machinery and improves wound healing in vitro and in vivo. PLoS One. 2013;8(11):e79325. https://doi.org/10.1371/journal.pone.0079325.

127. Hung YW, Lee LT, Peng YC, Chang CT, Wong YK, Tung KC. Effect of a nonthermal-atmospheric pressure plasma jet on wound healing: an animal study. J Chin Med Assoc. 2016;79(6):320–8. https://doi.org/10.1016/j.jcma.2015.06.024.

128. Bender CH, N-O, Weltmann K-D, Scharf C, Kramer A. Plasma for bio- decontamination, medicine and food security. Dordrecht: Springer; 2012. p. 321–4.

129. Kos S, Blagus T, Cemazar M, Filipic G, Sersa G, Cvelbar U. Safety aspects of atmospheric pressure helium plasma jet operation on skin: in vivo study on mouse skin. PLoS One. 2017;12(4):e0174966. https://doi.org/10.1371/journal.pone.0174966.

130. Keddam M, Nóvoa XR, Vivier V. The concept of floating electrode for contact-less electrochemical measurements: application to reinforcing steel-bar corrosion in concrete. Corros Sci. 2009;51(8):1795–801. https://doi.org/10.1016/j.corsci.2009.05.006.

131. Stoffels E, Flikweert AJ, Stoffels WW, Kroesen GMW. Plasma needle: a non-destructive atmospheric plasma source for fine surface treatment of (bio)materials. Plasma Sources Sci Technol. 2002;11(4):383–8. https://doi.org/10.1088/0963-0252/11/4/304.

132. Shimizu T, Steffes B, Pompl R, Jamitzky F, Bunk W, Ramrath K, et al. Characterization of microwave plasma torch for decontamination. Plasma Process Polym. 2008;5(6):577–82. https://doi.org/10.1002/ppap.200800021.

133. Hasse S, Hahn O, Kindler S, Woedtke TV, Metelmann H-R, Masur K. Atmospheric pressure plasma jet application on human oral mucosa modulates tissue regeneration. Plasma Med. 2014;4(1–4):117–29. https://doi.org/10.1615/PlasmaMed.2014011978.

134. Daeschlein G, Napp M, Lutze S, Arnold A, von Podewils S, Guembel D, et al. Skin and wound decontamination of multidrug-resistant bacteria by cold atmospheric plasma coagulation. J German Soc Dermatol. 2015;13(2):143–50. https://doi.org/10.1111/ddg.12559.

135. Daeschlein G, Scholz S, Ahmed R, von Woedtke T, Haase H, Niggemeier M, et al. Skin decontamination by low-temperature atmospheric pressure plasma jet and dielectric barrier discharge plasma. J Hosp Infect. 2012;81(3):177–83. https://doi.org/10.1016/j.jhin.2012.02.012.

136. Isbary G, Morfill G, Schmidt HU, Georgi M, Ramrath K, Heinlin J, et al. A first prospective randomized controlled trial to decrease bacterial load using cold atmospheric argon plasma on chronic wounds in patients. Br J Dermatol. 2010;163(1):78–82. https://doi.org/10.1111/j.1365-2133.2010.09744.x.

137. Emmert S, Brehmer F, Hänßle H, Helmke A, Mertens N, Ahmed R, et al. Atmospheric pressure plasma in dermatology: ulcus treatment and much more. Clin Plasma Med. 2013;1(1):24–9. https://doi.org/10.1016/j.cpme.2012.11.002.

138. Emmert S, Brehmer F, Hanssle H, Helmke A, Mertens N, Ahmed R, et al. Treatment of chronic venous leg ulcers with a hand-held DBD plasma generator. Plasma Med. 2012;2(1–3):19–32. https://doi.org/10.1615/PlasmaMed.2013005914.

139. Isbary G, Shimizu T, Zimmermann JL, Thomas HM, Morfill GE, Stolz W. Cold atmospheric plasma for local infection control and subsequent pain reduction in a patient with chronic post-operative ear infection. New Microbes New Infect. 2013;1(3):41–3. https://doi.org/10.1002/2052-2975.19.

140. Isbary G, Stolz W, Shimizu T, Monetti R, Bunk W, Schmidt HU, et al. Cold atmospheric argon plasma treatment may accelerate wound healing in chronic wounds: results of an open retrospective randomized controlled study in vivo. Clin Plasma Med. 2013;1(2):25–30. https://doi.org/10.1016/j.cpme.2013.06.001.

141. Ulrich C, Kluschke F, Patzelt A, Vandersee S, Czaika VA, Richter H, et al. Clinical use of cold atmospheric pressure argon plasma in chronic leg ulcers: a pilot study. J Wound Care. 2015;24(5):196, 8-200, 2-3. https://doi.org/10.12968/jowc.2015.24.5.196.
142. Stratmann B, Costea TC, Nolte C, Hiller J, Schmidt J, Reindel J, et al. Effect of cold atmospheric plasma therapy vs standard therapy placebo on wound healing in patients with diabetic foot ulcers: a randomized clinical trial. JAMA Netw Open. 2020;3(7):e2010411. https://doi.org/10.1001/jamanetworkopen.2020.10411.
143. Heinlin J, Zimmermann JL, Zeman F, Bunk W, Isbary G, Landthaler M, et al. Randomized placebo-controlled human pilot study of cold atmospheric argon plasma on skin graft donor sites. Wound Repair Regen. 2013;21(6):800–7. https://doi.org/10.1111/wrr.12078.
144. Heinlin J, Isbary G, Stolz W, Zeman F, Landthaler M, Morfill G, et al. A randomized two-sided placebo-controlled study on the efficacy and safety of atmospheric non-thermal argon plasma for pruritus. J Eur Acad Dermatol Venereol. 2013;27(3):324–31. https://doi.org/10.1111/j.1468-3083.2011.04395.x.
145. Li Y-F, Taylor D, Zimmermann J, Bunk W, Monetti R, Isbary G, et al. In vivo skin treatment using two portable plasma devices: comparison of a direct and an indirect cold atmospheric plasma treatment. Clin Plasma Med. 2013;1(2):35–9.
146. Hartwig S, Doll C, Voss JO, Hertel M, Preissner S, Raguse JD. Treatment of wound healing disorders of radial forearm free flap donor sites using cold atmospheric plasma: a proof of concept. J Oral Maxillofac Surg. 2017;75(2):429–35. https://doi.org/10.1016/j.joms.2016.08.011.
147. Kisch T, Helmke A, Schleusser S, Song J, Liodaki E, Stang FH, et al. Improvement of cutaneous microcirculation by cold atmospheric plasma (CAP): results of a controlled, prospective cohort study. Microvasc Res. 2016;104:55–62. https://doi.org/10.1016/j.mvr.2015.12.002.
148. Kisch T, Schleusser S, Helmke A, Mauss KL, Wenzel ET, Hasemann B, et al. The repetitive use of non-thermal dielectric barrier discharge plasma boosts cutaneous microcirculatory effects. Microvasc Res. 2016;106:8–13. https://doi.org/10.1016/j.mvr.2016.02.008.
149. Chuangsuwanich A, Assadamongkol T, Boonyawan D. The healing effect of low-temperature atmospheric-pressure plasma in pressure ulcer: a randomized controlled trial. Int J Low Extrem Wounds. 2016;15(4):313–9. https://doi.org/10.1177/1534734616665046.
150. Assadian O, Ousey KJ, Daeschlein G, Kramer A, Parker C, Tanner J, et al. Effects and safety of atmospheric low-temperature plasma on bacterial reduction in chronic wounds and wound size reduction: a systematic review and meta-analysis. Int Wound J. 2019;16(1):103–11. https://doi.org/10.1111/iwj.12999.

Suggested Reading

Plasma Sources

Reuter S, von Woedtke T, Weltmann KD. The kINPen – a review on physics and chemistry of the atmospheric pressure plasma jet and its applications. J Phys D Appl Phys. 2018;51:23300. https://doi.org/10.1088/1361-6463/aab3ad.

Plasma-Driven ROS Therapies

Privat-Maldonado A, Schmidt A, Lin A, Weltmann KD, Wende K, Bogaerts A, Bekeschus S. ROS from physical plasmas: redox chemistry for biomedical therapy. Oxidative Med Cell Longev. 2019;2019:9062098. https://doi.org/10.1155/2019/9062098. eCollection 2019

Safety

Bekeschus S, Schmidt A, Weltmann KD, von Woedtke T. The plasma jet kINPen – a powerful tool for wound healing. Clin Plasma Med. 2016;4(11):19–28. https://doi.org/10.1016/j.cpme.2016.01.001.

Schmidt A, von Woedtke T, Stenzel J, Lindner T, Polei S, Vollmar B, Bekeschus S. One year follow-up risk assessment in SKH-1 mice and wounds treated with an argon plasma jet. Int J Mol Sci. 2017;18(4):pii E868. https://doi.org/10.3390/ijms18040868.

Wende K, Bekeschus S, Schmidt A, Jatsch L, Hasse S, Weltmann KD, Masur K, von Woedtke T. Risk assessment of a cold argon plasma jet in respect to its mutagenicity. Mutat Res Genet Toxicol Environ Mutagen. 2016;798–799:48–54. https://doi.org/10.1016/j.mrgentox.2016.02.003.

Standardization

5

Mann MS, Tiede R, Gavenis K, Daeschlein G, Bussiahn R, Weltmann KD, Emmert S, von Woedtke T, Ahmed R. Introduction to DIN-specification 91315 based on the characterization of the plasma jet kINPen® MED. Clin Plasma Med. 2016;4(2):35–45. https://doi.org/10.1016/j.cpme.2016.06.001.

The Patient's View at Basic Clinical Principles

Contents

The Patient's View at Basic Clinical Principles

Christian Seebauer,
Hans-Robert Metelmann,
and Philine H. Doberschütz

Contents

© Springer Nature Switzerland AG 2022
H.-R. Metelmann et al. (eds.), *Textbook of Good Clinical Practice in
Cold Plasma Therapy*, https://doi.org/10.1007/978-3-030-87857-3_6

◉ **Core Messages**

- An innovative treatment opportunity like cold atmospheric plasma (CAP) requires extended information of the patient.
- The personal medical consultation should be accompanied by a written document.
- Since the document is targeted at the patient, the wording speaks to the patient.

6.1 Introduction

As in every medical specialty, successful plasma medicine requires the understanding and cooperation between the medical practitioner and the patient. The basis for patient compliance is informed consent. An innovative treatment like cold atmospheric plasma (CAP) medicine requires extended information of the patient.

This part of the textbook is intended to serve the medical practitioner as a template for medical briefing of patients. The personal medical consultation should be accompanied by a written document. The line of thoughts adopts the patient's perspective and provides text modules to facilitate the preparation of a consent form. Since such documents are targeted at the patient, the wording speaks to the patient:

» "Dear Patient,

You are consulting your doctor because of a medical or aesthetical problem, and the key term *plasma medicine* has been mentioned. It became obvious to you, that plasma medicine has nothing to do with blood plasma. Now, you are interested to learn about plasma medicine and why it makes sense to consider it for treating your problem.

The purpose of this document is to make you familiar with the basic clinical principles of plasma medicine. Please read this information carefully. Your doctor will inform you about treatment options with cold atmospheric plasma, typical risks and possible consequences, and the details of the medical intervention regarding your case. When you feel adequately informed and expressly wish to undergo plasma medicine treatment, please confirm your consent with your signature.

…"

6.2 General Aspects of Plasma Medicine

"Colloquially, the term "plasma medicine" often refers to tools that generate physical plasma or to products activated by physical plasma, mainly used for cosmetic purposes and by laypersons. Your doctor, on the other hand, is talking about cold physical atmospheric pressure plasma, abbreviated to CAP, generated by officially approved medical devices, and indicated with particular relevance for the medical therapy of chronic wounds and infected skin.

If you suffer from a severe skin infection or wound that is not healing, you have experienced the heavy burden on your health and well-being. These problems can sometimes be difficult to handle by established therapeutic procedures, calling for innovative treatment like CAP medicine.

A wound by itself is not a disease, and wound healing is just a natural process that does not require a targeted treatment. However, problems may arise due to the following reasons:

- When open wounds become severely infected by pathogens
- When wound healing is retarded and the risk of infection is rapidly increasing
- When wounds cannot heal because of consuming illness and show massive infection
- When pain or general risk prevention require rapid healing of open wounds and infected skin
- When wounds and skin infections are health-threatening skin abscesses
- When infected wounds contaminated with certain bacteria are causing smell and odor

CAP medicine covers all of these indications.

You might be interested to learn that CAP is ionized gas, generated by physical energy. CAP induces biochemical reactions and releases molecules that interact with human wound cells and with microbial cells, such as infectious bacteria and viruses. CAP therefore accelerates wound healing in two ways: by killing harmful germs at the wound surface (antisepsis) and by promoting the growth of healing cells (tissue regeneration and microcirculation). This double effect is a unique advantage of CAP treatment compared to conventional and established wound care measures.

CAP may look, if visible, like bluish little flames, but with a temperature not higher than 40 °C, it works on the cells without causing thermal damage, ensuring a painless treatment.

Moreover, jet-plasma application is a touch-free treatment that avoids unpleasant contact of the device with your wound or irritated skin and prevents the risk of unintentionally injuring numb wounds."

6.3 Selection of Patients

"You have learned that CAP treatment is useful for you, in case you are suffering from problematic wounds or infected skin and mucosa. This includes patients with the following:

- Chronic and infected wounds
- Wounds with standstill of healing but without infection
- Skin and mucosa lesions at risk of serious progression
- Non-healing wounds by other reasons
- Skin and mucosa with certain local infections and purulent focuses

Patients suffering from infective and inflammatory skin and mucosa diseases like herpes zoster, atopic eczema, or acne may soon benefit from CAP application.

You may also belong to a group of patients considered at risk of poor wound healing, who benefit from CAP treatment as preventive measure. This includes patients with the following criteria:

- With wounds that are not closing within 28 days
- Aged 60 years or older
- After menopause
- Under systemic steroid medication
- With cancer or a history of previous impaired wound healing

You see that CAP application can be used to support the healing of lesions and acute surgical wounds in cases where the patient's difficult health-status, biographic condition, or medication pushes the risk of problematic wounds. Accelerating the wound healing can also help to reduce scar formation. Together with the potential to prevent wound infection, CAP treatment is a promising option to control the risk of surgical site infections in the field of plastic surgery and aesthetic medicine."

6.4   Choice of Plasma Device

"Your individual medical problem calls for individual treatment, and your doctor will propose and choose the most appropriate CAP device for your treatment task. You might be interested to learn that there are two types of medical devices in use, approved by the competent authorities since 2013.

One type is called plasma jet or plasma torch device: CAP is generated by electrical tension within a slim tubular handpiece or a cylindrical tube located at the end of a flexible arm. The resulting ionized gas is driven out by a propellant gas and looks like a flame. This "plasma cocktail" consists of atmospheric air, noble gases (argon, helium), and gas mixtures of the working gases.

The other type of medical device is based upon dielectric barrier discharges (DBD): CAP is generated either within a small gap between the large surface of a flat handpiece and the surface to be treated (e.g., skin, wound), or on the surface of a specifically designed electrode structure which is positioned in close vicinity to the surface to be treated. This "plasma cocktail" looks like a carpet and consists of atmospheric air.

Jet plasma devices with plasma flames shaped like the tip of a lancet are very suitable for precise interventional procedures under visual inspection. They are used on wound craters and rugged tissue, on regions with undercut, and for intraoral application. Torch-like as well as DBD plasma devices with larger flames or plasma carpets are very convenient for the quick treatment of large and flat wounds and infected skin areas.

Rest assured that your doctor is only using CAP devices with CE certification as medical devices class-IIa according to the European Council Directive 93/42/EEC. These devices work with plasma sources that have been extensively examined for their biological and physical properties and have been tested in detailed pre-clinical and clinical investigations."

6.5 Handling of Complications

"You might have experienced that standard treatment of wounds and skin infections does not succeed in some cases. This is also true for CAP therapy. Even with well-proven healing effectiveness of CAP medicine, there are some patients with insufficient treatment results. Especially in chronic wounds, plasma medicine plays an important role – but it is not the only player. Continuous debridement, proper wound dressings, and keeping relevant co-morbidities and current medication under control are important as well.

First CAP medical devices had been approved in 2013 and still there are no known serious side effects or complications of therapy. Any enhanced risk of geno-toxic and mutagenic effects of CAP treatment has been excluded by well-established in vitro tests as well as by a long-term animal trial and long-term clinical observations.

In principle, complications in medical procedures are due to the general health and medical condition of the patient. Please help your doctor to identify any risk of complications by carefully reporting your health status and medical history."

Conclusion

"Dear Patient,

To sum up this information, we would like to answer some of the frequently asked questions:

Is the clinical efficacy of CAP treatment proven?

Yes, there is a number of plasma sources with comprehensive physical and biological characterization and detailed preclinical and clinical investigations to prove efficacy. The application for treatment purposes is authorized by CE certification as medical devices class-IIa according to the European Council Directive 93/42/EEC. These devices are approved for the treatment of chronic wounds and pathogen-associated skin diseases.

This statement does not include several other plasma tools on the market that claim to be suitable for "plasma medicine" but have no or very inadequate physical, technical, biological, or clinical references to prove this.

How is the risk of local or systemic side effects and complications?

Approved plasma devices are in clinical use since 2013. There are no case observations or clinical studies in the literature that report severe side effects of any kind, including carcinogenesis or genetic damage.

Slight local effects have to be considered, such as minor pinprick or irritation related to the tip of the plasma plume when using plasma jets. In very rare cases and unclear connection, a brief and mild redness of the skin following unintended touch might occur.

Is the medical effect in my case reliable?

The effectiveness of CAP in wound healing and treatment of infected skin is well documented. However, there are always a couple of patients without positive treatment results for unknown reasons. Plasma medicine plays an important role in wound healing – but it is not the only player. Steady debridement, proper wound dressings, restoration and perfusion of vessels, lymphatic drainage, and keeping relevant co-morbidities under control are important as well. This is especially true for chronic wounds.

Is the medical effect well controllable?

In wound healing, the medical effect can easily be controlled by measuring the regain of skin cover and the shrinking of the wound surface. On-going photo documentation is important. Documents will include scale and date and follow the very basic requirements of scientific medical photography.

Will I see a quick medical effect?

Wound healing is never quick. You have to know that it takes stamina by all persons involved and sometimes many weeks of repeated treatment to reach a reasonable result.

Can bacteria become resistant when treated by plasma?

One of the significant advantages of plasma medicine compared to other antimicrobial therapies is its effectiveness against multi-resistant skin and wound germs. From the opposite point of view, the development of new resistances when treating germs with plasma has never been described – neither in clinical cases and studies, nor in pre-clinical and basic research.

Is there an inhibitory effect on my normal flora?

There are no case reports or pre-clinical and basic research studies mentioning problematic effects on the normal flora in clinical plasma medicine.

Is plasma therapy cost-effective?

Currently, there are no thorough treatment-related economic or organizational studies available that compare the cost of plasma therapy to standard procedures.

Clinical experience shows that personnel costs are a greater factor than the costs of material consumption. Depending on the complexity and size of the wound and the optimal number of treatments, plasma therapy can be a time-consuming process. Several case reports, however, mention a faster overall healing and a shortened time of hospitalization when plasma therapy is conducted. The purchase price of medical plasma devices varies considerably but is well below medical laser devices.

Could it be done easier? Are there no alternative solutions?

Patients suffering from problematic wounds usually have experience with many alternative but fruitless solutions. The crucial point should therefore not be whether there is a simpler option, but which option is the most effective.

How is the acceptance of plasma therapy and compliance?

By common clinical experience, most patients are appreciative for plasma medicine as an innovative and pleasant treatment procedure. The compliance usually is extraordinarily high because of the burden of suffering that problematic wounds pose. However, there are no studies available in present literature that investigate the acceptance of CAP therapy from a socio-medical and health-economic perspective.
…"

Concluding Remark

The text modules proposed in this chapter make no claim to provide all the information that might be necessary for the patient to reach a decision. This chapter does not provide a legally guaranteed information sheet but aims to serve as orientation and support as to how the patient's information can be structured.

Treatment Tailored to Indications

Contents

Cold Plasma Treatment for Chronic Wounds

Steffen Emmert, Thoralf Bernhardt,
Mirijam Schäfer, Marie Luise Semmler,
Sander Bekeschus, Kai Masur,
Torsten Gerling, Philipp Wahl,
Tobias Fischer, and Lars Boeckmann

Contents

© Springer Nature Switzerland AG 2022
H.-R. Metelmann et al. (eds.), *Textbook of Good Clinical Practice in Cold Plasma Therapy*, https://doi.org/10.1007/978-3-030-87857-3_7

💬 **Core Messages**

- Chronic wounds comprise a very heterogeneous group of diseases.
- The most common causes of skin wounds are venous and/or arterial circulation disorders, diabetes, or constant tissue pressure (decubitus).
- The physiological process of wound healing can be divided into three phases: Hemostasis and inflammation (cleaning phase), re-epithelialization, and remodeling.
- Wound treatment depends on the stage of wound healing. It is also based on the extent of the wound exudation, the extent of the bacterial colonization, as well as the location, size, and depth of the wound.
- Restoration of blood and lymph flow is critical for proper wound healing according to the individual situation.
- Standard modern wound care includes debridement, disinfection, modern wound dressings, and compression therapy.
- Plasma medicine is a promising and innovative approach to treat chronic wounds.
- Cold atmospheric pressure plasma has an antibacterial effect, can promote tissue generation, and enhance dermal blood flow.
- Plasma treatment is applied for up to 90 seconds per cm^2 wound area per day after wound cleaning and disinfection at a mean frequency of every second day.

7.1 Introduction

Due to the high prevalence in the elderly population and the high treatment costs, chronic ulcers comprise a considerable socio-economic burden for the health system. In Europe, about 1–2% of the total health care budget is spent on treatment of venous diseases, which adds up to 600–900 million Euro for the Western European countries [1, 2]. Mean costs of leg ulcer treatment are calculated to be 9560 Euro per patient per year [3]. In Germany, total costs for the treatment of decubital ulcers, diabetic foot syndrome, and leg ulcers are estimated above 5 billion Euro per year [4]. Furthermore, indirect costs such as fitness for employment or early retirement, which additionally hamper patients' quality of life as well as the high risk for relapse, add to this problem. Venous diseases in Germany cause about 1.2% of all nonproductive days due to sick leave. Moreover, about 1% of all in-patients' hospital costs relate to the treatment of venous leg ulcers [5]. In addition, a rise in these costs for the public health system can be expected due to the demographic development with an increase in the elderly population. Therefore, there is a great need for and high interest in developing novel and innovative therapeutic approaches to accelerate the wound healing process and optimize wound treatment.

7.2 Diagnosis

In general, a wound can be defined as any tissue destruction, which is paralleled by the loss of tissue. Thus, wounds comprise a very heterogeneous group which is indicated by a plethora of wound classifications. The consequence of this heterogeneity is that no uniform and clear wound definition exists; the definition rather depends on the specialist's perspective. For example, the German guideline "wounds and wound treatment" defines chronic wounds as wounds that persist for more than 2–3 weeks [6]. The German guideline "local therapy of chronic wounds", however, defines chronic wounds as a loss of skin integrity, including one or more subcutaneous structures with no healing signs within 8 weeks [7]. A variety of classifications of wounds exist (▶ Box 7.1).

Wounds can be classified according to their form or structure, as open or closed wounds, or according to their depth. A skin erosion is a wound that only affects the epidermis and heals without any residues. An excoriation is defined as skin tissue damage down to the epidermal-dermal barrier, where the papillary valleys are still present. From these keratinocyte reservoirs, re-epithelialization can occur resulting in scar-free healing of excoriations. However, pigmentary changes with hyper- and hypo-pigmentation often remain as visible signs of former excoriations. An ulcer or skin ulceration is defined as a deep skin tissue damage down to at least the subcutaneous tissue, which always heals with a scar due to complete loss of basal keratinocytes. There is no limitation to the depth of an ulceration; an ulcer can expose muscles, tendons, and even bone tissue [8]. Causes of such ulcers include circulation disorders, infections, immunological phenomena, and tumors or combinations thereof.

Another wound categorization classifies acute and chronic wounds depending on the duration of the tissue damage. Often, a combination of the above-mentioned classifications of wounds is used: Acute wounds – according to their structure – can be classified as scrapes, lacerations, contused wounds, lacerated and bite wounds, stab wounds, bullet wounds, and others. Chronic wounds that persist for several weeks up to years are often classified in combination with their cause: mechanical, pressure, thermal, chemical burn, radiation-induced, or infectious [6, 7]. The most common causes of skin wounds are venous and/or arterial circulation disorders, diabetes, or constant tissue pressure.

In the following, we will focus on skin wounds that basically result from malnutrition of skin cells and on the effects of cold atmospheric plasma on those wounds. Malnutrition of skin cells results from reduced perfusion of the papillary capillaries, which results in a reduced nutrient supply by epidermal keratinocytes by diffusion. Constant tissue pressure can lead to impaired perfusion of the papillary capillaries, which is the cause of decubital ulcers (◻ Fig. 7.1). Constant tissue pressure can occur when someone is bedridden. Typical pressure points such as the buttocks or the heels then experience a reduced microcirculation in the papillary capillaries due to the body weight. Another cause of reduced microcirculation and malnutrition of the epidermis is the peripheral arterial occlusive disease. Here,

■ **Fig. 7.1** Decubitus at the heel due to constant tissue pressure

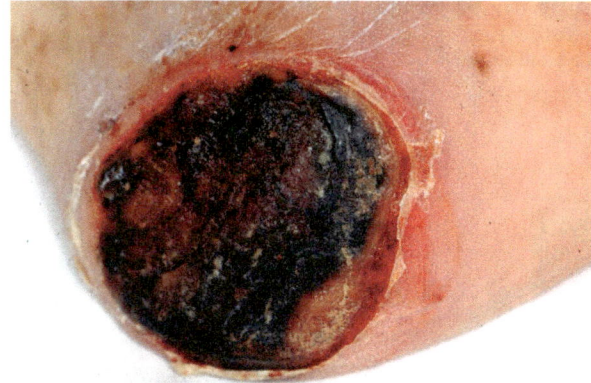

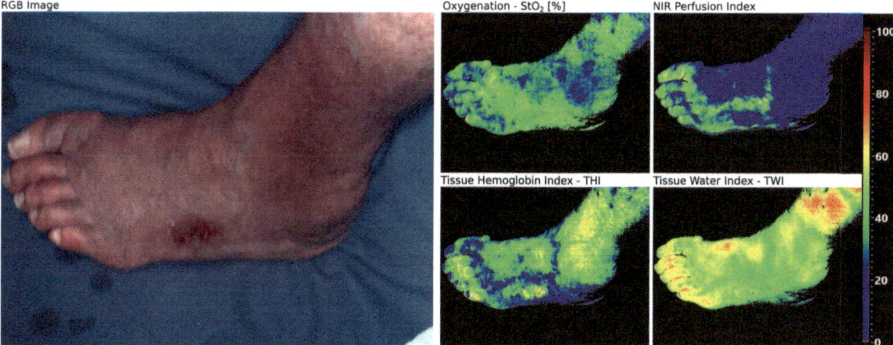

■ **Fig. 7.2** Arterial ulcer due to peripheral arterial occlusive vascular disease at typical location on the lateral foot. The ulcer is documented with a new hyperspectral imaging device (TIVITA®, Diaspective Vision GmbH, Am Salzhaff OT Pepelow, Germany). With this device, important wound parameters, including tissue oxygenation, (near infrared) perfusion, hemoglobin content, and water content (edema), can be quantified as early biomarkers for wound healing

occlusion of arteries that deliver oxygenized blood to the leg results in reduced perfusion of terminal vessels and malnutrition of the skin affecting the forefoot or the tips of the toes. This is also called the "principle of the last meadow", describing necrosis when the oxygenized blood stream runs dry. The results are visible as typical skin ulcerations at the outer ankle or foot (■ Fig. 7.2).

The molecular causes of skin ulcerations due to diabetes are quite comparable to ulcers due to arterial occlusive diseases. Diabetes leads to neuropathic angiopathy, i.e., constriction of small arterial vessels (microangiopathy), also resulting in reduced perfusion of the papillary capillaries and skin ulcerations (■ Fig. 7.3). Varicose veins caused by dilated vessels finally also lead to venous ulcers at the lower leg due to reduced perfusion of the papillary capillaries (■ Fig. 7.4). This is a process taking place over decades. As a consequence of the venous stasis, the bloodstream back to the trunk is impeded and a "backwater" of the blood down to

■ **Fig. 7.3** Plantar diabetic ulcer due to microangiopathy and diabetic neuropathy

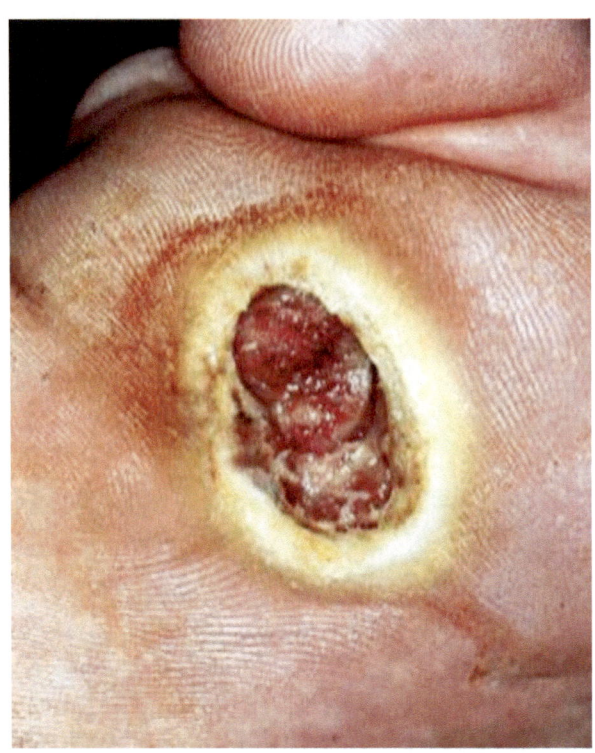

the skin capillaries develops which reduces the arterial afflux and, thus, sufficient nutrient supply to the epidermis [1].

Eighty percent of lower leg ulcers are due to venous diseases [9]. Reports on the prevalence of leg ulcers vary between 0.3% and 1%, i.e., between 240,000 and 800,000 patients in Germany [2, 4]. The prevalence of leg ulcers rises with increasing age and in most cases, ulcers develop in 60- to 80-year-olds [10]. On average, venous ulcers require about 24 weeks to heal. However, 15% of the ulcers never heal completely and the recurrence rate is about 15–71% after complete healing [11, 12]. The lifetime prevalence is up to 2% [9]. Depending on the definition, the prevalence of peripheral arterial circulatory diseases is estimated at 3–10% of the population. The percentage of patients with arterial circulatory disorders among 70-year-olds and older people rises to 15–20% [13]. For diabetic foot syndrome and diabetic ulcers, the prevalence is estimated – according to country and study – at 2–6% of all people with diabetes with an annual incidence ranging between 2% and 6% [14]. The quality report 2009 of the disease management program diabetes mellitus type II of the Association of Statutory Health Insurance Physicians in Nordrhein-Westfalen/Germany reports that 3.4% of 424,000 diabetic patients suffer from diabetic foot syndrome and a foot amputation is necessary in 0.8% of these cases [15].

Fig. 7.4 Venous ulcer at the typical location on the inner malleolus, the area of highest venous pressure due to insufficiency of the Vena saphena magna

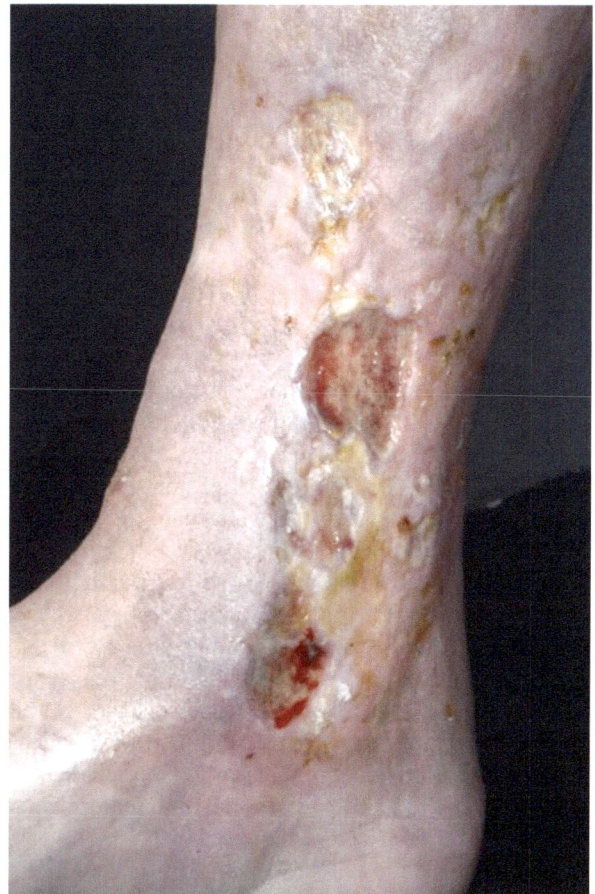

Box 7.1 Classification of Wounds

- Form/structure
- Open/closed wound
- Acute/chronic wound
- According to type:
    - Scrape: tangential pressure (excoriation)
    - Laceration: blunt force
    - Contused wound: blunt force
    - Lacerated wound: frayed wound edges
    - Cut: sharp
    - Stab wound: spiky
    - Bite: often bacterially colonized
    - Gun-shot wound

- According to cause:
  - Infected wound
  - Mechanical pressure
  - Thermal
  - Chemical burn
  - Radiation-induced

7.3 Physiology and Pathology

The human skin is one of the largest organs and serves as an important barrier to the exterior world. The skin protects our body from external environmental influences like ultraviolet (UV) radiation, chemical substances, and microorganisms. If the skin is damaged, skin cells and immunological defense mechanisms are activated almost immediately, which initiate the process of wound healing. Small and superficial wounds usually heal very quickly within weeks. Larger and deeper wounds may need some more time to heal, but can be, in general, well coped if other diseases do not further impair the body.

The standard process of wound healing is based on a variety of different mechanisms, including coagulation, inflammation, synthesis of extracellular matrix, and deposition as well as angiogenesis, fibrosis, and tissue remodeling [16]. The physiological process of wound healing can be divided into three phases: Hemostasis and inflammation (cleaning phase), re-epithelialization, and remodeling. In the following, the biologic course and the main components of the three wound-healing phases will be described in more detail.

7.3.1 Hemostasis and Inflammation

If blood vessels are injured, thrombocytes are recruited to the damaged wound area. These thrombocytes then come in contact with connective tissue components such as collagen and consequently activate blood coagulation, which stops the bleeding, a process also defined as hemostasis. The activated thrombocytes eventually release different signaling molecules like blood-clotting factors or cytokines, the latter of which initiate the inflammatory process within the wound. Here, the signaling molecule platelet-derived growth factor (PDGF) plays an important role. Upon PDGF release from the thrombocytes, neutrophils, macrophages, fibroblasts, and muscle cells are attracted and migrate into the wound milieu. Additional growth factors like transforming growth factor-beta (TGF-β) lead to further chemotaxis of macrophages, fibroblasts, and muscle cells. TGF-β also activates macrophages, which then secrete additional signaling molecules like fibroblast growth factor (FGF), PDGF, tumor necrosis factor-alpha (TNF-α), or interleukins (IL). TGF-β furthermore activates the expression of collagens and suppresses the collagenase activity [17]. During the later phases of this inflammatory process, neutrophils become active which clean the wounds from germs, destroyed tissue matrix, and dead cells by secreting matrix metalloproteinases (MMPs) and elastases [18–20]. Mast cells release amines and enzymes, which digest surrounding vessels to allow an accelerated transport of new cells into the wound milieu. This results in cellular and edematous swelling and the typical inflammatory symptoms as calor and rubor [17, 21]. In parallel, monocytes differentiate into special wound macrophages and support the cleaning process of the wound due to phagocytosis. They also release PDGF and TGF-β to intensify chemotaxis of fibroblasts and muscle cells [22].

7.3.2 Re-epithelialization

During the re-epithelialization phase, keratinocytes play a dominant role in reconstituting the normal epidermal skin layers and the skin barrier to prevent transepidermal water loss. For that, keratinocytes must migrate over the wound area and proliferate there. In the intact skin, basal keratinocytes are connected via hemidesmosomes with the basal membrane, whereas in suprabasal epidermal layers, cell-cell contacts of adjacent keratinocytes are formed by desmosomes. These cell contacts have to be decomposed during re-epithelialization to allow the migration of keratinocytes into the wound and their proliferation as well as their differentiation to reconstitute the epidermal layers [23, 24]. Besides keratinocytes, other cell types like fibroblasts, immune cells, or macrophages are active during this re-epithelialization phase. Each cell type releases a distinct set of signaling molecules, including growth factors, integrins, chemokines, or metalloproteinases. These factors mediate the strictly-directed epidermal remodeling at the wound site. Fibroblasts, for example, play an important role because they release high concentrations of TGF-β, which trigger the expression of metalloproteinases, collagen, proteoglycans, and fibronectin. Additionally, protease inhibitors are stimulated and simultaneously, the release of proteases is reduced. Thus, for proper wound healing, a balance of matrix metalloproteinases and their inhibitors is necessary [25, 26]. Further details regarding the biologic mechanisms of wound healing mediated by keratinocytes can be found in the review of Pastar et al. [24].

7.3.3 Remodeling

During the last phase of wound healing, skin layers are remodeled, including cellular connective tissue and blood vessels. Macrophages produce IL-10 that inhibits the chemotactic invasion of granulocytes as well as the release of IL-1β, monocyte chemoattractant protein 1 (MCP-1), macrophage inflammatory protein 1 alpha (MIP-1α), IL-6, and TNF-α [27]. Additional growth factors are released from fibroblasts, macrophages, keratinocytes, endothelial cells, and thrombocytes (epidermal growth factor (EGF), TGF-α, vascular endothelial growth factor (VEGF, bFGF, TGF-β). Together, these processes lead to remodeling of connective tissue, neo-angiogenesis, and renewal of the skin layers. Surrounding cofactors, like a reduced pH value and partial oxygen pressure as well as increased lactate levels, play important roles in the remodeling and the recruitment of blood vessels [22, 28, 29].

In any stage, the healing process of a wound can be disturbed and may lead to a chronic wound condition.

7.4 Standard Treatment Principles

The therapy of chronic venous ulceration includes the symptomatic therapy of the wound in addition to causal therapy. The local wound treatment depends on the stage of wound healing. It is also based on the extent of the wound exudation, the extent of the bacterial colonization, and the location, size, and depth of the wound. The most common and promising standard therapy of ulcerations includes repetitive debridements of the wound, i.e., removing biofilms of micro-organisms as well as necrotic and dead tissue. This can be done in different ways. The gold standard is surgical removal with a sharp scalpel [30]. Other debridement techniques, e.g., use ultrasonic waves for cleaning, or the pulse-lavage system, with a mechanical wound rinse with saline solution being sprayed directly into the wound and onto tissue parts. Enzymatic ointments are also used for debridements [30]. After successful removal of dead and necrotic tissue, the wound is washed out with physiological saline solution and modern wound dressings are applied to keep the wound moist. In venous ulcers, which are caused by hypertension of the veins, a continuous compression treatment with compression stockings is usually used [31]. The greatest challenge in chronically infected wounds is to control the multipathogenic overload. Here, active dressings such as antibiotic- or antiseptic-containing dressings (e.g., Fucidine ® or Betaisodona® gaze) can be used to prevent a wound infection. In case of excessive use, however, resistance or allergies may develop. Further active dressings include ions such as silver ions (i.e., Silvercel®, Urgosorb® Silver, Aquacel® Ag), which have antimicrobial activity, or growth factors (e.g., Regranex®) that are intended to stimulate the proliferation of skin cells. Furthermore, operations or skin transplantations may be necessary.

7.5 Treatment Rationale

Plasma medicine is a very promising and innovative approach to treat chronic wounds. In physical terms, plasma is defined as partial or completely ionized gas and is considered the fourth state of matter. In partially ionized gas, free charge carriers (ions and electrons), neutral molecules, and short-lived radicals (reactive nitrogen and oxygen species RONS) are present. As a result of the directed movement of the charge carriers, plasma contains electric current. Furthermore, different types of radiations are generated in the plasma by spontaneous emission of excited atoms, ions, or molecules over a wide spectral range, reaching from vacuum ultraviolet (VUV) over UV and visible radiation to infrared (IR), which leads to the characteristic glow of the plasma. It can be generated at different temperatures and pressures so that a variety of different plasma sources are available [32–34].

Because of the bactericidal effect, the use of hot plasma has proved to be an effective method not only for the sterilization of medical devices and implants but also for the cauterization and cutting of tissue [35–38]. The sterilization or disinfecting effect is based on the interaction of the individual plasma components with the contaminant [39]. Furthermore, plasmas have been used for a long time for coagulation purposes [36, 40].

So-called biocompatible, cold plasma sources, operating with temperatures of less than 40 °C, allowed the direct application on biological tissues [38, 41, 42]. Many research groups started to investigate this promising technology. These groups needed an interdisciplinary approach, including researchers from plasma physics, chemistry, engineering, microbiology, biochemistry, biophysics, medicine, and hygiene in order to address different aspects of plasma application. In particular, many research groups focused on interactions between plasma and biological materials [38, 42, 43].

Current research mainly investigated the application of cold plasma under atmospheric pressure. Numerous in vitro and in vivo studies demonstrated the antimicrobial potential of plasma not only against individual pathogens but also against resistant microorganisms as well as biofilms [44–50]. Daeschlein et al. [51] demonstrated the efficacy of plasma against most pathogens of wound infections in vitro. Cultured bacterial mixtures taken from the human skin were inactivated within a few seconds by dielectric barrier discharge (DBD) treatment [52]. The bactericidal effect of plasma was also shown in vivo; the skin of mice was sterilized by the application of plasma without harming the animals [38]. The treatment of artificially contaminated pig's eyes led to a significant reduction in bacterial load without any histological damages detectable [53]. Wound antiseptic treatments are crucial for infected wounds because the wound healing process is impaired and therefore cannot proceed correctly. It is generally acknowledged that microbial colonization of wounds delays or prevents the wound healing process [54], resulting in the development of a chronic wound. Plasmas are very good superficial antibiotics/antiseptics due to the previously described properties, and thus, it is obvious that these properties are already used for treatments of superficial disease, especially chronic wounds, which are negatively affected by bacteria.

So far, the standard therapy of infected ulcerations is based on topical or systemic antibiotic therapy. Besides the allergic potential which can be developed by patients against the antibiotics, an additional major drawback is the development of resistance. Here, plasma therapy combines two advantages: (i) the effective elimination of multi-resistant germs and (ii) it is extremely unlikely that microorganisms will develop resistance against plasma due to its diverse physicochemical properties. Further advantages of plasma treatments are the non-invasive, localized, and painless application, as well as its gaseous state, which allows the penetration into the smallest areas, e.g., the marginal area of fistulated ulcers. Recently, it could be shown that plasma even promotes proliferation of endothelial cells by stimulating angiogenesis through the release of growth factors [55]. Furthermore, there is evidence that the use of plasma influences the pH value [56, 57], which also may be of advantage in wound therapy. It is well known that the body naturally responds with acidification of wounds upon skin injury [58]. Moreover, the pH value in the environment of chronic wounds influences numerous factors of wound healing. This is utilized in therapeutically induced acidosis within the wound bed.

Arndt et al. [59] showed that atmospheric low-temperature plasma (MicroPlaSter β) positively influences the expression of several factors relevant to wound healing. In vitro, pro-inflammatory cytokines and growth factors such as IL-6, IL-8, MCP-1, TGF-β1, and TGF-β2 were stimulated or activated. Furthermore, migration rates of fibroblasts were increased by plasma, whereas the proliferation rate of fibroblasts was unaffected in the study. Pro-apoptotic and anti-apoptotic markers remained unchanged. However, expression rates of type I collagen and alpha-smooth muscle actin (alpha-SMA) were increased. Similar observations were made in in vitro and in vivo experiments on keratinocytes [60]. Increased expression rates of IL-8, TGF-β1, and TGF-β2 were induced by plasma (MicroPlaSter β). Here, the proliferation and migration of keratinocytes were unaffected.

So far, no side effects were reported for plasma applications. Experiments with mice, ex vivo studies on pig skin and human skin biopsies, as well as in vitro experiments on living human cells showed no cell damage (necrosis) after plasma treatments with doses typically used for wound treatment. Higher doses used for cancer treatment may induce apoptosis, necrosis, or senescence [38, 49, 61–63].

In two randomized controlled clinical phase II trials, patients with chronically infected wounds of different etiology received plasma treatments, in addition to the daily modern wound treatment [64, 65]. The patients acted as their control. Plasma was applied using one of two different indirect plasma devices (MicroPlaSter α and MicroPlaSter β) over 2 or 5 min. Irrespective of the device used and the treatment duration, significantly higher reduction rates of bacteria were achieved in plasma-treated wounds without any side effects for the patients in both studies.

A retrospective randomized controlled trial demonstrated the beneficial effect of indirect plasma treatment (MicroPlaSter α) in a patient group with chronically infected ulcers of different etiology [32]. The patients were divided into three groups and treated with plasma between 3 and 7 min. In the most heterogeneous group (different ulcers and different treatment times), no significant differences in wound width or length were measured. However, in the more homogenous two groups (chronic venous ulcers treated with different application times and chronic venous ulcers treated for 5 min), significant reductions in wound width were detected. Despite the limitations of this retrospective study, these results suggest for the first time that plasma can accelerate wound healing in patients with chronic ulcers.

These results were supported by a prospective randomized placebo-controlled clinical trial on acute wounds [66]. Forty patients with skin graft donor sites on the upper leg were randomized and either treated with plasma (MicroPlaSter β) or placebo (argon gas) for 2 min. Positive effects were observed in terms of improved re-epithelialization, fewer fibrin layers, and blood crusts, whereas wound surroundings were always normal, independent of the type of treatment. In general, the treatment was well tolerated and no side effects occurred. This trial on acute wounds demonstrated that cold, biocompatible plasma has beneficial effects even in the absence of pathogens and is therefore not limited to infected or chronic wounds.

In the meantime, some devices that generate cold atmospheric pressure plasma are approved for the treatment of chronic wounds as a medical device and gained a CE certification; i.e., the kINPen MED® device (INP Greifswald/neoplas tools GmbH, Greifswald) and the PlasmaDerm® device from CINOGY GmbH in Duderstadt. Clinical trials were also conducted with these devices, demonstrating positive effects related to wound healing [67, 68].

The aim of the study by Brehmer et al. [67] was to demonstrate the safety and efficacy of plasma application in chronic venous ulceration in the clinic as add-on therapy in addition to standard wound therapy. In the monocentric, two-arm, randomized, and controlled pilot study, seven patients with venous leg ulcers were treated over 8 weeks, three times a week, for 45 seconds per cm^2 wound area with the PlasmaDerm® device and in addition to the standard care. Seven other patients only received standard wound therapy. The standard therapy included repeated debridements of the wound, wound washing with physiological saline solution, and application of a modern wound dressing (Mepitel® or Mepilex®) to keep the wound moist, as well as a continuous compression treatment with compression stockings (Ulcer X®) to prevent hypertension of the veins [31].

Regarding the efficacy of the plasma application, there was a significant reduction in bacterial load in the wound immediately after plasma application. Besides the significantly higher reduction of bacterial load immediately after the plasma application, there was no difference detectable in the relative wound sizes between the two patients groups compared. However, the mean initial wound size was larger in the plasma group and plasma-treated wounds showed a greater absolute decrease until the end of the treatment period. In three patients, the ulcer size was reduced by about 50%. The only patient with a complete cure of the ulcer was in the plasma group. It is important to mention that patients of the plasma group reported less pain during the therapy and the plasma therapy received a positive assessment by doctors, too. Despite the low number of patients, it can be stated that the plasma treatment with the PlasmaDerm® device was safe and feasible.

Another clinical pilot study used a plasma jet device (kINPen® MED) on patients with multiple chronic venous ulcers [68]. Results demonstrated that the wound healing was not negatively influenced by the plasma jet, but the device was only partially suitable for large ulcers. Due to the thin plasma effluent streaming out of the device, the application is very spot-like with a small exposure area. Therefore, small-size wounds were chosen for plasma treatments, which, however, makes the interpretation of the results challenging. Upcoming clinical studies are intended to re-evaluate the effect with a device adapted for larger wound surfaces.

In a study assessing the antibacterial effects of cold plasma, conventional liquid antiseptic octenidine dihydrochloride (ODC) and a combination of both revealed that the sequential application of plasma and ODC presents the most efficient antiseptic treatment strategy for chronic wounds [69].

In a randomized, prospective, and controlled study with 50 patients, the size reduction of pressure-induced decubita was evaluated. Here, a statistically signifi-

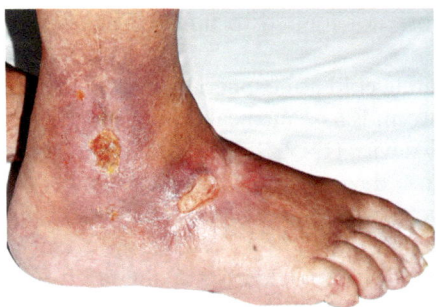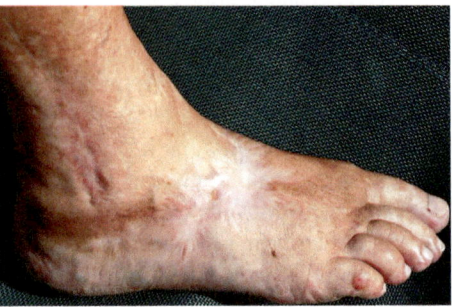

☐ Fig. 7.5   Chronic ulcers of mixed origin (CVI, trauma, osteomyelitis) that persisted for 14 years (left). The patient spent 2 weeks in our Clinic for Dermatology of the University Medical Center Rostock as an in-patient where he received a complex wound treatment including plasma. A standard wound treatment was then continued at home without plasma. Three months later, all ulcers on the right foot and leg healed completely for the first time in 14 years (right). (Bernhardt et al. [71])

cant improvement of wound healing was found in the plasma treatment group compared to the control group treated with a modern standard wound care [70].

In our wound clinic at the University Medical Center in Rostock, plasma treatment has been applied routinely for the last 4 years. In our registry with more than 300 patients, no side effects of the plasma treatment are recorded. In terms of efficacy, beneficial effects are noted in the majority of patients. For example, a patient who had leg ulcers of mixed origin, including trauma and osteomyelitis, suffered from wounds over 14 years. He visited our clinic for 2 weeks where we initiated a complex modern wound treatment including plasma. At home, he continued this treatment without plasma and 3 months later, all wounds on his right foot healed completely for the first time in 14 years (☐ Fig. 7.5) [71].

Further examples of positive effects of cold atmospheric plasma in chronic wound treatment are summarized in the compendium Wound Treatment with Cold Atmospheric Plasma – Examples and operation guidelines from clinical practice [72] and demonstrate the beneficial effects of plasma treatment. Nevertheless, prospective clinical trials with large patient groups and sufficient statistical power are still necessary to further confirm these demonstrated positive clinical effects of the plasma on accelerated wound healing.

7.6   Cold Plasma Therapy

7.6.1   Pre-Treatment Assessment

For plasma treatment of chronic wounds, the same careful wound treatment assessment should be performed as recommended for all wound treatments. This includes most importantly the elucidation of the wound cause (arterial, venous, diabetic, pressure). To this end, Doppler/Duplex ultrasound examinations may be necessary as well as a punch biopsy from the wound edge to exclude squamous cell carcinoma or any other malignancy. Then, the clinical examination of the wound and its depth is important: Is the wound clean, or is fibrin or dead tissue present? How deep is the wound? Are wound caves present? Are tendons or even bones visible or does granulation tissue fully cover the wound base? Finally, the germ colonization should be assessed by taking swabs for smears.

> **Important to Know**
> No specific pre-treatment wound assessment is necessary for plasma therapy.

7.6.2 Timing

Based on the existing experience and the standard wound treatment algorithms used, plasma treatment of chronic wounds is applied every 2–3 days daily for a maximum of 90 seconds per cm^2 wound area. In general, the plasma treatment is performed for 6–12 weeks; however, it may vary considerably according to the wound size, course of healing, and type of wound care setting (outdoor, indoor, day-care setting).

> **Important to Know**
> - Treatment for max. 90 sec/cm^2 wound area
> - Treatment for every 2–3 days
> - Mean treatment duration 6–12 weeks, depending on the course of healing

7.6.3 Diagnosis and Treatment Planning

As mentioned above, no specific pre-treatment assessment is necessary for plasma treatment. No side effects are expected, even if tendons or bones are visible in wounds. Within a complex wound treatment regimen, plasma treatment is usually performed before the application of a modern wound dressing. First, cleaning of the wound should be done. This includes wound debridement if necessary. Then wound disinfection for several minutes is advisable. After that, plasma treatment can be performed followed by the application of wound dressings and other topical treatments. As a last step, bandages are applied including compression therapy in case of venous ulcers.

> **Important to Know**
> Wound cleaning, debridement, and disinfection are followed by plasma treatment.
> Afterwards, wound dressings are applied.

7.6.4 Anesthesia

As plasma treatment usually is non-invasive and contact-free (jet devices) or nearly contact-free (DBD devices), no specific anesthesia for a plasma treatment is necessary. On the contrary, the plasma treatment may be able to reduce pain caused by the ulcer or the wound dressing by itself as several studies reported reduction of pain and itching by plasma treatment. However, for wound debridement, local anesthesia often is necessary to tolerate the mechanical removal of dead tissue on the wound surface. Another advantage of plasma is the beneficial effect on odor of skin ulcerations [73].

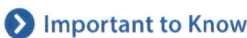 **Important to Know**

Plasma reduces pain; thus, no anesthesia is necessary for plasma treatment.

7.6.5 Post-Treatment Care

Plasma treatment can be quickly performed within complex wound treatment algorithms. Usually, plasma treatment is followed by the application of a modern wound dressing, topical ointments, and compression bandages. A special post-treatment care after the plasma treatment is not necessary as the treatment is well tolerated.

> **Important to Know**
>
> A special post-treatment care after plasma treatment is not necessary as the treatment is well tolerated.

7.6.6 Handling of Complications

The most common complications of wound treatment are pain and wound/tissue infections as well as erysipelas. Wound experts are familiar with such complications and easily counteract them if detected early. With respect to plasma therapy and due to its good tolerability, no specific complication may occur. This is based on a 7-year clinical experience with plasma wound treatment as well as the data from the plasma device-producing companies that are obliged to document all complications with the use of their devices.

> **Important to Know**
>
> Over 7 years of clinical application, no severe complications of plasma treatment have been reported.

Conclusion

Application of cold atmospheric plasma for disinfection and wound treatment has already moved into routine clinical practice. Within 90 seconds of plasma treatment, different medical effects like germ reduction, enhanced blood flow and skin oxygenation, and tissue stimulation are exerted in one application. According to the clinical experience of 7 years, plasma wound treatment is effective and safe. No relevant short-term or long-term side effects have been observed. Plasma devices should be further developed with large-area electrodes and combined with, e.g., wound dressings. To this end, specific international guidelines for medical plasma devices seem, therefore, mandatory.

7

Acknowledgments   This work is partly supported by the European Social Fund (ESF), reference: ESF/14-BM-A55-0001/18, ESF/14-BM-A55-0005/18, ESF/14-BM-A55-0006/18, and the Ministry of Education, Science and Culture of Mecklenburg-West Pomerania, Germany. S.E. is supported by the Deutsche Forschungsgemeinschaft (DFG EM 63/13-1) and the Damp Foundation. S.B. is supported by the German Federal Ministry of Education and Research (BMBF), grant number 03Z22DN11. Similar content may be found in the textbook Comprehensive Clinical Plasma Medicine. Metelmann R., von Woedtke T., Weltmann KD. (eds.), Springer, Heidelberg, 2018.

References

1. German Society for Phlebology. Leitlinien zur Diagnostik und Therapie des Ulcus cruris venosum. AWMF-Leitlinien-Register Nr. 037/009 2008.
2. Etufugh CN, Phillips TJ. Venous ulcers. Clin Dermatol. 2007;25:121–30.
3. Purwins S, Herberger K, Debus ES, Rustenbach SJ, Pelzer P, Rabe E, et al. Cost-of-illness of chronic leg ulcers in Germany. Int Wound J. 2010;7:97–102.
4. Nord D. Kosteneffektivität in der Wundbehandlung. Zentralbl Chir. 2006. https://doi.org/10.1055/s-2006-921433.
5. Bosanquet N, Franks P. Venous disease: the new international challenge. Phlebology. 1996;11:6–9.
6. German Society for Pediatric Surgery. Leitlinie zu Wunden und Wundbehandlung. AWMF-Leitlinienregister Nr. 006/129 2014.
7. German Society for Wound Healing and Wound Treatment e.V. Lokaltherapie chronischer Wunden bei Patienten mit den Risiken periphere arterielle Verschlusskrankheit, Diabetes mellitus, chronische venöse Insuffizienz. AWMF-Leitlinienregister Nr. 091/001 2012.
8. Moll I. Duale Reihe Dermatologie. 8th ed. Stuttgart: Thieme; 2016.
9. Valencia IC, Falabella A, Kirsner RS, Eaglstein WH. Chronic venous insufficiency and venous leg ulceration. J Am Acad Dermatol. 2001;44:401–24.
10. De Araujo T, Valencia I, Federman DG, Kirsner RS. Managing the patient with venous ulcers. Ann Intern Med. 2003;138:326–34.
11. Heit JA. Venous thromboembolism epidemiology: implications for prevention and management. Semin Thromb Hemost. 2002;28:3–13.
12. Kurz X, Kahn SR, Abenhaim L, et al. Chronic venous disorders of the leg: epidemiology, outcomes, diagnosis and management. Summary of an evidence-based report of the VEINES task force. Venous Insufficiency Epidemiologic and Economic Studies. Int Angiol. 1999;18:83–102.
13. German Society for Angiology and Society for Vascular Medicine e.V. Leitlinien zur Diagnostik und Therapie der peripheren arteriellen Verschlusskrankheit (PAVK). AWMF-Leitlinienregister Nr. 065/003 2009.
14. Programm für Nationale Versorgungs-Leitlinien. Nationale Versorgungs-Leitlinie Typ-2-Diabetes: Präventions- und Behandlungsstrategien für Fußkomplikationen. AWMF-Leitlinienregister Nr nvl/001c Version 2.8 2010.
15. Nordrheinische Gemeinsame Einrichtung Disease Management Programme. Qualitätssicherungsbericht 2009. Disease-Management-Programme in Nordrhein-Westfalen, Düsseldorf 2010.
16. Robson MC. Wound infection: a failure of wound healing caused by an imbalance of bacteria. Surg Clin North Am. 1997;77:637–50.
17. Diegelmann RF, Evans MC. Wound healing: an overview of acute, fibrotic and delayed healing. Front Biosci. 2004;9:283–9.
18. Hart CA, Scott LJ, Bagley S, Bryden AA, Clarke NW, Lang SH. Role of proteolytic enzymes in human prostate bone metastasis formation: in vivo and in vitro studies. Br J Cancer. 2002;86:1136–42.

19. Sylvia CJ. The role of neutrophil apoptosis in influencing tissue repair. J Wound Care. 2003;12: 13–6.
20. Broughton IG, Janis JE, Attinger CE. The basic science of wound healing. Plast Reconstr Surg. 2006;117:12–34.
21. Artuc M, Hermes B, Steckelings UM, Grützkau A, Henz BM. Mast cells and their mediators in cutaneous wound healing - active participants or innocent bystanders? Exp Dermatol. 1999;8: 1–16.
22. Diegelmann RFPD, Cohen IKMD, Kaplan AMPD. The role of macrophages in wound repair: a review. Plast Reconstr Surg. 1981;68:107–13.
23. Heng MCY. Wound healing in adult skin: aiming for perfect regeneration. Int J Dermatol. 2011;50:1058–66.
24. Pastar I, Stojadinovic O, Yin NC, Ramirez H, Nusbaum AG, Sawaya A, et al. Epithelialization in wound healing: a comprehensive review. Adv Wound Care. 2014;3:445–64.
25. Roberts AB, McCune BK, Sporn MB. TGF-β: regulation of extracellular matrix. Kidney Int. 1992;41:557–9.
26. Hall MC, Young DA, Waters JG, Rowan AD, Chantry A, Edwards DR, Clark IM. The comparative role of activator protein 1 and Smad factors in the regulation of Timp-1 and MMP-1 gene expression by transforming growth factor-beta1. J Biol Chem. 2003;278:10304–13.
27. Peranteau WH, Zhang L, Muvarak N, Badillo AT, Radu A, Zoltick PW, Liechty KW. IL-10 overexpression decreases inflammatory mediators and promotes regenerative healing in an adult model of scar formation. J Invest Dermatol. 2008;128:1852–60.
28. Knighton D, Hunt T, Scheuenstuhl H, Halliday B, Werb Z, Banda M. Oxygen tension regulates the expression of angiogenesis factor by macrophages. Science. 1983;221:1283–5.
29. LaVan FB, Hunt TK. Oxygen and wound healing. Clin Plast Surg. 1990;17:463–72.
30. Steed DL, Attinger C, Brem H, et al. Guidelines for the prevention of diabetic ulcers. Wound Repair Regen. 2008;16:169–74.
31. Dissemond J. Moderne Wundauflagen für die Therapie chronischer Wunden. Hautarzt. 2006;57:881–7.
32. Isbary G, Shimizu T, Li Y-F, Stolz W, Thomas HM, Morfill GE, Zimmermann JL. Cold atmospheric plasma devices for medical issues. Expert Rev Med Devices. 2013;10:367–77.
33. Tiede R, Hirschberg J, Daeschlein G, von Woedtke T, Vioel W, Emmert S. Plasma applications: a dermatological view. Contrib Plasma Phys. 2014;54:118–30.
34. Tiede R, Mann M, Viöl W, Welz C, Daeschlein G, Wolff HA, et al. New therapeutic options: plasma medicine in dermatology. HAUT. 2014;6:283–9.
35. Baxter HC, Campbell GA, Richardson PR, Jones AC, Whittle IR, Casey M, et al. Surgical instrument decontamination: efficacy of introducing an argon: oxygen RF gas-plasma cleaning step as part of the cleaning cycle for stainless steel instruments. IEEE Trans Plasma Sci. 2006;34:1337–44.
36. Raiser J, Zenker M. Argon plasma coagulation for open surgical and endoscopic applications: state of the art. J Phys D Appl Phys. 2006;39:3520–3.
37. Koban I, Holtfreter B, Hübner NO, Matthes R, Sietmann R, Kindel E, et al. Antimicrobial efficacy of non-thermal plasma in comparison to chlorhexidine against dental biofilms on titanium discs in vitro - proof of principle experiment. J Clin Periodontol. 2011;38:956–65.
38. Fridman G, Friedman G, Gutsol A, Shekhter AB, Vasilets VN, Fridman A. Applied plasma medicine. Plasma Process Polym. 2008;5:503–33.
39. Shimizu T, Steffes B, Pompl R, et al. Characterization of microwave plasma torch for decontamination. Plasma Process Polym. 2008;5:577–82.
40. Farin G, Grund KE. Technology of argon plasma coagulation with particular regard to endoscopic applications. Endosc Surg Allied Technol. 1994;2:71–7.
41. Stoffels E, Flikweert AJ, Stoffels WW, Kroesen GMW. Plasma needle: a non-destructive atmospheric plasma source for fine surface treatment of (bio)materials. Plasma Sources Sci Technol. 2002;11:383–8.
42. Moreau M, Orange N, Feuilloley MGJ. Non-thermal plasma technologies: new tools for bio-decontamination. Biotechnol Adv. 2008;26:610–7.

43. Dobrynin D, Fridman G, Friedman G, Fridman A. Physical and biological mechanisms of direct plasma interaction with living tissue. New J Phys. 2009;11:115020. (26pp)
44. Joaquin JC, Kwan C, Abramzon N, Vandervoort K, Brelles-Marino G. Is gas-discharge plasma a new solution to the old problem of biofilm inactivation? Microbiology. 2009;155:724–32.
45. Ehlbeck J, Schnabel U, Polak M, Winter J, von Woedtke T, Brandenburg R, et al. Low temperature atmospheric pressure plasma sources for microbial decontamination. J Phys D Appl Phys. 2011;44:013002. (18pp)
46. Daeschlein G, Scholz S, von Woedtke T, Niggemeier M, Kindel E, Brandenburg R, et al. In vitro killing of clinical fungal strains by low-temperature atmospheric-pressure plasma jet. IEEE Trans Plasma Sci. 2011;39:815–21.
47. Zimmermann JL, Dumler K, Shimizu T, Morfill GE, Wolf A, Boxhammer V, et al. Effects of cold atmospheric plasmas on adenoviruses in solution. J Phys D Appl Phys. 2011;44:505201. (9pp)
48. Klämpfl TG, Isbary G, Shimizu T, Li YF, Zimmermann JL, Stolz W, et al. Cold atmospheric air plasma sterilization against spores and other microorganisms of clinical interest. Appl Environ Microbiol. 2012;78:5077–82.
49. Maisch T, Shimizu T, Li YF, Heinlin J, Karrer S, Morfill G, Zimmermann JL. Decolonisation of MRSA, S. aureus and E. coli by cold-atmospheric plasma using a porcine skin model in vitro. PLoS One. 2012;7:1–9.
50. Daeschlein G, Napp M, von Podewils S, et al. In vitro susceptibility of multidrug resistant skin and wound pathogens against low temperature atmospheric pressure plasma jet (APPJ) and dielectric barrier discharge plasma (DBD). Plasma Process Polym. 2014;11:175–83.
51. Daeschlein G, von Woedtke T, Kindel E, Brandenburg R, Weltmann K-D, Jünger M. Antibacterial activity of an atmospheric pressure plasma jet against relevant wound pathogens in vitro on a simulated wound environment. Plasma Process Polym. 2010;7:224–30.
52. Fridman G, Peddinghaus M, Ayan H, Fridman A, Balasubramanian M, Gutsol A, et al. Blood coagulation and living tissue sterilization by floating-electrode dielectric barrier discharge in air. Plasma Chem Plasma Process. 2006;26:425–42.
53. Hammann A, Huebner NO, Bender C, et al. Antiseptic efficacy and tolerance of tissue-tolerable plasma compared with two wound antiseptics on artificially bacterially contaminated eyes from commercially slaughtered pigs. Skin Pharmacol Physiol. 2010;23:328–32.
54. Edwards R, Harding KG. Bacteria and wound healing. Curr Opin Infect Dis. 2004;17:91–6.
55. Kalghatgi S, Friedman G, Fridman A, Clyne AM. Endothelial cell proliferation is enhanced by low dose non-thermal plasma through fibroblast growth factor-2 release. Ann Biomed Eng. 2010;38:748–57.
56. Fridman G, Shereshevsky A, Jost MM, Brooks AD, Fridman A, Gutsol A, et al. Floating electrode dielectric barrier discharge plasma in air promoting apoptotic behavior in melanoma skin cancer cell lines. Plasma Chem Plasma Process. 2007;27:163–76.
57. Helmke A, Hoffmeister D, Mertens N, Emmert S, Schuette J, Vioel W. The acidification of lipid film surfaces by non-thermal DBD at atmospheric pressure in air. New J Phys. 2009;11:115025. (10pp)
58. Schneider LA, Korber A, Grabbe S, Dissemond J. Influence of pH on wound-healing: a new perspective for wound-therapy? Arch Dermatol Res. 2007;298:413–20.
59. Arndt S, Unger P, Wacker E, et al. Cold atmospheric plasma (CAP) changes gene expression of key molecules of the wound healing machinery and improves wound healing in vitro and in vivo. PLoS One. 2013;8:e79325. (9pp)
60. Arndt S, Landthaler M, Zimmermann JL, Unger P, Wacker E, Shimizu T, et al. Effects of cold atmospheric plasma (CAP) on defensins, inflammatory cytokines, and apoptosis-related molecules in keratinocytes in vitro and in vivo. PLoS One. 2015;10:1–16.
61. Sosnin EA, Stoffels E, Erofeev MV, Kieft IE, Kunts SE. The effects of UV irradiation and gas plasma treatment on living mammalian cells and bacteria: a comparative approach. IEEE Trans Plasma Sci. 2004;32:1544–50.
62. Awakowicz P, Bibinov N, Born M, et al. Biological stimulation of the human skin applying healthpromoting light and plasma sources. Contrib Plasma Phys. 2009;49:641–7.

63. Wende K, Landsberg K, Lindequist U, Weltmann K-D, von Woedtke T. Distinctive activity of a nonthermal atmospheric-pressure plasma jet on eukaryotic and prokaryotic cells in a cocultivation approach of keratinocytes and microorganisms. IEEE Trans Plasma Sci. 2010;38:2479–85.

64. Isbary G, Morfill G, Schmidt HU, et al. A first prospective randomized controlled trial to decrease bacterial load using cold atmospheric argon plasma on chronic wounds in patients. Br J Dermatol. 2010;163:78–82.

65. Isbary G, Heinlin J, Shimizu T, et al. Successful and safe use of 2 min cold atmospheric argon plasma in chronic wounds: results of a randomized controlled trial. Br J Dermatol. 2012;167:404–10.

66. Heinlin J, Isbary G, Stolz W, Zeman F, Landthaler M, Morfill G, et al. A randomized two-sided placebo-controlled study on the efficacy and safety of atmospheric non-thermal argon plasma for pruritus. J Eur Acad Dermatol Venereol. 2013;27:324–31.

67. Brehmer F, Haenssle HA, Daeschlein G, Ahmed R, Pfeiffer S, Görlitz A, et al. Alleviation of chronic venous leg ulcers with a hand-held dielectric barrier discharge plasma generator (Plasma-Derm ® VU-2010): results of a monocentric, two-armed, open, prospective, randomized and controlled trial (NCT01415622). J Eur Acad Dermatol Venereol. 2015;29:148–55.

68. Ulrich C, Kluschke F, Patzelt A, et al. Clinical use of cold atmospheric pressure argon plasma in chronic leg ulcers: a pilot study. J Wound Care. 2015;24:196–203.

69. Klebes M, Ulrich C, Kluschke F, Patzelt A, Vandersee S, Richter H, et al. Combined antibacterial effects of tissue-tolerable plasma and a modern conventional liquid antiseptic on chronic wound treatment. J Biophotonics. 2014;8:382–91.

70. Chuangsuwanich A, Assadamongkol T, Boonyawan D. The healing effect of low-temperature atmospheric-pressure plasma in pressure ulcer: a randomized controlled trial. Int J Low Extrem Wounds. 2016;15:313–9.

71. Bernhardt T, Semmler ML, Schäfer M, Bekeschus S, Emmert S, Boeckmann L. Plasma medicine: applications of cold atmospheric pressure plasma in dermatology. Oxidative Med Cell Longev. 2019;3873928:1–10.

72. Emmert S, editor. Wound treatment with cold atmospheric plasma – examples and operation guidelines from clinical practice. Munich: Springer Medizin; 2019. p. 1–93.

73. Metelmann H-R, Seebauer C, Miller V, Fridman A, Bauer G, Graves DB, et al. Clinical experience with cold plasma in the treatment of locally advanced head and neck cancer. Clin Plasma Med. 2018;9:6–13.

7

Cold Plasma Treatment for Acute Wounds

Karrer Sigrid and Arndt Stephanie

Contents

© Springer Nature Switzerland AG 2022
H.-R. Metelmann et al. (eds.), *Textbook of Good Clinical Practice in Cold Plasma Therapy*, https://doi.org/10.1007/978-3-030-87857-3_8

Core Messages

- CAP is able to accelerate acute wound healing.
- CAP could be used as preventive measure for acute wound infection without known side effects.
- CAP could be an alternative for conventional antiseptics or antibiotics.
- CAP could improve the patient's quality of life.

8.1 Introduction

The use of cold atmospheric plasma (CAP) has mainly focused on the treatment of chronic and hard-to-heal wounds. Since most acute wounds heal without special aid, studies on the treatment of acute wounds with CAP are still scarce. Nevertheless, there is a rationale to improve wound healing also in acute wounds. Bacterial contamination or wound infection can delay or even prevent wound healing and CAP could be used as a prophylactic or therapeutic disinfectant. As compared to the most commonly used antiseptics (chlorhexidine digluconate, polyhexanide, octenidine dihydrochloride), short exposure to CAP (60s) has been shown to be at least as effective regarding microbiostatic activity and thus could be used as an alternative to conventional antiseptics [1]. The use of antibiotics for prevention or treatment of wound infection on the other hand bears the risk of microbial resistance and other side effects such as allergies or intolerances. Thus, preventive measures, that do not exhibit these side effects, would be highly beneficial. Since in vitro and in vivo studies suggest that CAP can also accelerate wound healing irrespectively of bacterial load, CAP could be useful to shorten the time until re-epithelialization of larger wounds. A shorter healing time can reduce costs, pain, shorten hospitalization, reduce the rate of complications during the healing period, and improve the patient's quality of life.

8.2 Diagnosis

Acute wounds result from a discontinuation of the surface of the skin, which heals within less than 8 weeks. Wounds that persist for more than 8 weeks despite optimal treatment are defined as chronic wounds [2]. Acute wounds can be a consequence of surgery or trauma. Traumatic wounds include burns, contusions, excoriations, lacerations, cut or stab wounds, bullet wounds, animal bites, or gunshot wounds. Surgery wounds can be created by using a scalpel, a laser, liquid nitrogen, or also chemicals like acid. Acute wounds can be classified as non-inflammatory, clean wounds, or clean-contaminated wounds with a low risk of developing infection [3]. Contaminated and dirty or infected wounds after surgery or trauma have a high potential of infection and may need therapeutic or prophylactic measures. Wounds can be also categorized depending on their depth. If only the epidermis is lost, the wound is referred to as an erosion. When the wound involves structures deep to the epidermis, it is termed an ulceration. Wounds involving the epidermis and parts of the dermis are called partial-thickness wounds and those involving the epidermis, all of the dermis and deeper structures are called full-thickness wounds. In partial-thickness wounds, where the deep dermis has not been completely lost, adnexal structures such as hair follicles are still present. These adnexal structures serve as a reservoir of epithelial cells, which can repopulate the epidermis by migrating to the wound surface. In full-thickness wounds, where adnexal structures are lost, epithelial cells can only migrate from the ulcer edge. Acute wounds created by surgery can heal by primary or secondary intention. Primary intention healing occurs when the surgeon closes the wound by approximating the wound edges with side to side closures, flaps, or skin grafts. In secondary intention healing, the wound is left to heal on its own and the time until complete re-epithelialization depends on the nature, depth, location, size, and shape of the wound, the status and age of the host and environmental factors. Uncomplicated and clean wounds usually show a normal healing of the injured site following the physiological phases of wound healing with hemostasis, inflammation, re-epithelialization, and remodeling.

❶ Caution
Different kinds of acute wounds heal differently and at different rates and may need adjuvant therapeutic approaches.

8.3 Physiology and Pathology

Wound healing is a dynamic process with partly overlapping phases of tissue repair. The phases of wound healing comprise hemostasis, inflammation, re-epithelialization, and remodeling [3, 4].

❶ Caution
Acute wounds progress through different phases of wound healing in an orderly and timely manner [5].

Any phase of the healing process of a wound can be disturbed and may lead to a chronic wound condition. Wound healing is characterized by the communication of various cell types, and this communication is the prerequisite for physiological wound closure. In addition to immune and endothelial cells, epidermal keratinocytes and dermal fibroblasts are cell types crucial for the various cellular and molecular processes during wound healing.

The repair process is initiated immediately after injury by the release of various growth factors and cytokines of injured blood vessels and from degranulating platelets. Disruption of blood vessels also leads to the formation of a blood clot, which is composed of cross-linked fibrin, and of extracellular matrix proteins such as fibronectin, vitronectin, and thrombospondin [6, 7]. During hemostasis, activated platelets release various signaling molecules and cytokines, which initiate the inflammatory process within the wound. Platelet-derived growth factor (PDGF) attract neutrophils and macrophages and promote their migration into the wound area to clean the wound and to act against microorganisms. Transforming growth factor-ß (TGF-ß) activates macrophages, which then secrete additional signaling molecules like fibroblast growth factor (FGF), tumor necrosis factor-alpha (TNF-α), or interleukins (IL). During the re-epithelialization phase keratinocytes play a dominant role in the reconstitution of the epidermal skin layer. Keratinocytes migrate over the wound area and proliferate there. Beside keratinocytes, fibroblasts are active during this phase. They release high concentrations of TGF-ß, which promotes the expression of collagens and further extracellular matrix (ECM) components [8]. Furthermore, wound fibroblasts transform into myofibroblasts, a cell type with elevated stress fibers, important for wound contraction [4]. During the last phase of wound healing, skin layers are remodeled and angiogenesis leads to the formation of new blood vessels. Additional growth factors are released from fibroblasts, macrophages, keratinocytes, and endothelial cells (e.g., epidermal growth factor (EGF), vascular endothelial growth factor (VEGF), Angiopoietin-2, keratinocyte growth factor (KGF)). Together, these factors contribute to transition from granulation tissue to mature scar, characterized by continued collagen synthesis [4]. Even after the functional barrier of the skin is restored, remodeling of the extracellular matrix continues to occur. Collagen type III is replaced by the stable, preinjury phenotype collagen type I. The tensile strength of the tissue is further increased for up to one year after injury when the scar strength reaches about 80% of that of unwounded skin [9, 10].

Acute healing wounds normally show low levels of bacteria, inflammatory cytokines, proteases, and reactive oxygen species compared to chronic wounds.

❶ Caution

Wound healing time depends on many factors, such as complexity of the wound, wound size and depth, location, patient age, gender, and comorbidities (diabetes, hypertension, venous disease, etc.).

Wound healing can also be affected by local hypoxia, malnutrition, smoking, mechanical stress, or wound infection. Also drugs, e.g., corticosteroids, can impair wound healing by blocking the inflammatory process and the mitotic activity of fibroblasts [11].

On the other hand, wound healing can be enhanced by a variety of interventions. In acute surgical wounds, wound edges can be brought together by sutures, thus reducing the distance that cells need to migrate [12]. Also skin grafts can accelerate the healing of acute wounds [13]. Aseptic surgical techniques minimize the risk of wound infection, which would prolong wound healing [14]. Larger, open wounds after surgery or trauma can be treated with vacuum-assisted closure (VAC) to enhance granulation tissue formation and shorten healing time [15]. Finally, a CAP treatment could also help to accelerate the acute wound healing.

8.4 Standard Treatment Principles

Surgical wounds or certain clean traumatic wounds can be closed by sutures, tapes, or staples and thus heal by primary intention. If this is not possible in larger or infected wounds, wounds with necrotic margins or elder traumatic wounds, wound healing takes place by secondary intention.

In general, necrotic tissue or foreign bodies within the wound must be removed, e.g., by surgical debridement. Wounds should be cleaned with a sterile cleaning solution to remove dirt and to reduce bacteria. For this purpose, either sterile NaCl 0.9% or Ringer solution can be used, in case of bacterial contamination or infection, antiseptics like octenidine or polyhexanide solution can be applied [16]. Thereafter, sterile dressing materials are applied to cover and protect the wound and to create a moist wound environment.

> ❗ Caution
> A large variety of dressing materials are available and the most appropriate material should be chosen depending on the wound's clinical appearance.

Depending on the etiology of the acute wound, other procedures might be applicable. The treatment of burn wounds depends much on the area and depth of the wound. In case of blistering, the blister roof is often removed. In larger superficial wounds, skin grafting might become necessary. In acute lacerations, bruise wounds, cuts or decollement wounds, an exact inspection of the wound should be performed since these wounds are often contaminated or polluted and foreign bodies in the wound must be removed. Depending on the depth of the wounding, damage of nerves, larger blood vessels or tendons should be excluded and, if present, adequately treated. Animal bite wounds are always contaminated with pathogenic germs and must be explored carefully invasively or non-invasively. They are at higher risk of wound infection or phlegmone and usually are left to heal by secondary intention. In high risk wounds, a prophylactic antibiosis should be considered. In addition, physical therapies such as negative pressure wound therapy (VAC) can help to stimulate the growth of new granulation tissue and help to close deeper wounds faster.

8.5 Treatment Rationale

A CAP treatment of acute wounds might have the rationale to speed wound closure, to prevent or treat wound infection and to contribute to a better quality of the resultant scar regarding strength and cosmetic appearance. Since microbial colonization can delay or prevent wound healing resulting in a chronic wound, plasma could be used in acute wounds as a prophylactic disinfectant instead of topical antiseptics or antibiotics.

Besides the efficacy and clinical outcome, safety is an important requirement when treating patients with CAP.

> ❶ **Caution**
>
> Plasma applications are contact-free and pain-free; treatment times are short, and no allergic reactions, bacterial resistances, or other side effects have been observed so far [17–21].

Various studies have been conducted to investigate CAP safety. These observations were made on the basis of cell culture analyses, ex vivo and in vivo studies in animals, and also in clinical studies in patients with acute or chronic wounds.

Ex vivo studies of different CAP compositions on skin surfaces have shown no damage to the underlying tissue concerning necrosis or enhanced apoptosis. Furthermore, with CE-certified plasma sources, thermal damage can be neglected if recommendations are respected [20, 22]. Mutagenicity studies with different plasma devices detected no increase in the mutation rate of V79 Chinese hamster cells [23–25]. Using the kINPen® MED (neoplas tools GmbH, Greifswald, Germany), absence of genotoxicity was shown by means of a micronucleus (MN) assay or in a hen's egg test model for micronuclei induction (HET-MN) [26]. Overall, toxicity experiments using the MicroPlaSter/Adtec SteriPlas (Adtec Healthcare, Hounslow, UK) according to clinical plasma treatment times (1 or 2 min) did not show any relevant effects on the viability of keratinocytes and fibroblasts [24].

In fact, there is enough rationale and evidence to support the use of CAP not only in chronic wounds but also in acute wounds. Wound healing seems to be influenced positively not only via germ reduction, but also by modifying the wound microenvironment. The molecular effects of CAP have been investigated in wound-relevant cells and in different animal models of acute wound healing. The most important wound-relevant cells are fibroblasts, keratinocytes, endothelial cells, and immune cells. During tissue injury, these cells communicate with each other via autocrine (same cell type) and paracrine (different cell type) mechanisms to coordinate the complex process of wound healing. In an open wound, CAP treatment affects these cells directly and also works via cell–cell communication and exchange of various wound healing-relevant cytokines (e.g., IL-6, IL-8, TNF-alpha) and growth factors (e.g., TGF-ß1/2, VEGF, EGF, FGF). These factors are induced by CAP [27–29] and activate intracellular signaling pathways, thus influencing cellular mechanisms such as migration, proliferation, contraction, or angiogenesis.

Different plasma devices have been shown to influence migration and proliferation of fibroblasts transiently [30]. Increased proliferation and migration of fibroblasts and keratinocytes are important mechanisms of wound healing and promote rapid re-epithelialization and collagen synthesis [31]. Multiple studies using different plasma devices and different animal models of wound healing could confirm accelerated wound closure and wound contraction. However, CAP can exert its effect in different phases of wound healing [28, 29, 32–40]. To promote wound contraction, fibroblasts differentiate into myofibroblasts. This differentiation process is also activated by CAP treatment and further promotes physiological tissue repair [28, 38, 41].

In addition, studies have shown that plasma modulates the body's immune system. An induction of antimicrobial peptides like ß-defensins (BD) in keratinocytes might contribute to the antibacterial effects of plasma treatment [27]. Furthermore, numerous studies have shown that plasma treatment stimulates and alters the redox balance of skin cells [29, 42–44]. Inflammation and antioxidant defense are intimately connected. Plasma-treated wounds show a modulated cytokine pattern (e.g., induction of interleukin 1β (IL-1β), IL-6, and tumor-necrosis factor α (TNFα)) with increased early myeloid cell infiltrate [29]. Concomitantly, CAP leads to an early activation of nuclear erythroid-related factor 2 (Nrf2) signaling pathway which controls cellular defense [29, 45].

Antioxidant defense and inflammation are necessary factors in wound healing but are insufficient without adequate blood supply. Several angiogenesis-related factors (e.g., keratinocyte growth factor (KGF), basic fibroblast growth factor (bFGF), vascular endothelial growth factor (VEGFA), heparin-binding EGF-like growth factor (HBEGF), colony stimulating growth factor (CSF2), angiopoietin-2 (Ang-2), angiostatin (PLG), amphiregulin (AR), endostatin, and angiogenic-involved receptor FGF R1 and VEGF R1) are modulated by CAP and convey a positive effect on angiogenesis during wound healing [29, 46–48].

Using a hyperspectral imaging technology (HIS), the influence of CAP on tissue microcirculation was analyzed in one patient with an acute, postoperative wound on the neck [49, 50]. HIS was performed before, right after, and 10 min after a treatment with the kINPen MED. A significant increase of superficial and deeper cutaneous oxygen saturation with elevated hemoglobin concentration in the treated and surrounding wound could be shown. This stimulating effect on blood perfusion and oxygenation might also contribute to an improved wound healing.

Of course, the biological response to plasma treatment depends on many variables, such as the plasma source used, the composition of the plasma components, the operation parameters, the treatment frequency, and the treatment intervals. Therefore, results from studies using different plasma sources and treatment parameters must be interpreted carefully.

However, it is remarkable that fundamental mechanisms of wound healing are influenced by plasma and have positive effects on the healing process (● Fig. 8.1).

❶ Caution

CAP mechanisms such as activation of immune cells, fibroblasts, and keratinocytes, induction of wound healing-relevant cytokines, growth factors, and protective mechanisms, induction of neovascularization, an increased blood perfusion and oxygenation in the wound area – altogether result in an accelerated re-epithelialization and wound closure.

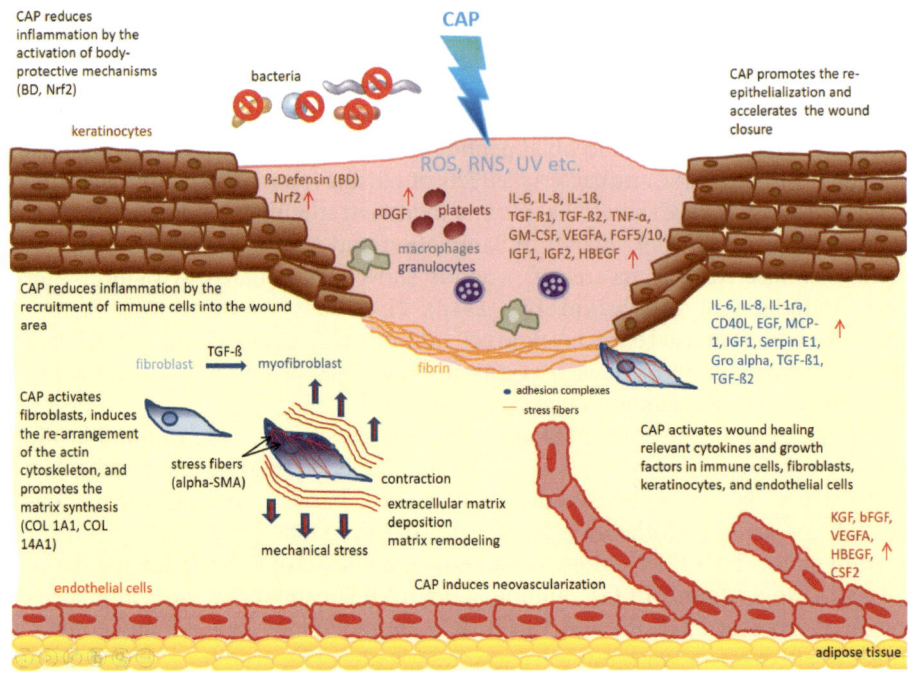

🔲 **Fig. 8.1** Molecular and cellular effects mediated by CAP during wound healing

8.6 Cold Plasma Therapy

Cold plasma therapy has been used for the treatment of chronic wounds in several studies, but only few clinical studies support the use of a plasma treatment also for acute wounds. Due to scarce published data, no established treatment protocols can be recommended so far.

Several publications describe positive effects of the kINPen MED on acute wounds. Six healthy volunteers with four standardized, vacuum-generated blister-wounds (10–18 mm^2) on the forearm received either no treatment (A), treatment with CAP for 60 s (B), treatment with octenidine (C) or sequential treatment with CAP and octenidine (D) [51]. The dynamics of wound area decline were assessed during 6 visits (V1-6) over the course of 2 weeks by photography and confocal laser scan microscopy (CLSM). Wounds showed a statistically more rapid wound area decline after CAP treatment (treatment arm B) as compared to the other wounds. Wound repair was accelerated especially in its early inflammatory phases and thus induced an earlier onset of the proliferative stage. This appears more likely than a solely antiseptic effect of CAP treatment, since treatment with octenidine (either alone or in combination with CAP) displayed no potential to speed tissue regeneration, probably due to cytotoxic effects.

Metelmann et al. investigated the potential of CAP to improve healing in acute wounds after laser skin resurfacing [52]. In five human subjects, four small CO_2-laser wounds (1×1 cm^2) were created on the lower arms and then treated by various patterns of plasma application. The results of healing were evaluated by aesthetic aspects such as the color and texture of the recovering skin as compared to surrounding untreated skin. One laser wounded site was treated with 10 seconds of plasma stimulation using the kINPen MED, the second site with 30 seconds of plasma stimulation, the third site with 10 seconds over three following days and the fourth site was left untreated. The outcome of the treatment was followed for ten days and was evaluated by blinded analysis of photographs by five independent examiners. Short-term plasma stimulation (10 s), repeatedly applied for 3 days, seemed to be the most effective treatment in regards to an early aesthetic recovery. Long-term (30 s) plasma stimulation with a single application followed the second place of ranking. The site that received no treatment was even better ranked that the site with single short-term (10 s) plasma stimulation. The authors state from this small case series that plasma stimulation positively influences the healing of superficial acute skin lesions. This is possibly caused not only by the antiseptic CAP effect but also by additional stimulation of tissue regeneration. In a subsequent publication, the results of a 6- and 12-month follow-up of these five patients were presented [21]. Also in later stages, CAP treatment showed better results in terms of avoiding post-traumatic skin disorders and revealed superior aesthetics during scar formation. Repeated plasma treatment was superior to the other groups in avoiding postoperative hyperpigmentation. In addition, there were no precancerous lesions in the skin up to 12 months after plasma treatment. However, to exclude any cancer risk from plasma treatment, much longer follow-up periods would be needed.

A recently published prospective, randomized controlled trial focused on the tissue-activating effects of CAP in acute phase wounds generated by a CO_2-laser in 12 healthy volunteers [53]. The subjects received a treatment with a fractional CO_2 laser in four similarly sized regions (1.5×2.0 cm) on their left forearm. Thereafter, each lesion received one of the following treatments: plasma treatment (kINPen MED for 60 seconds), a betamethasone valerate and gentamicin sulfate ointment, basic fibroblast growth factor (Fibroblast® Spray), or no treatment (control group). For evaluation, a three-dimensional dermal analysis device (ANTERA 3DTM, Miravex Co., Ltd., Ireland) was used to measure the process of wound healing, redness, roughness, and pigmentation immediately before and after the laser treatment and at days 1, 3, 7, 14, and 28 after treatment. The day after therapy, the a*index (indicating redness) of the plasma-treated areas was significantly improved as compared to the control group ($p = 0.03$). From day 3 on, these two groups showed similar tendencies in all evaluated items. CAP, the ointment and the bFGF spray, did not show significant differences regarding all items at any time. In this study, the significant improvement in redness after CAP treatment, compared with the control, demonstrated an anti-inflammatory effect of plasma, which was equivalent to that of conventional therapies. No complications, such as pain, infections, or bleeding were observed in all treatment groups.

With the aim to assess the impact of CAP on the process of donor site healing, 40 patients with skin graft donor sites (SGDS) on the upper leg were enrolled in a pilot study [54]. All patients had a previous standardized harvesting of a split-thickness graft (thickness 4 mm) on the thigh as part of a reconstructive surgical intervention. The trial was planned as a self-controlled study. The skin graft donor site was divided into two equally sized areas that were randomly assigned to receive either CAP treatment or a placebo treatment (using the chemically inert noble gas argon). The treatment device was the MicroPlaSter ß (Adtec Healthcare, Hounslow, UK), a plasma torch, using argon gas. Treatment lasted 2 min (per treatment area of 5 cm^2) and was performed daily except for the weekends. Treatment started on the first postoperative day. If possible, plasma treatment was performed until complete re-epithelialization, but this was only possible in one-third of the patients. Between the study treatments, the wounds were covered with an absorbent foam dressing. Standardized photographs of each wound area were taken and were rated independently by two blinded investigators. The investigators compared the wound areas with regard to re-epithelialization, blood crusts, fibrin layers, and wound surroundings. From the second treatment onwards, the donor site areas treated with CAP showed significantly improved healing in terms of enhanced re-epithelialization and fewer fibrin layers and blood crusts as compared with the placebo-treated areas. The interrater agreement of the blinded investigators was very high. Surroundings of the wounds were always normal with no signs of inflammation or maceration. No relevant side effects of the treatment were observed and treatments were well tolerated. This study was able to show the benefits of CAP to standardized acute wounds, in which bacteria should not play a major role for wound healing.

Larger, prospective, controlled clinical studies are still needed to prove the positive effects of CAP treatment in acute wounds. Also, the optimal treatment parameters and protocols have to be defined, since plasma dose, treatment time, and frequency certainly will influence treatment outcome.

8.6.1 Pre-Treatment Assessment

Pre-treatment, a standardized wound documentation should be performed and bacterial swabs might be useful to document pre-treatment bacterial load and composition and to look for multiresistant strains.

❶ Clinical Tip
Photo documentation prior to and during plasma treatment could help to visualize treatment results objectively.

8.6.2 Timing

Treatment with CAP should be performed after cleaning the wound with sterile NaCl 0.9% or Ringer solution to remove detritus and wound exudate. An antiseptic pretreatment with octenidine or polyhexanide solution is not necessary due to the antibacterial effects of CAP. When treating acute wounds, CAP treatment is usually applied as an add-on treatment to standard wound therapy and should begin as soon as possible after wounding in order to prevent wound infection. Additionally, studies suggest that CAP accelerates wound healing already in its early inflammatory phase. However, there is not enough evidence from the literature to state which treatment frequency, application time, and treatment duration might be optimal to enhance wound healing. It is not known yet if daily treatments are superior to one, two, or three treatments per week and if patients profit from a treatment until complete re-epithelialization has taken place. These parameters will also depend on the plasma device used for treatment. Further clinical studies should clarify optimal timing for CAP therapy.

8.6.3 Diagnosis and Treatment Planning

Treatment with CAP can be easily performed in an ambulatory setting without need of a special planning.

8.6.4 Anesthesia

For the treatment of acute wounds with CAP, no anesthesia is needed, since treatment is usually not painful.

8.6.5 Post-Treatment Care

No special post-treatment care is needed. Standard wound management can be performed as usual, with CAP as an add-on treatment.

8.6.6 Handling of Complications

Up to now, no relevant acute complications or side effects occurred when using cold plasma for the treatment of wounds. Clinical studies suggest that CAP is well tolerated and causes no significant pain when certified plasma devices are used and the recommended application times are abided.

8.7 Conclusion

Patients with wounds, whatever their cause, may suffer from physical, mental, and social consequences of their wounds and the care of them [55]. The healing time, the frequency of dressing change, and possible complications such as infections during wound healing do not only affect the patient's well-being but are also important cost drivers. At the end, unaesthetic or functionally impairing scars might further reduce the patients' quality of life. Therefore, cost-efficient and practicable modern technologies that contribute to a more rapid wound healing, decrease the frequency of complications, and contribute to more aesthetic scarring without causing relevant side effects are needed. Further studies are necessary to prove if CAP would be able to fulfill all or part of these requirements.

References

1. Langner I, Kramer A, Matthes R, Rebert F, Kohler C, Koban I, et al. Inhibition of microbial growth by cold atmospheric plasma compared with the antiseptics chlorhexidine digluconate, octenidine dihydrochloride, and polyhexanide. Plasma Processes and Polymers. 2019;16(4).
2. German Society for Wound healing and wound treatment e.V. Lokaltherapie chronischer Wunden bei Patienten mit den Risiken periphere arterielle Verschlusskrankheit, Diabetes mellitus, chronische venöse Insuffizienz. AWMF-Leitlinienregister Nr. 091/0001.2012.
3. Falabella A, Kirsner R. Wound Healing. CRC Press 2019;ISBN 9780367392338.
4. Werner S, Grose R. Regulation of wound healing by growth factors and cytokines. Physiol Rev. 2003;83(3):835–70.
5. Morton LM, Phillips TJ. Wound healing and treating wounds: differential diagnosis and evaluation of chronic wounds. J Am Acad Dermatol. 2016;74(4):589–606.
6. Martin P. Wound healing--aiming for perfect skin regeneration. Science. 1997;276(5309):75–81.
7. RAF C. Wound repair. Overview and general considerations. The Molecular and Cellular Biology of Wound Repair (2nd ed). 1996:3–50.
8. Diegelmann RF, Evans MC. Wound healing: an overview of acute, fibrotic and delayed healing. Front Biosci. 2004;9:283–9.
9. Ireton JE, Unger JG, Rohrich RJ. The role of wound healing and its everyday application in plastic surgery: a practical perspective and systematic review. Plast Reconstr Surg Glob Open. 2013;1(1):e10–e9.
10. Levenson SM, Geever EF, Crowley LV, Oates JF 3rd, Berard CW, Rosen H. The healing of rat skin wounds. Ann Surg. 1965;161(2):293–308.
11. Guo S, Dipietro LA. Factors affecting wound healing. J Dent Res. 2010;89(3):219–29.
12. Waheed A, Council M. Wound closure techniques. StatPearls. Treasure Island (FL): StatPearls Publishing; 2020.
13. Bystrzonowski N, Hachach-Haram N, Kanapathy M, Richards T, Mosahebi A. Epidermal graft accelerates the healing of acute wound: a self-controlled case report. Plast Reconstr Surg Glob Open. 2016;4(11):e1119–e.
14. Bowler PG, Duerden BI, Armstrong DG. Wound microbiology and associated approaches to wound management. Clin Microbiol Rev. 2001;14(2):244–69.
15. Sinha K, Chauhan VD, Maheshwari R, Chauhan N, Rajan M, Agrawal A. Vacuum assisted closure therapy versus standard wound therapy for open musculoskeletal injuries. Adv Orthop. 2013;2013:245940.
16. Rüttermann M, Maier-Hasselmann A, Nink-Grebe B, Burckhardt M. Local treatment of chronic wounds in patients with peripheral vascular disease, chronic venous insufficiency, and diabetes. Dtsch Arztebl Int. 2013;110(3):25–31.
17. Daeschlein G, Scholz S, Ahmed R, Majumdar A, von Woedtke T, Haase H, et al. Cold plasma is well-tolerated and does not disturb skin barrier or reduce skin moisture. Journal der Deutschen Dermatologischen Gesellschaft. J German Society Dermatol: JDDG. 2012;10(7):509–15.
18. Fridman G, Friedman G, Gutsol A, Shekhter A, Vasilets V, Fridman A. Applied Plasma Medicine Plasma Process Polym. 2008;5:503–33.
19. Isbary G, Zimmermann J, Shimizu T, Li Y-F, Morfill G, Thomas H. Nonthermal plasma – More than five years of clinical experience. Clin Plasma Med J. 2013;1(1):19–23.

8

20. Lademann J, Ulrich C, Patzelt A, Richter H, Kluschke F, Klebes M, et al. Risk assessment of the application of tissue-tolerable plasma on human skin. Clinical Plasma Medicine. 2013;1(1):5–10.
21. Metelmann H, Vu T, Do H, Le T, Hoang T, Phi T, et al. Scar formation of laser skin lesions after cold atmospheric pressure plasma (CAP) treatment: a clinical long term observation. Clinical Plasma Medicine. 2013;1(1):30–5.
22. Weltmann KD, Kindel E, Brandenburg R, Meyer C, Bussiahn R, Wilke C, et al. Atmospheric pressure plasma jet for medical therapy: plasma parameters and risk estimation. Contribut Plasma Phy 4. 2009;9(9):631–40.
23. Boxhammer V, Li YF, Koritzer J, Shimizu T, Maisch T, Thomas HM, et al. Investigation of the mutagenic potential of cold atmospheric plasma at bactericidal dosages. Mutat Res. 2013;753(1):23–8.
24. Maisch T, Bosserhoff AK, Unger P, Heider J, Shimizu T, Zimmermann JL, et al. Investigation of toxicity and mutagenicity of cold atmospheric argon plasma. Environ Mol Mutagen. 2017;58(3):172–7.
25. Wende K, Bekeschus S, Schmidt A, Jatsch L, Hasse S, Weltmann K, et al. Risk assessment of a cold argon plasma jet in respect to its mutagenicity. Mutat Res-Gen Tox En. 2016;798:48–54.
26. Kluge S, Bekeschus S, Bender C, Benkhai H, Sckell A, Below H, et al. Investigating the mutagenicity of a cold argon-plasma jet in an HET-MN model. PLoS One. 2016;11(9):e0160667.
27. Arndt S, Landthaler M, Zimmermann JL, Unger P, Wacker E, Shimizu T, et al. Effects of cold atmospheric plasma (CAP) on ss-defensins, inflammatory cytokines, and apoptosis-related molecules in keratinocytes in vitro and in vivo. PLoS One. 2015;10(3):e0120041.
28. Arndt S, Unger P, Wacker E, Shimizu T, Heinlin J, Li YF, et al. Cold atmospheric plasma (CAP) changes gene expression of key molecules of the wound healing machinery and improves wound healing in vitro and in vivo. PLoS One. 2013;8(11):e79325.
29. Schmidt A, von Woedtke T, Vollmar B, Hasse S, Bekeschus S. Nrf2 signaling and inflammation are key events in physical plasma-spurred wound healing. Theranostics. 2019;9(4):1066–84.
30. Arndt S, Schmidt A, Karrer S, von Woedtke T. Comparing two different plasma devices kINPen and Adtec SteriPlas regarding their molecular and cellular effects on wound healing. Clin Plasma Med. 2018;9:24–33.
31. Werner S, Krieg T, Smola H. Keratinocyte-fibroblast interactions in wound healing. J Invest Dermatol. 2007;127(5):998–1008.
32. Choi J, Song Y, Lee H, Kim G, Hong J. The topical application of low-temperature argon plasma enhances the anti-inflammatory effect of Jaun-ointment on DNCB-induced NC/Nga mice. BMC Complement Altern Med. 2017;27(17(1)):340.
33. Garcia-Alcantara E, Lopez-Callejas R, Morales-Ramirez P, Pena-Eguiluz R, Fajardo-Munoz R, Mercado-Cabrera A, et al. Accelerated mice skin acute wound healing in vivo by combined treatment of argon and helium plasma needle. Arch Med Res. 2013;44(3):169–77.
34. Hirata T, Kishimoto T, Tsutsui C, Kanai T, Mori A. Healing burns using atmospheric pressure plasma irradiation. Japanese J Appl Physics. 2014;53:010302.
35. Kim HY, Kang SK, Park SM, Jung HY, Choi BH, Sim JY, et al. Characterization and effects of Ar/air microwave plasma on wound healing. Plasma Process Polym. 2015;12:1423–34.
36. Kubinova S, Zaviskova K, Uherkova L, Zablotskii V, Churpita O, Lunov O, et al. Non-thermal air plasma promotes the healing of acute skin wounds in rats. Sci Rep. 2017;7:45183.
37. Lee OJ, Ju HW, Khang G, Sun PP, Rivera J, Cho JH, et al. An experimental burn wound-healing study of non-thermal atmospheric pressure microplasma jet arrays. J Tissue Eng Regen Med. 2016;10(4):348–57.
38. Nasruddin YN, Mukai K, Rahayu HSE, Nur M, Ishijima T, Enomoto H, et al. Cold plasma on full-thickness cutaneous wound accelerates healing through promoting inflammation, re-epithelialization and wound contraction. Clin Plasma Med. 2014;2:28–35.
39. Nasruddin YN, Nakajima T, Mukai K, Komatsu E, Rahayu HSE, Nur M, et al. A simple technique to improve contractile effect of cold plasma jet on acute mouse wound by dropping water. Plasma Process Polym. 2015;12:1128–38.

40. Xu GM, Shi XM, Cai JF, Chen SL, Li P, Yao CW, et al. Dual effects of atmospheric pressure plasma jet on skin wound healing of mice. Wound repair and regeneration : official publication of the wound healing society [and] the European tissue repair. Society. 2015;23(6):878–84.

41. Schmidt A, Bekeschus S, Wende K, Vollmar B, von Woedtke T. A cold plasma jet accelerates wound healing in a murine model of full-thickness skin wounds. Exp Dermatol. 2017;26(2):156–62.

42. Bekeschus S, Schmidt A, Bethge L, Masur K, von Woedtke T, Hasse S, et al. Redox stimulation of human THP-1 monocytes in response to cold physical plasma. Oxidative Med Cell Longev. 2016;2016:5910695.

43. Bekeschus S, Schmidt A, Napp M, Kramer A, Kerner W, von Woedtke T, et al. Distinct cytokine and chemokine patterns in chronic diabetic ulcers and acute wounds. Exp Dermatol. 2017;26(2):145–7.

44. Bekeschus S, Winterbourn CC, Kolata J, Masur K, Hasse S, Broker BM, et al. Neutrophil extracellular trap formation is elicited in response to cold physical plasma. J Leukoc Biol. 2016;100(4):791–9.

45. Schmidt A, Dietrich S, Steuer A, Weltmann KD, von Woedtke T, Masur K, et al. Non-thermal plasma activates human keratinocytes by stimulation of antioxidant and phase II pathways. J Biol Chem. 2015;290(11):6731–50.

46. Arndt S, Unger P, Berneburg M, Bosserhoff AK, Karrer S. Cold atmospheric plasma (CAP) activates angiogenesis-related molecules in skin keratinocytes, fibroblasts and endothelial cells and improves wound angiogenesis in an autocrine and paracrine mode. J Dermatol Sci. 2017;

47. Kalghatgi S, Friedman G, Fridman A, Clyne AM. Endothelial cell proliferation is enhanced by low dose non-thermal plasma through fibroblast growth factor-2 release. Ann Biomed Eng. 2010;38(3):748–57.

48. Kalghatgi SUFG, Fridman A, Friedman G, Clyne AM. Non-thermal dielectric barrier discharge plasma treatment of endothelial cells. Conf Proc IEEE Eng Med Biol Soc. 2008:3578–81.

49. Rutkowski R, Schuster M, Unger J, Seebauer C, Metelmann HR, V. Woedkte T, et al. Hyperspectral Imaging for in vivo monitoring of cold atmospheric plasma effects on microcirculation in treatment of head and neck cancer and wound healing. Clin Plasma Med. 2017(7–8).

50. Daeschlein G, Rutkowski R, Lutze S, von Podewils S, Sicher C, Wild T, et al. Hyperspectral imaging: innovative diagnostics to visualize hemodynamic effects of cold plasma in wound therapy. Biomed Tech (Berl). 2018;63(5):603–8.

51. Vandersee S, Richter H, Lademann J, Beyer M, Kramer A, Knorr F, et al. Laser scanning microscopy as a means to assess the augmentation of tissue repair by exposition of wounds to tissue tolerable plasma. Laser Phys Lett. 2014;11(11):115701.

52. Metelmann HR, von Woedtke T, Bussiahn R, Weltmann KD, Rieck M, Khalili R, et al. Experimental recovery of CO2-laser skin lesions by plasma stimulation. Am J Cosmetic Surg. 2012;29:52–6.

53. Nishijima A, Fujimoto T, Hirata T, Nishijima J. Effects of cold atmospheric pressure plasma on accelerating acute wound healing: a comparative study among 4 different treatment groups modern plastic. Surgery. 2019;9:18–31.

54. Heinlin J, Zimmermann JL, Zeman F, Bunk W, Isbary G, Landthaler M, et al. Randomized placebo-controlled human pilot study of cold atmospheric argon plasma on skin graft donor sites. Wound repair and regeneration : official publication of the Wound Healing Society [and] the European Tissue Repair Society. 2013;21(6):800–7.

55. Lindholm C, Searle R. Wound management for the 21st century: combining effectiveness and efficiency. Int Wound J. 2016;13(Suppl 2):5–15.

8

Plasma Treatment of the Diabetic Foot Syndrome

Bernd Stratmann, Tania-Cristina Costea, and Diethelm Tschoepe

Contents

© Springer Nature Switzerland AG 2022
H.-R. Metelmann et al. (eds.), *Textbook of Good Clinical Practice in Cold Plasma Therapy*, https://doi.org/10.1007/978-3-030-87857-3_9

🗨 **Core Messages**
- DFU require highly individualized and wound adapted therapy. Beside standard care procedures, a plethora of applications exist, mainly based on empirical values.
- Polymicrobial infections are common in DFU, skin derived microbes are often present in wounds.
- Main objective in chronic wound treatment is to reactivate the avital wound area and to induce the healing process.
- Primary wound closure needs to be achieved to reconstitute the natural barrier for (re)infection and to create optimal conditions for secondary healing.

9.1 Introduction

Cold atmospheric plasma (CAP) has been applied in several chronic wound situations as diabetic foot ulcers, surgical wounds, burning wounds, etc [1–3]. It has shown beneficial effects on wound healing which mostly were accounted to the antimicrobial effects of plasma. Recently, evidence arose from in vitro and in vivo studies that CAP treatment may stimulate microcirculation and cellular proliferation, resulting in activation of chronic wounds [4]. Up to now, clinical evidence from prospective randomized placebo-controlled trials was lacking and reports were based on case-controlled studies or case reports. Very recently, this evidence was underlined by applying CAP in a well-defined placebo-controlled trial [5]. Now it is evident that CAP stimulates wound healing by different pathways with the antimicrobial effect – due to its properly short activity – being less relevant.

9.2 Diagnosis

Treatment of diabetic foot ulcers requires highly individualized and patient focused regimes considering wound staging and evaluation of vascular situation [6]. In stages where perfusion is diminished by peripheral arterial disease (PAD), arterial blood flow has to be restored by appropriate vascular procedures [7]. Therefore, wound therapy should be guided by provisioning blood flow to the affected limb as only perfused wound areas support sustainable wound healing. Screening for peripheral artery disease (PAD) is thus obligatory and can easily be performed by evaluation of the ankle-brachial-index, whereas local perfusion can be assessed by measurement of transcutaneous oxygen pressure or comparable measurements.

Regarding the wound itself, the identification of microbial colonization and focused systemic instead of local, surficial antibiotic treatment is of importance to overcome the chronic inflammatory state [8]. Regularly performed debridement for removal of avital tissue and refreshment of wound ground and margins in combination with moisture wound dressings best describe standard care treatment of DFU. Consequent off-loading procedures for prevention of recurrence of trauma are mandatory for successful wound healing.

Depending on wound stage, which is precisely characterized via Wagner-Armstrong scaling considering wound depth and infection status, different wound care strategies may be applied [9]. Osteomyelitis and neuropathic arthropathy can be can be assessed by MRI techniques or X-ray analysis. In suspicion of osteomyelitis, best practice is to treat it like osteomyelitis as long as the diagnosis is not available.

It is beyond the scope of this chapter to describe DFU therapy by detail, therefore current published guidelines are recommended for further information [6].

9.3 Physiology and Pathology

Diabetic foot ulcers (DFU) are associated with significant impairment in quality of life, increased morbidity and mortality, as well as amplified health care burden [10]. DFU is one of the common causes of hospital inpatient admission in Western countries. The prevalence of DF in Europe is 5.1%, with an annual incidence of 2–4% in developed countries [11, 12]. Its prevalence is estimated between 2% and 10% in Germany [13, 14]. Patients with type 2 (T2DM) are more affected than those with type 1 DM (T1DM) [15]. The life time risk of a diabetic patient developing a foot ulcer (DFU) has been estimated to be 19–34% [16, 17]. A major problem in treatment of DFU is the high annual recurrence rate of 50% that often is due to impaired healing. Between 20 and 40% of all chronic diabetic foot ulcers are supposed to heal within 12 weeks, and 50% of the ulcers are healed by 6 months. Around 30% of the patients require surgical intervention [18, 19].

Foot ulcers are defined as lesions involving a skin break with loss of epithelium extending into the dermis and deeper layers, sometimes involving bone and muscle. Non-traumatic amputation is regarded as "the removal of a terminal, nonviable portion of the limb" and seen as an allowed curative intervention [20].

The etiology of DFUs often relies on a combination of factors, most commonly diabetic peripheral neuropathy (DPN, loss of pain sensation, >60% of cases) associated with unperceived trauma, peripheral arterial disease (PAD, loss of nutritive blood flow, 35% of cases), and infection as well as foot deformations (e.g., neuropathic arthropathy, 5% of cases) [21]. In middle- and high-income countries, up to 50% of patients with diabetes and foot ulceration have underlying peripheral artery disease (PAD) [22]. DM is a known risk factor for certain infectious diseases because diabetic individuals are in an immunocompromised state, especially if metabolic control is insufficient but even in a well-controlled state [23, 24].

DFU are characterized by chronic arrest in an inflammatory phase which suppresses the switch to the next phase of wound healing – the proliferation phase that precedes the maturation episode. Therefore, the wound is lacking effective triggers to overcome stagnation, which is caused by biofilm deposition or reduced anti-inflammatory signaling [25].

9.4 Standard Treatment Principles

Hallmarks of successful healing in DFU are adequate arterial inflow, aggressive management of infection, and offloading, yielding in pressure relief from the wound and its margins. Early multifactorial assessment and treatment of DFU is crucial for therapeutic success. The earlier the chronic status of a wound described by chronic infection, inflammation, and lack of epithelialization can be resolved, the more efficient wound therapy can be applied and wound closure can be achieved. Therapy is guided by the MOIST-concept comprising moisture balance, oxygen balance, infection control, support of healing, and tissue management [26]. Treatment of DFU is highly individualized, based on common recommendation, a plethora of wound dressings, debridement procedures, and stage-dependent interventions exist, and again the reader is referred to local guidelines for appropriate choice of standard wound care.

9.5 Treatment Rationale

Treatment of DFU is a highly individualized patient- and wound-oriented treatment – there is no one-for-all concept that guarantees therapeutic success. Wound healing requires an active wound that presents with a self-healing tendency. Chronic wounds are arrested in the inflammatory state [25]. To overcome this stagnation, activation has to be achieved by either physical or biological debridement or other procedures to remove avital tissue and biofilm that hamper cell proliferation. This opens the wound for reinitiating of the wound healing process. Support to activate involved cells is needed in long-standing chronic wounds to achieve primary wound closure. Primary wound closure is the basis for secondary healing and fits as a barrier for microbial reinfection, even as a barrier for skin-derived microbes [6].

Cold atmospheric plasma has shown to activate several cell types like keratinocytes and epithelial cells in vitro and in vivo that are essential for healing and thus is able to support wound healing at a cellular level [27].

9.6 Cold Atmospheric Plasma Treatment

Cold atmospheric plasma has been proposed as a tool for various biological and medical applications, relying on its capacity to reduce bacterial load in the wound and to initiate wound healing by cellular activation [2, 28]. CAP has proven beneficial effects in the treatment of chronic wounds described in several case reports and preliminary studies since 2007 [29]. In a small study performed later on, Isbary et al. were able to prove the antimicrobial effect in chronic ulcer wounds and showed significant infection reduction without side effects in a second study even after 2 minutes instead of 5 minutes exposure to CAP [30]. Both Isbary-studies included wounds of different origins (venous, arterial, diabetic, and traumatic ulcers) and proved effects on bacterial infection regardless of bacterial type. This finding was confirmed in several other studies.

Beside the often-described antimicrobial effects [31], CAP activates cell proliferation in different types of cells like keratinocytes [27], endothelial cells [32], peripheral blood mononuclear cells [33], and fibroblasts [34], while, on the other hand, plasma has been shown to induce apoptosis in a number of different cell types calling interest in anti-cancer therapy [35, 36]. Of these, keratinocytes and fibroblasts are of great importance in the later wound-healing phases. A recent study examined the cross-talk between CAP activated keratinocytes and fibroblasts with consequences mainly on the expression of growth factors in fibroblasts [37–39]. Different types of plasma devices are available ranging from contact free, plasma jet-based systems to surface contacting patch-derived devices.

First clinical evidence from randomized blinded prospective studies is available now, sustaining previously observed effects [5, 40].

The first randomized, placebo-controlled patient-blinded trial evaluated 62 wounds of 43 patients in a controlled hospitalized environment [5]. Wounds included in the trial were superficial or those that permeated to tendon and presented with infection but no signs of ischemia. CAP and placebo treatments were added to standard wound care, which included systemic antibiotic treatment if indicated, regular wound debridement, local disinfection, off-loading, and moist wound care. It was conducted as a bi-center trial and randomization took patient's age, gender, and smoking status into account. Wounds were randomized separately and, during analysis, wound size and patient were considered as potentially influencing factors. CAP was applied for 5 days on a daily basis and for three more applications every second day following manufacturer's recommendation on a wound-individualized fashion (30 seconds per cm^2 of wound surface). An approved and certified argon plasma jet (KINPen Med, neoplas tools GmbH) was used as active treatment, whereas the same device without plasma generation but only argon gas was used as placebo in the same way. Patient's blindness was kept by sound imitation in the switched off-mode. Wound surface regression during treatment was documented and evaluated by a blinded investigator. Clinical and microbial infection was assessed at each change of dressings, right before wound treatment and CAP application.

This is a statistically significant result ($p = 0.03$). CAP therapy had a remaining wound area of only 30.5% after the treatment period, compared with 55.2% for those on placebo ($P = 0.03$). Thus, the amount of wound surface closed under cold plasma treatment was 55% higher than the amount closed under the standard treatment alone [5] (◘ Fig. 9.1).

The CAP treatment was painless and well tolerated. None of the study patients experienced any CAP therapy-related side effects throughout the course of the treatment. This effect is mainly attributable to the earlier induction of wound healing, which was proven by an earlier achievement of a 10% (CAP vs. placebo, $P = 0.009$) surface reduction with CAP [5] (◘ Fig. 9.2).

The authors were not able to prove the antimicrobial effect of CAP treatment. Although the CAP group was in favor and obviously started from a higher amount of microbial load, superiority was not significantly shown. In contrast to previous reports, this study evaluated microbial status before each CAP treatment and not directly after. This might indicate that CAP acutely diminishes microbial load, but wounds over the course of time get reinfected. Obviously, CAP does not eradicate germs completely during the treatment, pointing to the importance of concurrent

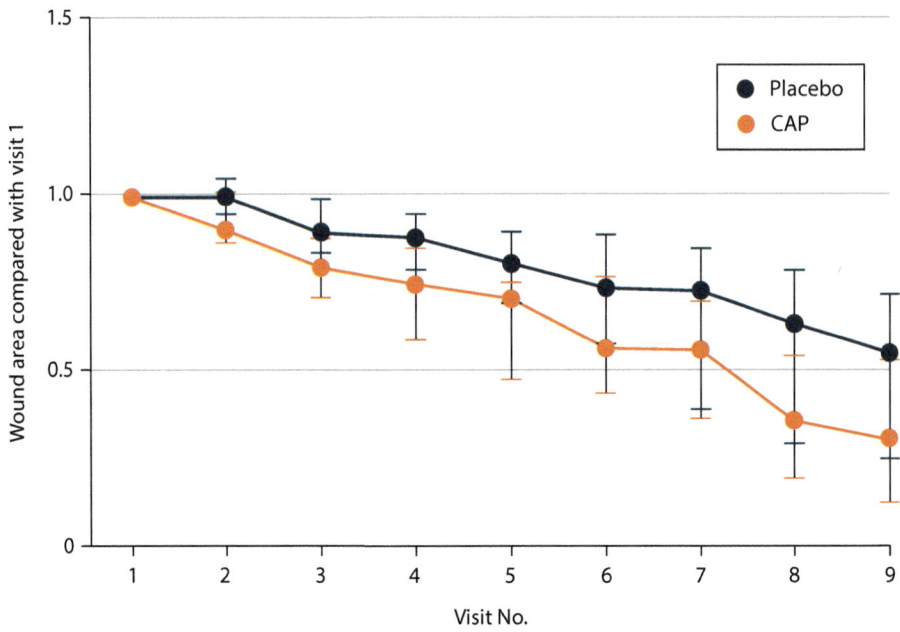

◨ Fig. 9.1 Wound size reduction during the KPW-trial, given as reduction in relation to start as medians with 95% CI, per endpoint analysis significant difference in wound size at V9 [5]

Proportion of DFU wounds with 10% reduction in wounds surface area

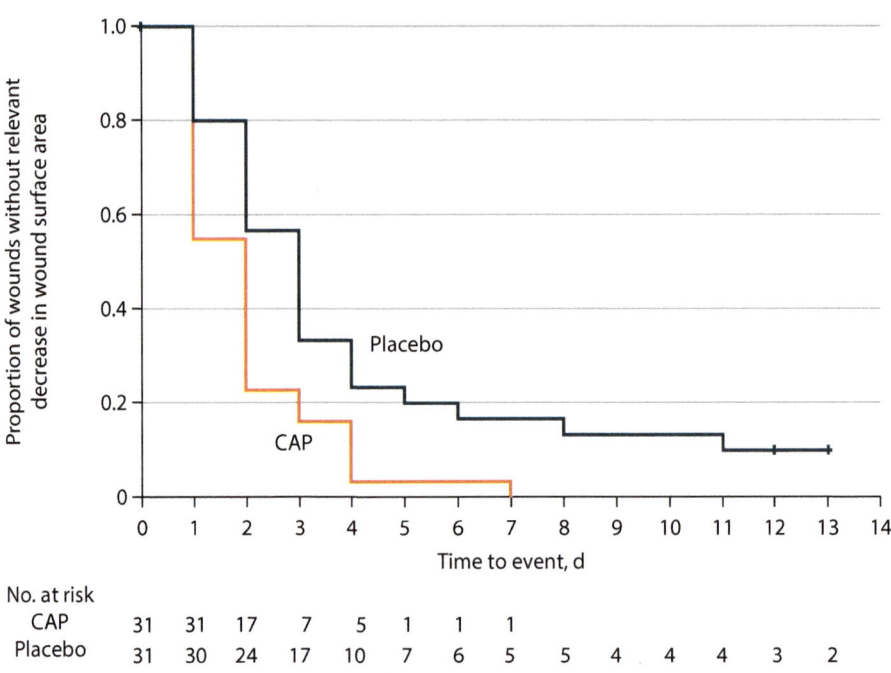

◨ Fig. 9.2 Proportion of wounds with 10% reduction in wound surface area during treatment [5]

antiseptic and antibiotic adjunctive therapy. The patients will be kept under observation for five more years for an assessment of the long-term safety of the treatment [5].

A second monocenter trial was recently published from Teheran, evaluating a helium-based CAP in a randomized but not placebo-controlled study [40]. Patients were block-randomized to receiving CAP or standard care. The authors analyzed 22 patient-wounds per group. Regarding wound surface regression, the authors achieved pretty comparable results to the trial mentioned above. All patients were treated with antibiotics in parallel. CAP was applied three times a week for 3 weeks resulting in nine treatments in total. Each application took 5 minutes, irrespective of the wound size. CAP resulted in a significantly more pronounced wound surface reduction and more patients in the CAP group reached the endpoint 50% wound surface reduction. The authors measured the bacterial load directly before and after CAP and were able to prove the preciously described direct antimicrobial effect as an immediate result of CAP treatment [40].

To summarize these early and new results, it now becomes obvious that CAP induces more than the reduction in microbial load and that the more important effect is the activation of the chronic wound on cellular basis and by improvement of microcirculation. Further biochemical analyses need to be performed to understand these beneficial effects of CAP.

9.6.1 Pre-treatment Assessment

For application of CAP in diabetic foot ulcer, standard wound care management best describes pre-treatment procedures. Routine wound management comprises mechanical debridement to remove avital tissue and to recondition wound margins, followed by antiseptic rinsing for surface cleaning. After this, CAP should be applied following manufacturer's advice.

The vascular status of the patient should be evaluated before, as wound healing strongly depends on perfusion – if indicated, revascularization procedures should be considered. Regarding infection, systemic antibiosis should be initiated following microbial analysis and antibiogram to improve wound healing. CAP treatment has local and time-dependent effects on microbial load, as shown by the studies outlined above [3, 5, 40].

9.6.2 Timing

CAP can be applied in each phase of wound healing. It shows beneficial effects on infection management, on cell activation in terms of chemokine and growth factor release, as well as cell proliferation on fibroblasts and keratinocytes which are main actors in late wound healing, and thus CAP stimulates wound healing in early and late stages. The duration of each treatment should follow the manufacturer's advice; for example, for the KINPen Med a treatment of $30s/cm^2$ of wound surface is recommended. Best time point for application of CAP is after debridement and rinsing of the wound, before new dressings are applied.

9.6.3 Diagnosis and Treatment Planning

CAP should be applied if perfusion of the wound area is guaranteed. It is able to reactivate chronic wounds and to support wound healing, but this strongly depends on perfusion. Debridement should precede CAP application to remove avital tissue, in order to uncover the wound basis to achieve a maximum effect. Wound disinfection is reasonable as supportive procedure and recommended by current guidelines. Treatment should be done at least every second day on occasion of change of wound dressing, but may be intensified to a once daily treatment. CAP is applied as long as wound healing is ongoing, there is no clear limitation for treatment duration.

9.6.4 Anesthesia

CAP does not require anesthesia; our study results and application during general treatment were reported to be painless; however, in patients with painful diabetic neuropathy associated with allodynia, caution should be taken to apply CAP contact-free, the plasma effluent per se is well tolerated even in these patients.

9.6.5 Post-Treatment Care

Following CAP wound dressings should be applied following standard care procedures, there is no limitation in the choice of dressing as no interactions are described up to now. In general, exudate management is required, and optimal wound healing conditions should be achieved by moist wound dressings.

9.6.6 Handling of Complications

Available studies indicate that CAP rarely leads to complications associated with the treatment [3, 5, 40]. CAP should be applied in a sterile environment as is usual for wound care procedures. Devices are equipped with single use sterile supplies to keep patient's safety. Mobile devices are preferable for use in clinical settings as it is easier and associated with lower risk to move the device than the patient.

Skin irritation, increased scar formation, or local side effects have not been observed, even in long-term follow-up of patients. One study (Stratmann et al.) will evaluate these effects in a follow-up period of five years.

> **Conclusion**
> Recently published clinical evidence exists that CAP can significantly improve wound healing in diabetic foot ulcers. The effect does not singularly rely on its antimicrobial effect, which has been proven directly after application of CAP, but is more attributable on the cell activation/proliferation impact that is associated with

improvements in microcirculation and faster wound closure. Given these beneficiary effects, CAP treatment improves patient's quality of life and is of socioeconomic value as it potentially reduces duration of hospitalization. CAP is easy to apply and safe and thus may be used even in an ambulatory environment.

References

1. Costea TC, Arbi A. Cold plasma in the treatment of burns. Diabetes Stoffwech H. 2019;28(5):245–50.
2. Weltmann KD, Kindel E, von Woedtke T, Hahnel M, Stieber M, Brandenburg R. Atmospheric-pressure plasma sources: prospective tools for plasma medicine. Pure Appl Chem. 2010;82(6):1223–37.
3. Ulrich C, Kluschke F, Patzelt A, Vandersee S, Czaika VA, Richter H, et al. Clinical use of cold atmospheric pressure argon plasma in chronic leg ulcers: A pilot study. J Wound Care. 2015;24(5):196–203.
4. Rutkowski R, Schuster M, Unger J, Seebauer C, Metelmann HR, von Woedtke T, et al. Hyperspectral imaging for in vivo monitoring of cold atmospheric plasma effects on microcirculation in treatment of head and neck cancer and wound healing. Clin Plasma Med. 2017;7-8:52–7.
5. Stratmann B, Costea TC, Nolte C, Hiller J, Schmidt J, Reindel J, et al. Effect of cold atmospheric plasma therapy vs standard therapy placebo on wound healing in patients with Diabetic foot ulcers: a randomized clinical trial. JAMA Netw Open. 2020;3(7):e2010411.
6. Schaper NC, van Netten JJ, Apelqvist J, Bus SA, Hinchliffe RJ, Lipsky BA, et al. Practical guidelines on the prevention and management of diabetic foot disease (IWGDF 2019 update). Diabetes Metab Res Rev. 2020;36(Suppl 1):e3266.
7. Rayman G, Vas P, Dhatariya K, Driver V, Hartemann A, Londahl M, et al. Guidelines on use of interventions to enhance healing of chronic foot ulcers in diabetes (IWGDF 2019 update). Diabetes Metab Res Rev. 2020;36(Suppl 1):e3283.
8. Lipsky BA, Senneville E, Abbas ZG, Aragon-Sanchez J, Diggle M, Embil JM, et al. Guidelines on the diagnosis and treatment of foot infection in persons with diabetes (IWGDF 2019 update). Diabetes Metab Res Rev. 2020;36(Suppl 1):e3280.
9. Armstrong DG, Lavery LA, Harkless LB. Validation of a diabetic wound classification system. The contribution of depth, infection, and ischemia to risk of amputation. Diabetes Care. 1998;21(5):855–9.
10. Boulton AJ, Vileikyte L, Ragnarson-Tennvall G, Apelqvist J. The global burden of diabetic foot disease. Lancet. 2005;366(9498):1719–24.
11. Reiber GE, Vileikyte L, Boyko EJ, del Aguila M, Smith DG, Lavery LA, et al. Causal pathways for incident lower-extremity ulcers in patients with diabetes from two settings. Diabetes Care. 1999;22(1):157–62.
12. Zhang P, Lu J, Jing Y, Tang S, Zhu D, Bi Y. Global epidemiology of diabetic foot ulceration: a systematic review and meta-analysis (dagger). Ann Med. 2017;49(2):106–16.
13. Heyer K, Herberger K, Protz K, Glaeske G, Augustin M. Epidemiology of chronic wounds in Germany: analysis of statutory health insurance data. Wound Repair Regen. 2016;24(2):434–42.
14. Kroger K, Berg C, Santosa F, Malyar N, Reinecke H. Lower limb amputation in Germany an analysis of data from the German Federal Statistical Office between 2005 and 2014. Dtsch Arztebl Int. 2017;114(8):130. −+.
15. Bohn B, Grunerbel A, Altmeier M, Giesche C, Pfeifer M, Wagner C, et al. Diabetic foot syndrome in patients with diabetes. A multicenter German/Austrian DPV analysis on 33 870 patients. Diabetes Metab Res Rev. 2018;34(6):e3020.
16. Singh N, Armstrong DG, Lipsky BA. Preventing foot ulcers in patients with diabetes. JAMA. 2005;293(2):217–28.

17. Weck M, Slesaczeck T, Paetzold H, Muench D, Nanning T, von Gagern G, et al. Structured health care for subjects with diabetic foot ulcers results in a reduction of major amputation rates. Cardiovasc Diabetol. 2013;12:45.
18. Falanga V. Wound healing and its impairment in the diabetic foot. Lancet. 2005;366(9498): 1736–43.
19. Jeffcoate WJ, Price P, Harding KG, International Working Group on Wound Healing and Treatments for People with Diabetic Foot Ulcers. Wound healing and treatments for people with diabetic foot ulcers. Diabetes Metab Res Rev. 2004;20(Suppl 1):S78–89.
20. Bowker JH, Pfeifer MA. Levin and O'Neal's the diabetic foot. Philadelphia: Mosby/Elsevier; 2008.
21. Clayton WE, T.A. A review of the pathophysiology, classification, and treatment of foot ulcers in diabetic patients. Clin Diabetes. 2009;27(2):52–8.
22. Peters EJG, Childs MR, Wunderlich RP, Harkless LB, Armstrong DG, Lavery LA. Functional status of persons with diabetes-related lower-extremity amputations. Diabetes Care. 2001;24(10):1799–804.
23. Shah BR, Hux JE. Quantifying the risk of infectious diseases for people with diabetes. Diabetes Care. 2003;26(2):510–3.
24. Muller LM, Gorter KJ, Hak E, Goudzwaard WL, Schellevis FG, Hoepelman AI, et al. Increased risk of common infections in patients with type 1 and type 2 diabetes mellitus. Clin Infect Dis. 2005;41(3):281–8.
25. Patel S, Srivastava S, Singh MR, Singh D. Mechanistic insight into diabetic wounds: pathogenesis, molecular targets and treatment strategies to pace wound healing. Biomed Pharmacother. 2019;112:108615.
26. Dissemond J, Assenheimer B, Engels P, Gerber V, Kroger K, Kurz P, et al. MOIST – a concept for the topical treatment of chronic wounds. J Dtsch Dermatol Ges. 2017;15(4):443–5.
27. Hasse S, Tran TD, Hahn O, Kindler S, Metelmann HR, von Woedtke T, et al. Induction of proliferation of basal epidermal keratinocytes by cold atmospheric-pressure plasma. Clin Exp Dermatol. 2016;41(2):202–9.
28. von Woedtke T, Schmidt A, Bekeschus S, Wende K, Weltmann KD. Plasma medicine: A field of applied redox biology. In Vivo. 2019;33(4):1011–26.
29. Isbary G, Morfill G, Schmidt HU, Georgi M, Ramrath K, Heinlin J, et al. A first prospective randomized controlled trial to decrease bacterial load using cold atmospheric argon plasma on chronic wounds in patients. Br J Dermatol. 2010;163(1):78–82.
30. Isbary G, Heinlin J, Shimizu T, Zimmermann JL, Morfill G, Schmidt HU, et al. Successful and safe use of 2 min cold atmospheric argon plasma in chronic wounds: results of a randomized controlled trial. Br J Dermatol. 2012;167(2):404–10.
31. Daeschlein G, Scholz S, Ahmed R, von Woedtke T, Haase H, Niggemeier M, et al. Skin decontamination by low-temperature atmospheric pressure plasma jet and dielectric barrier discharge plasma. J Hosp Infect. 2012;81(3):177–83.
32. Kalghatgi S, Friedman G, Fridman A, Clyne AM. Endothelial cell proliferation is enhanced by low dose non-thermal plasma through fibroblast growth factor-2 release. Ann Biomed Eng. 2010;38(3):748–57.
33. Bekeschus S, Masur K, Kolata J, Wende K, Schmidt A, Bundscherer L, et al. Human mononuclear cell survival and proliferation is modulated by cold atmospheric plasma jet. Plasma Process Polym. 2013;10(8):706–13.
34. Ngo MHT, Liao JD, Shao PL, Weng CC, Chang CY. Increased fibroblast cell proliferation and migration using atmospheric N-2/Ar micro-plasma for the stimulated release of fibroblast growth factor-7. Plasma Process Polym. 2014;11(1):80–8.
35. Partecke LI, Evert K, Haugk J, Doering F, Normann L, Diedrich S, et al. Tissue tolerable plasma (TTP) induces apoptosis in pancreatic cancer cells in vitro and in vivo. Bmc. Cancer. 2012;12:473.
36. Schmidt A, Bekeschus S, von Woedtke T, Hasse S. Cell migration and adhesion of a human melanoma cell line is decreased by cold plasma treatment. Clin Plasma Med. 2015;3(1):24–31.

9

37. Schmidt A, Bekeschus S, Jarick K, Hasse S, von Woedtke T, Wende K. Cold physical plasma modulates p53 and mitogen-activated protein kinase signaling in keratinocytes. Oxidative Med Cell Longev. 2019;2019:7017363.

38. Schmidt A, von Woedtke T, Bekeschus S. Periodic exposure of keratinocytes to cold physical plasma: an in vitro model for redox-related diseases of the skin. Oxidative Med Cell Longev. 2016;2016:9816072.

39. Zhao B, Ye X, Yu JD, Li L, Li WQ, Li SM, et al. TEAD mediates YAP-dependent gene induction and growth control. Genes Dev. 2008;22(14):1962–71.

40. Mirpour S, Fathollah S, Mansouri P, Larijani B, Ghoranneviss M, Tehrani MM, et al. Cold atmospheric plasma as an effective method to treat diabetic foot ulcers: A randomized clinical trial. Sci Rep. 2020;10(1):1–9.

Cold Plasma Palliative Treatment of Cancer

Christian Seebauer, Hans-Robert Metelmann, Thomas von Woedtke, Kerstin Böttger, Runa Tschersche-Mondry, Benjamin Schade, and Sander Bekeschus

Contents

© Springer Nature Switzerland AG 2022
H.-R. Metelmann et al. (eds.), *Textbook of Good Clinical Practice in Cold Plasma Therapy*, https://doi.org/10.1007/978-3-030-87857-3_10

🔵 **Core Messages**

- From a scientific point of view and on the basis of significant experimental and preclinical research, cold atmospheric plasma (CAP) is suitable for the treatment of cancer.
- Nevertheless, clinical CAP treatment of cancer at present is largely off-label use of approved plasma medical devices.
- There is a small range of indications to use CAP for the benefit of patients in palliative cancer treatment.
- The antimicrobial efficacy of CAP can play a key role in palliative care of tumor patients with infected ulcerations.

10.1 Introduction

From a scientific point of view and on the basis of significant experimental and preclinical research, cold atmospheric plasma (CAP) is suitable for the treatment of cancer [5, 24]. From a clinical point of view, however, clinical plasma treatment of cancer is still off-label use of the approved medical devices.

Randomized clinical trials are needed to add plasma medicine to the guidelines of evidence-based medicine [2, 15] and CAP medical devices to the toolbox of cancer treatment. A major impediment is the fact that cancer is a deadly disease, and cancer treatment is strictly limited to measures at the top of the pyramid of evidence-based medicine. A randomized clinical trial with cancer patients suffering, for example, from head and neck cancer, requires a comparison of an innovative treatment like CAP application with standard treatment like surgery, radiation, or cytostatic chemotherapy. To achieve necessary comparability, the long way to evidence-based medicine starts with collecting and evaluating clinical data of case reports and pilot studies [21].

There are already clinical case reports since several years demonstrating the healing results of CAP therapy [6, 12, 16]. Small cancer cell clusters like in early skin cancer (🔲 Fig. 10.1) and in lymph node metastases (🔲 Fig. 10.2) can be inactivated by focused application of CAP. First clinical investigations indicate a promising healing tendency of premalignant mucosa lesions (🔲 Fig. 10.3) suspected to be caused partly by infection and inflammation [23].

Anyhow, there is already a certain range of indications to use CAP for the benefit of cancer patients. It is based on long-established microbial decontamination of wounded body surfaces [10].

10.2 Diagnosis

The antimicrobial efficacy of CAP can play a key role in palliative care of tumor patients with infected ulcerations [16, 22].

The main goal and first intention of cancer therapy is curative treatment, that is, the permanent removal of the tumor. If this is beyond reach, palliative care

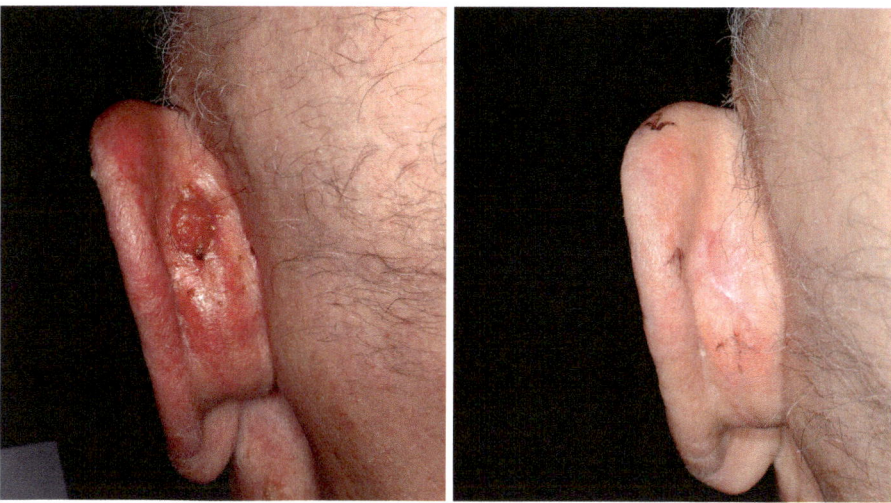

🔲 **Fig. 10.1** A patient with a suspected small skin cancer cell clusters behind the ear. Experimental CAP application prior to standard treatment with written consent of the patient. Status before (left side) and 5 month after several interventions (right side) without evidence of disease

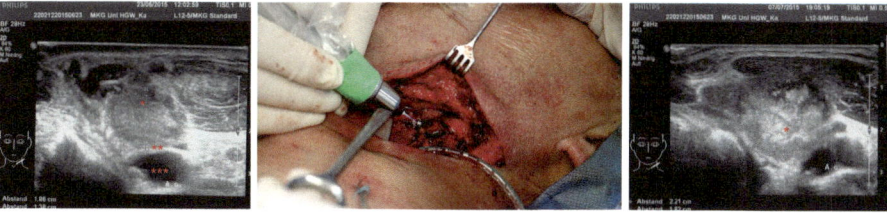

🔲 **Fig. 10.2** A patient with suspected lymph node metastasis of an oral cavity squamous cell carcinoma, located at the neck. The pre-operative sonogram (above) presents the lymph node (*), inseparably grown into the wall (**) of the Arteria carotis communis (***), a main artery of the head. The operative situation (in the middle) presents the metastasis as unresectable, experimental treatment occurs by targeted application of jet plasma. The post-operative sonogram 10 days after the single intervention (below) unveils disaggregation of the lymph node metastasis. (Reprinted with kind permission: Seebauer et al. [26], p. 105)

becomes the focus of care. Treatment goals now are managing pain, taking care of nutrition and open airways, and facilitating social contacts, to alleviate the symptoms and emotional issues of cancer eventually.

In some cancer patients suffering from advanced incurable tumors, open contaminated ulcerations are part of the disease progression. These ulcerations are caused by necrotic tissue due to progressive tumor growth, weak systemic and local immunological response, and various accompanying illnesses. The wounds may be associated with pain, exudate, bleeding, and especially an offensive smell caused by anaerobe microbial pathogens. This may adversely affect self-esteem, causing patients to isolate themselves at a time when social support is critically needed. Due to the high wound vulnerability, local antiseptic wound care of microbial con-

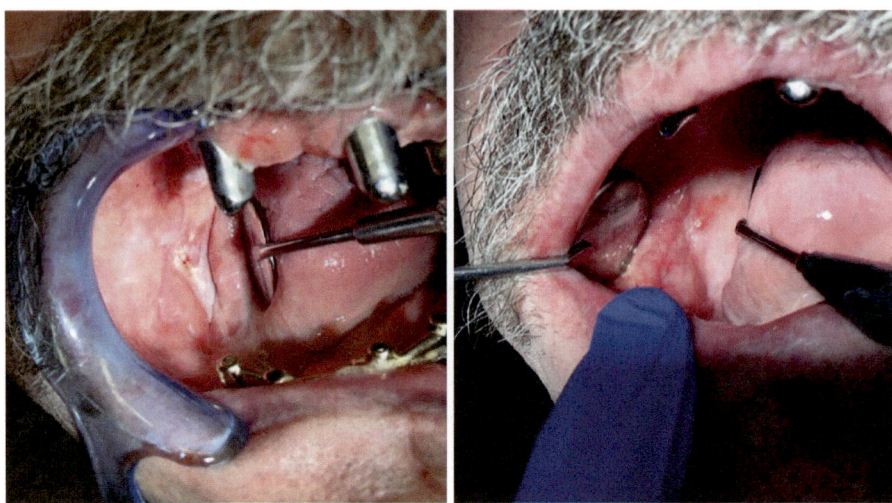

□ Fig. 10.3 A patient with histologically proven precancerous lesion of the oral cavity mucosa. Experimental CAP application prior to standard treatment with written consent of the patient. Status before (left side) and 3 weeks after several jet plasma interventions (right side)

10

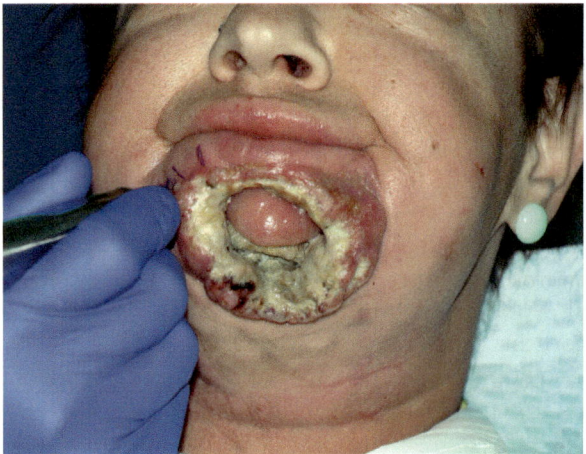

□ Fig. 10.4 A patient with a locally advanced squamous cell carcinoma of the oral cavity is presenting the typical diagnosis for CAP treatment. Tumor progression has broken the wall to the chin. The options of standard tumor treatment and curative care are exhausted. The patient is suffering from intensive bad odor caused by contaminated necrotic and rotten tumor tissue. CAP application for decontamination as part of palliative care is obviously appreciated, as wearing earrings is an expression of her self-confidence. (Reprinted with kind permission: Seebauer et al. [26], p. 100)

taminated tumor areas is frequently complicated by bleeding, pain, and patient dissatisfaction.

There is a consensus of experts that contamination of cancer ulcerations with microbial pathogens makes a diagnosis for palliative CAP treatment, as shown in □ Fig. 10.4.

> **Tip**
>
> It is the antimicrobial effectiveness of plasma that is mainly used in palliative plasma oncology.

10.3 Physiology and Pathology

10.3.1 Antimicrobial Effect

Decontamination [7], treatment of superficial infections [9], and bacterial reduction [1] have been among the first clinical findings of CAP effectiveness.

By reducing microbial colonization of cancer ulcerations, inflammatory response, and the related symptoms, for example, pain, bleeding, and wound odor, the emotional and physical burden of cancer can be reduced, and quality of life improved [16, 20, 22].

10.3.2 Anti-Cancer Effect

CAP application focuses on microbial pathogens, but it is evident that cancer cells just below the layer of microbial pathogens are affected to some extent as well. The physiological and pathological background of these effects might be different. Plasma-induced immunogenic cell death has to be considered [3, 11, 14, 18], and modulation of inflammation, too [4]. Combination of CAP treatment with palliative cytostatic chemotherapy [8, 13, 25] may confer additive cytotoxicity, as well as palliative radiotherapy [19].

In a clinical pilot study with six cancer patients, it has been shown that CAP treatment for decontamination noticeably inhibited the growth of tumors in some patients and caused a reduction in odor and need for pain medication. Partial remission was achieved for at least 9 months in two patients after CAP treatment. Incisional biopsies found apoptotic tumor cells and a desmoplastic reaction within the surrounding tumor tissue [17].

10.4 Standard Treatment Principles

Curatively intended cancer treatment is an off-label use of CAP medical devices. Palliative intended application for decontamination of cancer lesions is an authorized use of CAP medical devices. The effectiveness of CAP treatment against not only microbes but also cancer cells is a highly welcomed side effect.

CAP application is a supplementary treatment. It has to be seen strictly in an overall context of palliative medicine that includes all measures of pain reduction, securing of the airways, adequate fluid intake, and sufficient nutrition. In the case of CAP-related side effects of any kind, the supplementary treatment should be stopped.

■ **Fig. 10.5** Anatomical difficulties of CAP treatment: A cancer patient in palliative care with an ulceration deeply in the former paranasal sinus. The most appropriate way to apply CAP is a jet plasma device

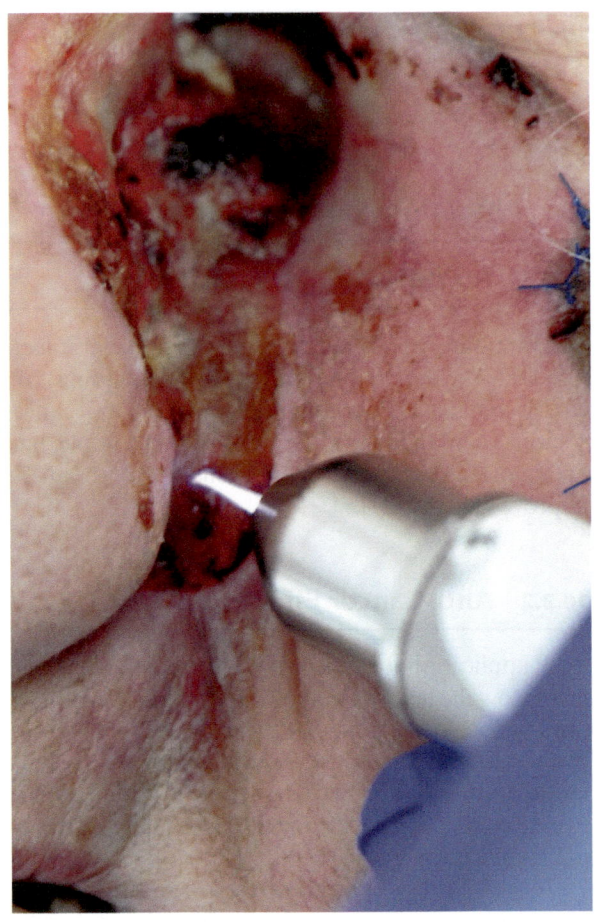

10

Medical devices generating a jet plasma facilitate application under visual control, an accurate motion of the plasma jet plume over the target tissue, and CAP application at deep tissue defects, extended fistula, undercut areas, and intra-oral or anatomically hard-to-access areas (■ Fig. 10.5).

CAP is used to treat oral cancer with very mild side effects such as bad taste during and after treatment and minimal discomfort during treatment. None of the known side effects are severe or life-threatening, and most are transient with full recovery. Another benefit of CAP treatment is that it leaves no residuals on the target tissue.

> **Tip**
>
> CAP application is an innovative addition to standard palliative tumor patient care.

10.5 Treatment Rationale

The target cells of CAP treatment are not the cancer cells but the microbial pathogens in the tumor wound bed. The treatment rationale is decontamination caused by CAP. The cancer cells might be inactivated by means of clinical aspects to some extent as well, but it is still unclear why some patients react to the CAP impact with tumor reduction and why some patients do not.

◘ Figure 10.6 illustrates the treatment rationale by a case report: A 51-year-old Caucasian male patient presented with an ulcerated and contaminated lymph node metastasis of the neck (◘ Fig. 10.6, left image). The patient was treated for decontamination due to offensive smell, pain, and recurrent bleeding.

After 2 months of CAP treatment (◘ Fig. 10.6, center image), the odor, pain, and bleeding were gone, and the formerly infected and necrotic tumor surface displayed a smooth surface topology. Microbiological examination revealed a reduction of bacterial colonization, especially of anaerobic bacteria like Bacteroides species, which led to decreased bacterial decomposition products and wound odor. Thus, due to the decrease of local and perifocal inflammation, wound vulnerability and algesia were significantly reduced.

After 4 months of CAP treatment (◘ Fig. 10.6, right image), a substantial decline of tumor tissue was observed, being a side effect of antimicrobial plasma application. The ulcerated tumor area was reduced to one-quarter of its original size. The wound margin and center were sclerosed and calloused. In parallel to plasma treatment, the wound bed was regularly covered by a physiological fibrin coating.

Worth mentioning, however, is the palliative result of the CAP treatment that was not sufficient to prevent the decease of the patient eventually.

10.6 Therapy

10.6.1 Identification of Suitable Patients

The final responsibility to identify the patients suitable for palliative CAP treatment lies in the hands of the cancer-treating medical specialist.

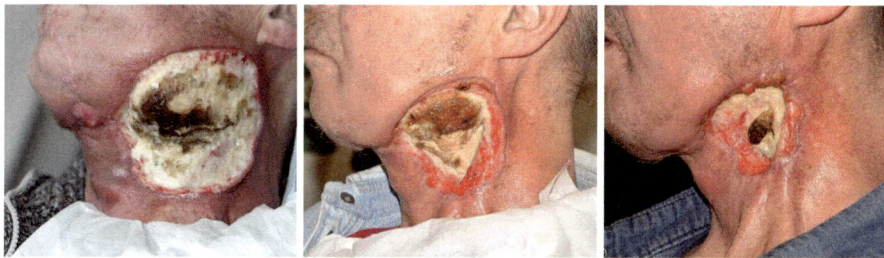

◘ **Fig. 10.6** A patient with a contaminated cancer ulceration before (left side), 2 months after (in the middle), and 4 months after (right side) palliative CAP treatment. (Reprinted with kind permission: Seebauer et al. [27])

10.6.2   Informing the Patient

CAP application as an innovative treatment requires extensive information of the patient and written consent to undergo the treatment. Most patients, for the time being, are not familiar with CAP medicine. They might have frequently asked questions.

— Is the clinical efficacy of CAP proven?

CAP therapy is based on randomized clinical studies and approved medical plasma devices. Their application for treatment purposes is authorized as medical devices class IIa for the treatment of pathogen-related diseases and wounds according to the European Council Directive 93/42/EEC by CE-certification.

— What are the undesirable local or systemic side effects?

Approved plasma devices are in clinical use since 2013. There are no case observations or clinical studies known reporting severe side effects of any kind, including carcinogenesis or genetic damage.

10.6.3   Obtain Written Consent

10

Written consent is self-evident in medical interventions and it is strongly recommended that (i) the patient understands the motivation and principles of the cold plasma application, (ii) there are no unwanted side effects known from standard medical applications of cold plasma, and (iii) it cannot be guaranteed that the palliative plasma-based care will fully satisfy the expectations of the patient, since biological processes are not always predictable.

> ⚠ **Caution**
> An innovative treatment like CAP requires vitally extensive information and written consent of the patient.

10.6.4   Treatment

Treatment of cancer ulcerations is multifaceted, challenging, and has to be performed on an individualized basis. The complexity and variability of different clinical situations require specific approaches.

Clinical experience in CAP oncology is mainly based on jet plasma devices. Jet plasma will be applied without touch of the device and does not cause pain in most patients. There is, in principle, no need for local anesthesia or cooling of the treatment area.

To prepare the tissue of application, it might be useful to remove the biofilm. However, drying the area is not recommendable because CAP Plasma is more active in wet tissue environments.

There is no scientific standard on how to apply CAP Plasma. Based on clinical experience, ulcerated tumor regions should receive treatment with jet plasma for 1 minute/cm^2 at a distance of approximately 10–15 mm in a meandering manner. Using the plasma jet, it is important to carefully follow the fissured, ragged, indented, and jagged surface of the ulceration, and to take care of undercuts. This is especially important in intraoral lesions (◘ Fig. 10.5). Plasma treatment should be performed every 2–3 days and might be terminated after the elimination of the offensive smell generated by the anaerobe pathogens.

The CAP treatment can be implemented in daily wound treatment and dressing changes. No special aftercare is needed related to the use of CAP.

In principle, treatment can be delegated to a qualified nurse. Supervision by the medical specialist is a matter of course.

Conclusion

From a scientific point of view and on the basis of significant experimental and pre-clinical research, cold atmospheric plasma (CAP) should be very useful for the treatment of cancer. From a clinical point of view, however, CAP treatment of cancer is at present largely off-label use of the approved plasma medical devices. Nevertheless, there is a small range of indications to use CAP for the benefit of patients, especially in palliative cancer treatment. The antimicrobial efficacy of CAP can play a key role in the care of tumor patients in very advanced stage of disease with infected ulcerations of the tumor, lymph node, and skin metastasis.

Decontamination, treatment of superficial infections, and bacterial reduction have been among the first clinical findings of CAP effectiveness and fruitful applications. The antimicrobial capacities are useful for patients suffering from contaminated cancer ulcerations.

CAP application is deactivating bacteria, viruses, and fungi, but it is evident that cancer cells just below the layer of microbial pathogens are affected to some extent as well. The physiological and pathological background of these effects might be different. Plasma-induced immunogenic cell death has to be considered and modulation of inflammation, too. A combination of CAP with palliative cytostatic chemotherapy may confer additive cytotoxicity, as well as palliative radiotherapy.

References

1. Assadian O, Ousey KJ, Daeschlein G, Kramer A, Parker C, Tanner J, Leaper DJ. Effects and safety of atmospheric low-temperature plasma on bacterial reduction in chronic wounds and wound size reduction: a systematic review and meta-analysis. Int Wound J. 2019;16:103–11.
2. AWMF – Guidelines of scientific medical societies in Germany. Rational therapeutic use of cold physical plasma. Reg-No 007-107, Classification S2k (2020/21) submitted.
3. Bekeschus S, Clemen R, Niessner F, Sagwal SK, Freund E, Schmidt A. Medical gas plasma jet technology targets murine melanoma in an immunogenic fashion. Adv Sci. 2020;7(10): 1903438.
4. Bekeschus S, Moritz J, Helfrich I, Boeckmann L, Weltmann KD, Emmert S, Metelmann HR, Stoffels I, von Woedtke T. Ex vivo exposure of human melanoma tissue to cold physical plasma elicits apoptosis and modulates inflammation. Appl Sci. 2020;10(6):1971.

5.   Berner J, Seebauer C, Sagwal SK, Boeckmann L, Emmert S, Metelmann HR, Bekeschus S. Medical gas plasma treatment in head and neck cancer – challenges and opportunities. Appl Sci. 2020;10(6):1944.

6.   Chen Z, Simonyan H, Cheng X, Gjika E, Lin L, Canady J, Sherman J, Young C, Keidar M. A novel micro cold atmospheric plasma device for glioblastoma both in vitro and in vivo. Cancers. 2017;9(6):61.

7.   Daeschlein G, Scholz S, Ahmed R, von Woedtke T, Haase H, Niggemeier M, Kindel E, Brandenburg R, Weltmann KD, Jünger M. Skin decontamination by low-temperature atmospheric pressure plasma jet and dielectric barrier discharge plasma. J Hosp Infect. 2012;81: 177–83.

8.   Gjika E, Pal-Ghosh S, Kirschner ME, Lin L, Sherman JH, Stepp MA, Keidar M. Combination therapy of cold atmospheric plasma (CAP) with temozolomide in the treatment of U87MG glioblastoma cells. Sci Rep. 2020;10:16495.

9.   Hilker L, von Woedtke T, Weltmann KD, Wollert HG. Cold atmospheric plasma: a new tool for the treatment of superficial driveline infections. Eur J Cardiothorac Surg. 2017;51:186–7.

10.   Isbary G, Heinlin J, Shimizu T, Zimmermann JL, Morfill G, Schmidt HU, Monetti R, Steffes B, Bunk W, Li Y, Klaempfl T, Karrer S, Landthaler M, Stolz W. Successful and safe use of 2 min cold atmospheric argon plasma in chronic wounds: results of a randomized controlled trial. Br J Dermatol. 2012;167(2):404–10.

11.   Khalili M, Daniels L, Lin A, Krebs FC, Snook AE, Bekeschus S, Bowne WB, Miller V. Non-thermal plasma-induced immunogenic cell death in cancer. J Phys D Appl Phys. 2019;52:423001.

12.   Keidar M, Yan D, Sherman JH. Cold plasma cancer therapy. 1st ed. California: Morgan & Claypool Publisher; 2019. p. 4–5.

13.   Liedtke KR, Freund E, Hermes M, Oswald S, Heidecke CD, Partecke LI, Bekeschus S. Gas plasma-conditioned ringer's lactate enhances the cytotoxic activity of cisplatin and gemcitabine in pancreatic cancer in vitro and in ovo. Cancers. 2020;12(1):123.

14.   Lin AG, Xiang B, Merlino DJ, Baybutt TR, Sahu J, Fridman A, Snook AE, Miller V, Lin AG, Xiang B, Merlino DJ, Baybutt TR, Sahu J, Fridman A, Snook AE, Miller V. Non-thermal plasma induces immunogenic cell death in vivo in murine CT26 colorectal tumors. Onco Targets Ther. 2018;7:e1484978.

15.   McCormick KA, Fleming B. Clinical practice guidelines. The Agency for Health Care Policy and Research fosters the development of evidence-based guidelines. Health Prog. 1992;73(10):30–4.

16.   Metelmann H-R, Nedrelow DS, Seebauer C, Schuster M, von Woedtke T, Weltmann K-D, Kindler S, Metelmann PH, Finkelstein SE, Von Hoff DD, Podmelle F. Head and neck cancer treatment and physical plasma. Clin Plasma Med. 2015;3(1):17–23.

17.   Metelmann HR, Seebauer C, Miller V, Fridman A, Bauer G, Graves DB, Pouvesle JM, Rutkowski R, Schuster M, Bekeschus S, Wende K, Masur K, Hasse S, Gerling T, Hori M, Tanaka H, Ha Choi E, Weltmann KD, Metelmann PH, Von Hoff DD, von Woedtke T. Clinical experience with cold plasma in the treatment of locally advanced head and neck cancer. Clin Plasma Med. 2018;9:6.

18.   Miller V, Lin A, Fridman A. Why target immune cells for plasma treatment of cancer. Plasma Chem Plasma Process. 2016;36(1):259–68.

19.   Pasqual-Melo G, Sagwal SK, Freund E, Gandhirajan RK, Frey B, von Woedtke T, Gaipl U, Bekeschus S. Combination of gas plasma and radiotherapy has immunostimulatory potential and additive toxicity in murine melanoma cells in vitro. Int J Mol Sci. 2020;21(4):1379.

20.   Rutkowski R, Daeschlein G, von Woedtke T, Smeets R, Gosau M, Metelmann HR. Long-term risk assessment for medical application of cold atmospheric pressure plasma. Diagnostics (Basel). 2020;10(4):210.

21.   Sackett DL. Evidence-based medicine. Semin Perinatol. 1997;21(1):3–5.

22.   Schuster M, Seebauer C, Rutkowski R, Hauschild A, Podmelle F, Metelmann C, Metelmann B, von Woedtke T, Hasse S, Weltmann KD, Metelmann HR. Visible tumor surface response to physical plasma and apoptotic cell kill in head and neck cancer. J Craniomaxillofac Surg. 2016;44(9):1445–52.

10

23. Seebauer C, Freund E, Haase S, Miller V, Segebarth M, Lucas C, Kindler S, et al. Effects of cold physical plasma on oral lichen planus: an in-vitro study. Oral Dis. 2020;27(7):1728–37. https://doi.org/10.1111/odi.13697.

24. Semmler ML, Bekeschus S, Schäfer M, Bernhardt T, Fischer T, Witzke K, Rebl H, Grambow E, Vollmar B, Nebe JB, Metelmann H-R, Emmert S, Boeckmann L. Molecular mechanisms for the efficacy of cold atmospheric pressure plasma (CAP) in cancer treatment. Cancers. 2020;12(2): 1–19.

25. Yao X, Lin L, Soni V, Gjika E, Sherman JH, Yan D, Keidar M. Sensitization of glioblastoma cells 579 to temozolomide by a helium gas discharge tube. Phys Plasma. 2020;27:114502.

26. Seebauer C, et al. Palliative Plasmabehandlung von Kopf-Hals-Tumoren und kurative Konzepte. In: Plasmamedizin. Berlin Heidelberg: Springer. https://doi.org/10.1007/978-3-662-52645-3_8.

27. Seebauer C, et al. Palliative treatment of head and neck cancer. In: Comprehensive clinical plasma medicine. Springer Nature; 2018. p. 187. https://doi.org/10.1007/978-3-319-67627-2_10.

Cold Atmospheric Plasma Treatment and Surgical Site Infections

Rico Rutkowski, Vu Thi Thom,
Nguyen Dinh Minh,
and Hans-Robert Metelmann

Contents

© Springer Nature Switzerland AG 2022
H.-R. Metelmann et al. (eds.), *Textbook of Good Clinical Practice in Cold Plasma Therapy*, https://doi.org/10.1007/978-3-030-87857-3_11

Core Messages

- Surgical site infections represent a significant epidemiological burden in both low-income developing countries and high-income industrialized countries, affecting millions of people.
- Pathogens directly related to SSI can be of endogenous or exogenous origin, with the risk of local pathogen entry both in the period between the surgical incision and wound closure and in the postoperative phase.
- Clinical advantages in the application of cold atmospheric plasma in the context of SSI include increased reduction of bacterial load, a reduction of the postoperative pain level, a shortening of the wound healing time, and an improved aesthetic outcome.

11.1 Introduction

Thermal atmospheric plasma has been established for several decades in medical applications (including surface conditioning, technical sterilization, disinfection, and electrosurgery) [1, 2]. Based on technological innovations, various concepts for the generation of cold atmospheric plasma (CAP) have been developed in recent years [3–5]. In a biomedical application horizon that is constantly growing in both theory and practice, wound therapy, similar as the handling of infectious skin diseases, is one of the best-investigated treatment indications. Despite the fact that the subcellular, immunological, and molecular biological signaling cascades, mechanisms and interactions between cold atmospheric plasma and tissue are not completely understood. Yet, a wide antimicrobial and wound healing promoting potential is demonstrated in several in vitro and in vivo studies [6–11]. The combination of antimicrobial efficacy and high biocompatibility within the scope of wound healing disorders and in skin and mucosa compromised infections suggests that the innovative technology of cold atmospheric plasma should not only be used to reduce an existing pathology but also as part of preventive strategies.

11.2 Diagnosis and Role of Surgical Site Infection (SSI)

Despite an enormous improvement in surgical techniques, sterilization methods, pharmacological prophylaxis, and an increasing pathophysiological understanding of wound healing in the last decades, surgical site infections (SSI) are among the most common healthcare-associated nosocomial infections [12, 13]. The US Center for Disease Control and Prevention (CDC) has declared antibiotic resistance to be among the world's most pressing public health concerns. However, despite differences in incidence and prevalence, SSI not only occur in low-income developing countries, but also represent a significant epidemiological burden in high-income countries affecting millions of people worldwide [14–16]. SSI are infections that occur in or next to the surgical incision during the first 30 days after surgery (if an implant is inserted up to 1 year), and can inter alia be classified clinically based on their anatomical depth (incisional (superficial or deep) or organ/space) [17]. The most important clinical signs include erythema, swelling, pain, local overheating, and, depending on the anatomical region, functional limitations. Early detection can be difficult, as it can take several days before the classic symptoms manifest themselves. SSI are directly associated with increased morbidity and mortality [12, 18, 19]. These circumstances are often associated with prolonged pain and impaired function, prolonged hospitalization, recurrent surgery, or, in the worst case, death due to a progressive, systemic infection. Demographic change and closely associated conditions like a rising number of surgical interventions (especially in the outpatient sector), multimorbidity, and polypharmacy, as well as the growing challenge of global microbial resistance problems are directly linked to an increased expenditure for diagnostics and treatment [20–23]. While there exists an undeniably estimated number of unknown SSI cases on the one hand and although there is no widely accepted method to evaluate healthcare costs due to complications on the other hand, it is highly evident that SSI are responsible for a substantial increase in healthcare-related costs [24–26].

11.3 Physiology and Pathology

Pathogens that are directly related to SSI can be of endogenous or exogenous origin. The most significant risk occurs in the time between the surgical incision and wound closure [27, 28]. Especially the resident flora (intra- and extraoral) is of particular importance [29, 30]. Regarding the most common pathogens, there is a distinct correlation with the type of surgical procedure performed. Considering the distribution shown in ◘ Table 11.1, it becomes clear that the physiological flora of the body, also called standard flora, carries a significant proportion of causative pathogens. Overall, the amount of multiresistant organisms associated with wound infections has been increasing for decades [31, 32]. Quantitatively, it could be shown that a microbial colonization of $>10^5$ microorganisms per gram of tissue significantly enhances the risk of developing a SSI [33]. In addition to the large microbiological risk component, there are various other predisposing factors that can also impact the risk of SSI [34–40]. Knowledge about certain dependent and independent risk factors allows the implementation of an adequate risk assessment as well as the conception and use of targeted prevention and therapeutic measures. ◘ Table 11.2 shows an overview of selected risk factors.

11.4 Standard Treatment Principles

Due to the enormous clinical and economic consequences of surgical site infections, the need for effective preventive and therapeutic strategies is increasing. It has been estimated that approximately half of SSI are preventable by the use of evidence-based strategies [13]. Considering individual and general risk factors, this requires a

◘ Table 11.1 Most common SSI-causing pathogens in Germany depending on the surgical area (Data from KISS-Surveillance-System (Modul OP KISS), 01/2012–12/2016) [59, 60]

Frequency #	Abdominal surgery		Traumatology		Gynecology		Overall	
	Pathogen	Ratio (%)	Pathogen	Ratio (%)	Pathogen	Ratio (%)	Pathogen	Ratio (%)
1	E. coli	31.39	S. aureus (MRSA ratio)	29.95 11.96	S. aureus (MRSA ratio)	19.96 11.05	S. aureus (MRSA ratio)	18.92 14.19
2	Enterococcus spp.	30.02	Koagulase neg. Staph.	21.25	E. coli	12.90	Enterococcus spp.	17.82
3	P. aeroguinosa	6.22	Enterococcus spp.	11.41	Enterococcus spp.	10.36	E. coli	15.61
4	Klebsiella spp.	6.20	E. coli	5.17	Koagulase neg. Staph.	8.38	Koagulase neg. Staph.	14.64
5	Bacteroides spp.	5.13	Enterobacter spp.	2.94	Proteus spp.	5.29	P. aeroguinosa	4.51

11

◘ Table 11.2 Selection of various risk factors that affect SSI occurrence [60]

Preoperative	Perioperative	Postoperative
General Low/high age Malnutrition Obesity Nicotine/alcohol Local and systemic infections ASA-score >2 Cortisone therapy **Comorbidities** Diabetes mellitus Renal insufficiency (requiring dialysis) Disease of blood-forming system Liver disease Cytotoxic therapy	**General** Insufficient disinfection of hands and operations area Deficient sterilization of instruments and implants Hypothermia Hypoxia Mismatching perioperative antibiotic therapy **Operation specific** High NNIS-score Delayed or extended operation time Type of operation (e.g., emergency, recurrence, contaminated, infected) Surgical technique Expertise of the surgeon	Inadequate wound care Drains Improperly prolonged parenteral nutrition Not indicated prolongation of systemic antibiotic therapy Stress ulcer Incorrectly adjusted blood glucose Pain Hypothermia Hypoxia Numerous preoperative risk factors

ASA Classification of the American Society of Anesthesiologists, *NNIS* National Nosocomial Infections Surveillance Score combination of different interdisciplinary preoperative, intraoperative, and postoperative approaches including risk reduction of bacterial colonization as a key challenge. Besides basic hygienic measures like hand disinfection, professional treatment of medical devices, weight reduction, smoking cessation, risk-adjusted screening and remediation measures, nutritional supplementation, pharmacological adjustments, as well as various measures to prepare the patient and the surgical site for the upcoming surgery are also important in the preoperative setting [41–45]. Furthermore, there was shown an increased significance for intraoperative factors such as skin antiseptic, antimicrobial prophylaxis, surgical techniques, measures for the reduction of dead space, and monitoring acid-base and electrolyte balance as well as blood and glycemic control under anesthesia [46–50]. Accordingly, there are various evidence-based strategies in the postoperative period which essentially comprise type and duration of antimicrobial prophylaxis as well as wound management [51–55]. Current recommendations originate from worldwide leading institutions such as World Health Organization (WHO) and the CDC [12, 13]. ◘ Table 11.3 provides an overview of actual recommended pre-, intra-, and postoperative strategies.

11.5 Treatment Rationale

The rationale for the use of cold atmospheric plasma is the possibility of multimodal therapy within a single treatment. Depending on the dosage, especially the lethal effect against numerous pathogens on the one hand and the influence of metabolic processes, cell migration, cell proliferation, and angiogenesis on cellular and subcellular level, which stimulate wound healing, on the other hand, seem promising. Summarizing all scientifically and clinically evidence-based findings, there is a considerable common intersection between preventative and therapeutic anti-SSI approaches and the indications and potentials of clinical use of cold atmospheric plasma. Particularly against the background of best possible reduction of bacterial load as a key challenge, different approaches result for plasma medicine.

11.6 Cold Plasma Therapy

In numerous surgical disciplines, a fundamental perioperative risk for the occurrence of SSI is closely related to the typically high proportion of facultative pathogens.

11.6.1 Case I

Besides the tumor resection, the removal of cervical lymph nodes is another important part of surgical first-line therapy of head and neck cancer. During surgery, a temporary connection between oral cavity, tumor mass, and neck wound is not

□ Table 11.3 In 2014, the Healthcare Infection Control Practices Advisory Committee (HICPAC) reviewed and suggested strong recommendations (mod.) of CDC (1999) that should be accepted as practice for preventing surgical site infections [61]

Preparation of the patient	Identify and treat all infections remote to the surgical site before elective operations and postpone elective operations on patients with remote site infections until the infection has resolved Do not remove hair preoperatively unless the hair at or around the incision site will interfere with the operation. If hair removal is necessary, remove immediately before the operation, with clippers Tobacco cessation for a minimum of at least 30 days before elective operations Skin around the incision site should be free of gross contamination before performing antiseptic skin preparation
Hand/forearm antisepsis for surgical team	Perform preoperative surgical hand/forearm antisepsis according to manufacturer's recommendations for the product being used
Operating room ventilation	Maintain positive pressure ventilation in the operating room and adjoining spaces Maintain the number of air exchanges, airflow patterns, temperature, humidity, location of vents, and use of filters
Cleaning and disinfection of environmental surfaces	Do not perform special cleaning or closing of operating rooms after contaminated or dirty operations
Reprocessing of surgical instruments	Sterilize all surgical instruments according to published guidelines and manufacturer's recommendations Immediate-use steam sterilization should never be used for reasons of convenience, as an alternative to purchasing additional instrument sets, or to save time (exception: patient care items that will be used immediately in emergency situations when no other options are available)
Surgical attire and drapes	Wear a surgical mask that fully covers the mouth and nose when entering the operating room if an operation is about to begin or already underway, or if sterile instruments are exposed (throughout the operation) Wear a new, disposable, or hospital laundered head covering for each case, when entering the operating room and ensure it fully covers all hair on the head and all facial hair not covered by the surgical mask Wear sterile gloves if serving as a member of the scrubbed surgical team and put on sterile gloves after donning a sterile gown Use surgical gowns and drapes that are effective barriers when wet (i.e., materials that resist liquid penetration) Change scrub suits that are visibly soiled, contaminated, and/or penetrated by blood or other potentially infectious materials
Sterile and surgical technique	Adhere to principles of sterile technique when performing all invasive surgical procedures If drainage is necessary, use a closed suction drain Place a drain through a separate incision distant from the operative incision and remove the drain as soon as possible
Post-op incision care	Protect primarily closed incisions with a sterile dressing for 24–48 hours postoperatively

11

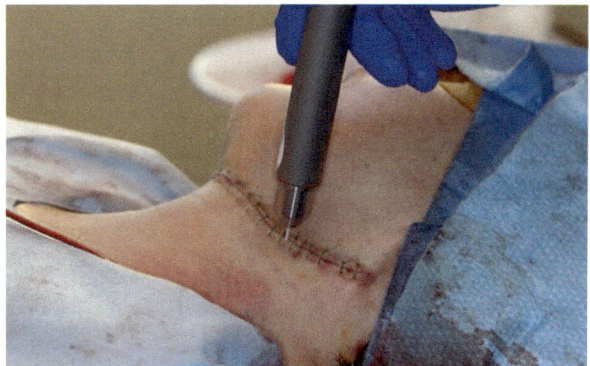

◘ **Fig. 11.1** Reducing microbial load and supporting wound healing in early wound healing period after neck dissection. CAP treatment was performed at 30 s/cm² within the intraoperative setting, immediately after wound closure

uncommon. Due to the high risk for spreading of microbiological colonization (intra- and postoperatively) with a subsequent increased hazard for SSI, we applied CAP with the intention of reducing the microbial load (◘ Fig. 11.1). CAP treatment was performed at 30 s/cm² within the intraoperative setting, immediately after wound closure, with continuous movement of the plasma torch. No SSI was observed in the neck dissection area in the 13 patients treated thus far.

11.6.2 Case II/III

Tracheotomy wounds, as well as the extensive wound surfaces after abdominoplasties, are occasionally associated with SSI. Following significant weight loss, patients show residual problems due to the redundant skin and functional restriction. Several studies identified independent risk factors for the development of SSI and consequential prolonged hospital stay [56, 57]. In addition to general risk factors resulting from different comorbidities (i.e., diabetes mellitus, immunosuppression, smoking), abdominoplasty-specific variables increase the overall risk. These include hygienic difficulties, insufficient microcirculation in fat tissue, and chronically recurring skin infections. Consequently, we started to support early wound healing by daily application of CAP (◘ Figs. 11.2 and 11.3). CAP treatment was performed at 30 s/cm² (once a day, for a total of 10 of respectively 14 days) postoperatively. No SSI was observed in the 21 patients treated thus far.

11.6.3 Case IV

Donor site wound healing disorders after raising of microvascular flaps for reconstructive surgery represents another indication for plasma treatment (◘ Fig. 11.4, currently treatment of five patients completed). Ideally suited for reconstruction of orofacial defects with good functional and cosmetic results, the radial forearm flap is often criticized for donor site complications and morbidity [58]. After subtotal loss of the split skin graft, CAP treatment was performed at 30 s/cm² (once a day, for a total of 10 days).

◘ Fig. 11.2 Application of CAP, directly after surgical tracheostomy wound closure. CAP treatment was performed at 30 s/cm² (once a day, for a total of 10 days) postoperatively

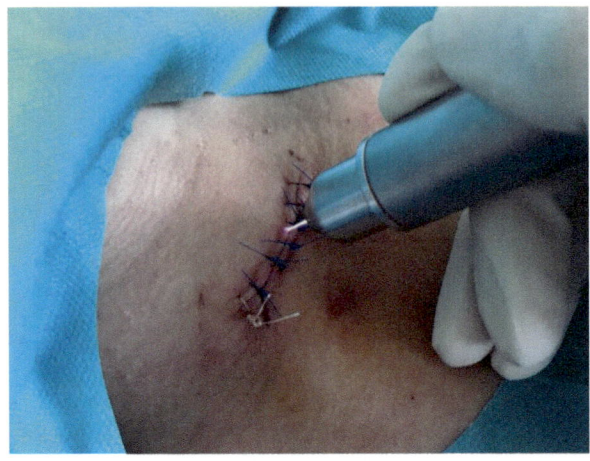

◘ Fig. 11.3 Application of CAP in the area of the right abdomen after abdominoplasty. CAP treatment was performed at 30 s/cm² (once a day, for a total of 14 days) along the infected scar, with continuous movement of the plasma torch as recommended by the manufacturer

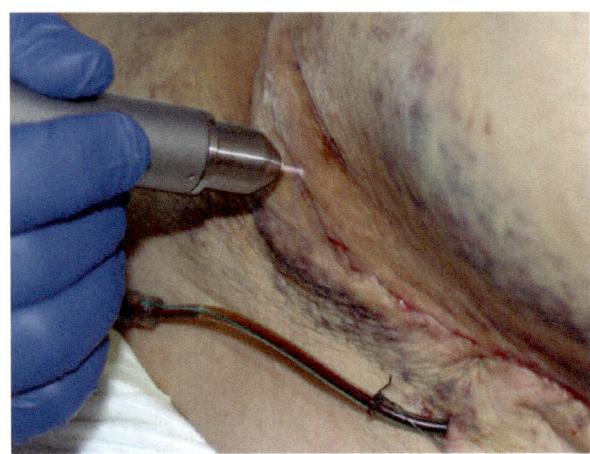

11

11.6.4 Case V

A Vietnamese adult patient was diagnosed with T-hemisphere cranial defect and after 1 year underwent brain traumatic surgery. The patient received antibiotics including vimotram and ciprofloxacin by vein infusion. During his hospital stay, the wound surface was directly treated with both CAP and prontosan (a type of wound gel) in combination. The wound area was continuously treated with CAP dose of 30 s/cm² once a day for 75 days. The result is presented in ◘ Fig. 11.5 showing the beneficial effect of CAP treatment with the large and complicated wound area. A questionnaire was provided to the patient during treatment and the day of discharge from the hospital concerning the pain feeling. The patient did not feel pain, itching, or discomfort during plasma treatment.

Fig. 11.4 CAP treatment for donor site wound healing disorder after raising of microvascular radial forearm flap. After subtotal loss of the split skin graft, CAP treatment was performed at 30 s/cm² (once a day, for a total of 10 days) in the area of the graft donor site, with continuous movement of the plasma torch. During CAP therapy, increasing wound bed granulation was observed in all treated cases without functional impairment of the forearm or hand

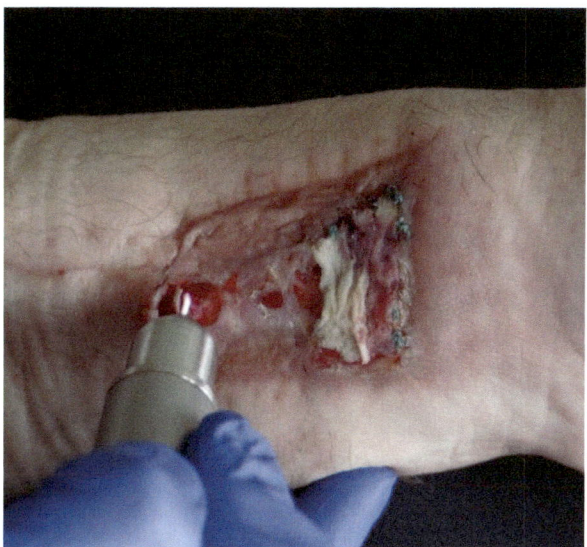

11.6.5 Case VI

A Vietnamese pediatric patient was admitted to the hospital for congenital heart defects surgery. After surgery, the patient suffered multiple ulcer lesions at the occipital knob that was continuously treated by CAP once a day for 40 days with dose of 30 s/cm² (Fig. 11.6). The wound site was examined to be infected with *A. baumannii*. Antibiotics, anti-inflammation drugs, and nutrition was provided to the patient during hospital stay. For this pediatric patient the questionnaire was not applied.

Plasma therapy was performed with kINPen© MED (neoplas tools GmbH, Greifswald, Germany) in cases I–IV. The CAP device used for case V and VI generated a cold gliding arc plasma under atmospheric pressure and a modulated DC power supplier with 5.9 kV peak voltage and 50 Hz frequency. Argon gas was used with a flow rate of 8 L/m which pushes the plasma column with a velocity of about 10 ms^{-1}. Evaluation of wound healing including CAP impact on local quantitative microbial load and the aesthetic-reconstructive result, both from the patient's and an observer's view, were collected. Hyperspectral imaging (HSI) was used to monitor and objectify the impact of CAP on microcirculation in and around plasma-treated area. Within the preoperative approach, analysis of microbial contamination was performed by quantitative microbiological tests. The collected data were evaluated against comparative data without CAP therapy. Concerning a still ongoing data collection, the evaluation could not be completed yet. However, an interim evaluation already indicates various clinical advantages in the patient group treated with CAP. These benefits include the following facts:

- Higher reduction of bacterial load in preoperative setting (added to normal skin antiseptic; publication under review)
- Efficient reduction of bacterial load in postoperative setting (quantitative comparison to the standard wound treatment still pending; publication under review)

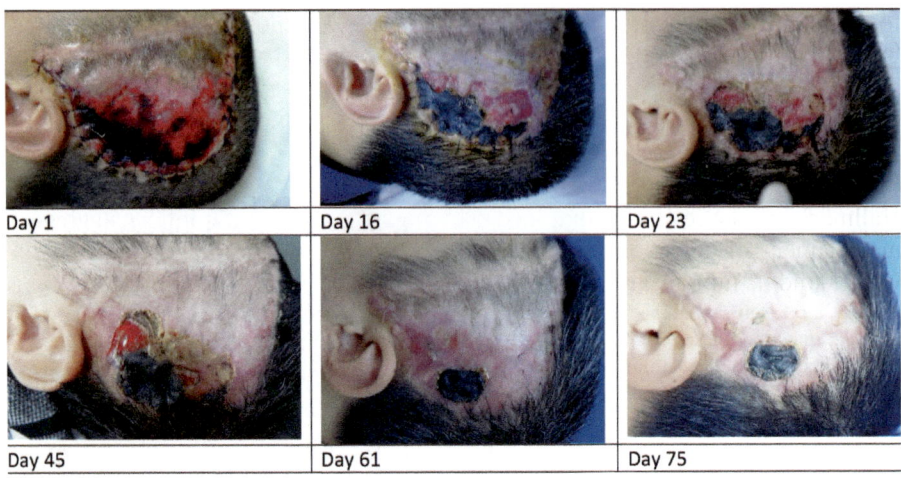

Fig. 11.5 CAP treatment for the wound diagnosis of T-hemisphere cranial defect in a patient with a history of brain traumatic injury surgery. The patient was treated with CAP (30 s/cm^2 once a day for 75 days). The plasma torch was moved continuously on the entire wound area

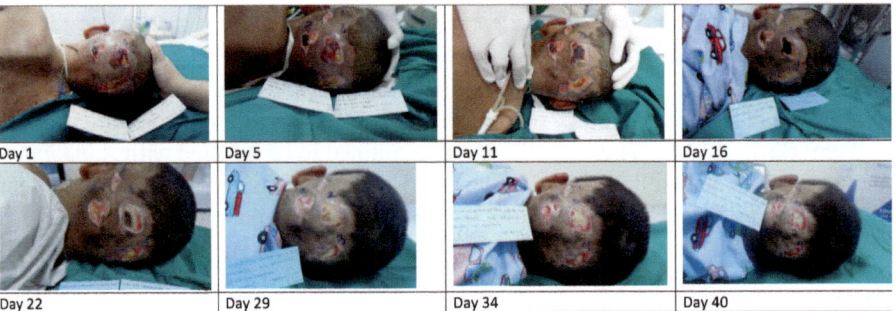

Fig. 11.6 A pediatric patient who had undergone congenital heart defects surgery had occipital multiple ulcer lesions treated with CAP (30 s/cm^2, once a day)

- Reduction of postoperative pain level
- Shortening the period of wound healing
- Significantly increased oxygen saturation superficially and deeply immediately after CAP treatment, lasting for a longer time (Plasma-associated impact on microcirculation exceeds the field of actual plasma application, publication under review)
- Decrease of functional rehabilitation time of the hand after CAP treatment on donor site of radial forearm flap
- Functional-aesthetic improvement of scars (analyzed by POSAS score)
- A sure indication of reduction of hospitalization (e.g., oncology patients could be treated more quickly with adjuvant therapy)

Both the preoperative as well as the postoperative CAP application could be performed without the occurrence of acute therapy-associated complications. Long-term follow-up examinations (6–60 months after the last CAP treatment) have thus far shown no signs of negative side effects or complications.

Conclusion

Surgical site infections are one of the most common nosocomial infections worldwide and impact the increase of morbidity and mortality as well as healthcare-related costs significantly. Exceeding the limit of the actual health care system, there is the urgent need for additional and new evidence-based anti-SSI strategies. Especially due to the central task of the best possible reduction of bacterial load within anti-SSI concept, CAP could be the missing key for this major challenge. Own research results as well as numerous external studies illustrate the enormous potential of plasma medicine in the context of SSI prevention and therapy. According to our clinical experience, CAP can easily be integrated into the preoperative and postoperative setting. Especially in postoperative care, there is the possibility of delegation, stationary as well as outpatient. Cross-sectional areas such as the interaction of plasma with liquids, for example, to increase the antiseptic effects, will expand current scientific and clinical questions. However, there is still a need for further evidence-based prospective research to improve the clinical use of CAP, extend existing indications, and fulfill the integration into daily clinical practice.

References

1. Moisan M, Barbeau J, Crevier M-C, Pelletier J, Philip N, Saoudi B. Plasma sterilization. Methods and mechanisms. Pure Appl Chem. 2002;74(3):349–58.
2. Von Woedtke T, Kramer A, Weltmann KD. Plasma sterilization: what are the conditions to meet this claim? Plasma Process Polym. 2008;5(6):534–9.
3. Bárdos L, Baránková H. Cold atmospheric plasma: sources, processes, and applications. Thin Solid Films. 2010;518(23):6705–13.
4. Bekeschus S, Schmidt A, Weltmann K-D, von Woedtke T. The plasma jet kINPen–A powerful tool for wound healing. Clin Plasma Med. 2016;4(1):19–28.
5. Conrads H, Schmidt M. Plasma generation and plasma sources. Plasma Sources Sci Technol. 2000;9(4):441.
6. Daeschlein G, Scholz S, Ahmed R, Von Woedtke T, Haase H, Niggemeier M, et al. Skin decontamination by low-temperature atmospheric pressure plasma jet and dielectric barrier discharge plasma. J Hosp Infect. 2012;81(3):177–83.
7. Daeschlein G, Scholz S, Arnold A, von Podewils S, Haase H, Emmert S, et al. In vitro susceptibility of important skin and wound pathogens against low temperature atmospheric pressure plasma jet (APPJ) and dielectric barrier discharge plasma (DBD). Plasma Process Polym. 2012;9(4):380–9.
8. Daeschlein G, von Woedtke T, Kindel E, Brandenburg R, Weltmann KD, Jünger M. Antibacterial activity of an atmospheric pressure plasma jet against relevant wound pathogens in vitro on a simulated wound environment. Plasma Process Polym. 2010;7(3–4):224–30.
9. Isbary G, Morfill G, Schmidt H, Georgi M, Ramrath K, Heinlin J, et al. A first prospective randomized controlled trial to decrease bacterial load using cold atmospheric argon plasma on chronic wounds in patients. Br J Dermatol. 2010;163(1):78–82.

10. Isbary G, Stolz W, Shimizu T, Monetti R, Bunk W, Schmidt H-U, et al. Cold atmospheric argon plasma treatment may accelerate wound healing in chronic wounds: results of an open retrospective randomized controlled study in vivo. Clin Plasma Med. 2013;1(2):25–30.
11. Tipa RS, Kroesen GM. Plasma-stimulated wound healing. IEEE Trans Plasma Sci. 2011;39(11):2978–9.
12. Allegranzi B, Zayed B, Bischoff P, Kubilay NZ, de Jonge S, de Vries F, et al. New WHO recommendations on intraoperative and postoperative measures for surgical site infection prevention: an evidence-based global perspective. Lancet Infect Dis. 2016;16(12):e288–303.
13. Berríos-Torres SI, Umscheid CA, Bratzler DW, Leas B, Stone EC, Kelz RR, et al. Centers for Disease Control and Prevention guideline for the prevention of surgical site infection, 2017. JAMA Surg. 2017;152(8):784–91.
14. Allegranzi B, Nejad SB, Combescure C, Graafmans W, Attar H, Donaldson L, et al. Burden of endemic health-care-associated infection in developing countries: systematic review and meta-analysis. Lancet. 2011;377(9761):228–41.
15. Magill SS, Edwards JR, Bamberg W, Beldavs ZG, Dumyati G, Kainer MA, et al. Multistate point-prevalence survey of health care–associated infections. N Engl J Med. 2014;370(13): 1198–208.
16. European Centre for Disease Prevention and Control, Suetens C, Hopkins S, Kolman J, Högberg LD. Point prevalence survey of healthcare-associated infections and antimicrobial use in European acute care hospitals: 2011–2012: Publications Office of the European Union; 2013.
17. Horan TC, Andrus M, Dudeck MA. CDC/NHSN surveillance definition of health care–associated infection and criteria for specific types of infections in the acute care setting. Am J Infect Control. 2008;36(5):309–32.
18. Jarvis WR. Selected aspects of the socioeconomic impact of nosocomial infections: morbidity, mortality, cost, and prevention. Infect Control Hosp Epidemiol. 1996;17(8):552–7.
19. Kirkland KB, Briggs JP, Trivette SL, Wilkinson WE, Sexton DJ. The impact of surgical-site infections in the 1990s: attributable mortality, excess length of hospitalization, and extra costs. Infect Control Hosp Epidemiol. 1999;20(11):725–30.
20. Barnett K, Mercer SW, Norbury M, Watt G, Wyke S, Guthrie B. Epidemiology of multimorbidity and implications for health care, research, and medical education: a cross-sectional study. Lancet. 2012;380(9836):37–43.
21. Laxminarayan R, Duse A, Wattal C, Zaidi AK, Wertheim HF, Sumpradit N, et al. Antibiotic resistance—the need for global solutions. Lancet Infect Dis. 2013;13(12):1057–98.
22. Maher RL, Hanlon J, Hajjar ER. Clinical consequences of polypharmacy in elderly. Expert Opin Drug Saf. 2014;13(1):57–65.
23. World Health Organization. Antimicrobial resistance: global report on surveillance. Geneva: World Health Organization; 2014.
24. Magill SS, Hellinger W, Cohen J, Kay R, Bailey C, Boland B, et al. Prevalence of healthcare-associated infections in acute care hospitals in Jacksonville, Florida. Infect Control Hosp Epidemiol. 2012;33(3):283–91.
25. Broex E, Van Asselt A, Bruggeman C, Van Tiel F. Surgical site infections: how high are the costs? J Hosp Infect. 2009;72(3):193–201.
26. Umscheid CA, Mitchell MD, Doshi JA, Agarwal R, Williams K, Brennan PJ. Estimating the proportion of healthcare-associated infections that are reasonably preventable and the related mortality and costs. Infect Control Hosp Epidemiol. 2011;32(2):101–14.
27. Bowler P, Duerden B, Armstrong DG. Wound microbiology and associated approaches to wound management. Clin Microbiol Rev. 2001;14(2):244–69.
28. Singh R, Singla P, Chaudhary U. Surgical site infections: classification, risk factors, pathogenesis and preventive management. Int J Pharma Res Health Sci. 2014;2(3):203–14.
29. Geffers C, Baerwolff S, Schwab F, Gastmeier P. Incidence of healthcare-associated infections in high-risk neonates: results from the German surveillance system for very-low-birthweight infants. J Hosp Infect. 2008;68(3):214–21.
30. Towfigh S, Cheadle WG, Lowry SF, Malangoni MA, Wilson SE. Significant reduction in incidence of wound contamination by skin flora through use of microbial sealant. Arch Surg. 2008;143(9):885–91.

11

31. Gjødsbøl K, Christensen JJ, Karlsmark T, Jørgensen B, Klein BM, Krogfelt KA. Multiple bacterial species reside in chronic wounds: a longitudinal study. Int Wound J. 2006;3(3):225–31.
32. Neu HC. The crisis in antibiotic resistance. Science. 1992;257(5073):1064–74.
33. Krizek TJ, Robson MC. Evolution of quantitative bacteriology in wound management. Am J Surg. 1975;130(5):579–84.
34. Chen S, Anderson MV, Cheng WK, Wongworawat MD. Diabetes associated with increased surgical site infections in spinal arthrodesis. Clin Orthop Relat Res. 2009;467(7):1670–3.
35. Gaynes RP, Culver DH, Horan TC, Edwards JR, Richards C, Tolson JS, et al. Surgical site infection (SSI) rates in the United States, 1992–1998: the National Nosocomial Infections Surveillance System basic SSI risk index. Clin Infect Dis. 2001;33(Supplement_2):S69–77.
36. Harrington G, Russo P, Spelman D, Borrell S, Watson K, Barr W, et al. Surgical-site infection rates and risk factor analysis in coronary artery bypass graft surgery. Infect Control Hosp Epidemiol. 2004;25(6):472–6.
37. Leong G, Wilson J, Charlett A. Duration of operation as a risk factor for surgical site infection: comparison of English and US data. J Hosp Infect. 2006;63(3):255–62.
38. Malone DL, Genuit T, Tracy JK, Gannon C, Napolitano LM. Surgical site infections: reanalysis of risk factors. J Surg Res. 2002;103(1):89–95.
39. ter Gunne AFP, Cohen DB. Incidence, prevalence, and analysis of risk factors for surgical site infection following adult spinal surgery. Spine. 2009;34(13):1422–8.
40. Vilar-Compte D, de Iturbe IÁ, Martín-Onraet A, Pérez-Amador M, Sánchez-Hernández C, Volkow P. Hyperglycemia as a risk factor for surgical site infections in patients undergoing mastectomy. Am J Infect Control. 2008;36(3):192–8.
41. Melling AC, Ali B, Scott EM, Leaper DJ. Effects of preoperative warming on the incidence of wound infection after clean surgery: a randomised controlled trial. Lancet. 2001;358(9285):876–80.
42. Hetem DJ, Bootsma MC, Bonten MJ. Prevention of surgical site infections: decontamination with mupirocin based on preoperative screening for Staphylococcus aureus carriers or universal decontamination? Clin Infect Dis. 2015;62(5):631–6.
43. Darouiche RO, Wall MJ Jr, Itani KM, Otterson MF, Webb AL, Carrick MM, et al. Chlorhexidine–alcohol versus povidone–iodine for surgical-site antisepsis. N Engl J Med. 2010;362(1):18–26.
44. Tanner J, Norrie P, Melen K. Preoperative hair removal to reduce surgical site infection. The Cochrane Library; 2011.
45. Parienti JJ, Thibon P, Heller R, Le Roux Y, von Theobald P, Bensadoun H, et al. Hand-rubbing with an aqueous alcoholic solution vs traditional surgical hand-scrubbing and 30-day surgical site infection rates: a randomized equivalence study. JAMA. 2002;288(6):722–7.
46. Obermeier A, Schneider J, Wehner S, Matl FD, Schieker M, von Eisenhart-Rothe R, et al. Novel high efficient coatings for anti-microbial surgical sutures using chlorhexidine in fatty acid slow-release carrier systems. PLoS One. 2014;9(7):e101426.
47. Kurz A, Sessler DI, Lenhardt R. Perioperative normothermia to reduce the incidence of surgical-wound infection and shorten hospitalization. N Engl J Med. 1996;334(19):1209–16.
48. Buchleitner AM, Martínez-Alonso M, Hernández M, Solà I, Mauricio D. Perioperative glycaemic control for diabetic patients undergoing surgery. The Cochrane Library; 2012.
49. Meyhoff CS, Wetterslev J, Jorgensen LN, Henneberg SW, Høgdall C, Lundvall L, et al. Effect of high perioperative oxygen fraction on surgical site infection and pulmonary complications after abdominal surgery: the PROXI randomized clinical trial. JAMA. 2009;302(14):1543–50.
50. Beldi G, Bisch-Knaden S, Banz V, Mühlemann K, Candinas D. Impact of intraoperative behavior on surgical site infections. Am J Surg. 2009;198(2):157–62.
51. Silva JM, de Oliveira AMR, Nogueira FAM, Vianna PMM, Pereira Filho MC, Dias LF, et al. The effect of excess fluid balance on the mortality rate of surgical patients: a multicenter prospective study. Crit Care. 2013;17(6):R288.
52. Masden D, Goldstein J, Endara M, Xu K, Steinberg J, Attinger C. Negative pressure wound therapy for at-risk surgical closures in patients with multiple comorbidities: a prospective randomized controlled study. Ann Surg. 2012;255(6):1043–7.

53. Dumville JC, Gray TA, Walter CJ, Sharp CA, Page T, Macefield R, et al. Dressings for the prevention of surgical site infection. The Cochrane Library; 2016.
54. Ata A, Lee J, Bestle SL, Desemone J, Stain SC. Postoperative hyperglycemia and surgical site infection in general surgery patients. Arch Surg. 2010;145(9):858–64.
55. Gyssens IC. Preventing postoperative infections: current treatment recommendations. Drugs. 1999;57(2):175–85.
56. Vu MM, Gutowski KA, Blough JT, Simmons CJ, Kim JY. Development of an individualized surgical risk calculator for abdominoplasty procedures. Plast Reconstr Surg. 2015;136(4S):95–6.
57. Massenburg BB, Sanati-Mehrizy P, Jablonka EM, Taub PJ. Risk factors for prolonged length of stay in abdominoplasty. Plast Reconstr Surg. 2015;136(4S):164–5.
58. Richardson D, Fisher SE, Vaughan DE, Brown JS. Radial forearm flap donor-site complications and morbidity: a prospective study. Plast Reconstr Surg. 1997;99(1):109–15.
59. Infektionen NRfrSvn. Modul OP-KISS, Referenzdaten Berechnungszeitraum: Januar 2012 bis Dezember 2016. 2017.
60. Rutkowski R, Schuster M, Unger J, Metelmann I, Chien TTT. Cold atmospheric plasma in context of surgical site infection. In: Comprehensive clinical plasma medicine. Cham: Springer International Publishing; 2018. p. 151–62.
61. U.S. Department of Health and Human Services CfDCaP. Meeting Minutes: Healthcare Infection Control Practices Advisory Committee (HICPAC). 2014.

11

Cold Plasma Treatment for an Artificial Fistula at Risk

*Lutz Hilker, Thomas von Woedtke,
Kai Masur, Klaus-Dieter Weltmann,
Hans-Georg Wollert,
and Alexander Kaminski*

Contents

© Springer Nature Switzerland AG 2022
H.-R. Metelmann et al. (eds.), *Textbook of Good Clinical Practice in
Cold Plasma Therapy*, https://doi.org/10.1007/978-3-030-87857-3_12

🏅 **Core Message**
- CAP has the potential for effective treatment of superficial artificial fistula infections, especially in patients with LVAD-associated drivelines.
- In patients with the need for surgical revision of ascending artificial fistula infections, CAP is a potent tool for intraoperative use during wound dressings and has a positive impact on the granulation and the epithelialization process.
- After wound closure in anatomically difficult areas, the use of CAP fastens the wound healing process and reduces the onset of wound infections.
- The combination of negative pressure wound therapy (NPWT) with the use of CAP has a positive effect on wound healing in patients with chronic wounds.

12.1 Introduction

Patients with implants that have contact points through the skin are generally at risk of infection at these points of contact. Unfavorable conditions can lead to an increase in infection of the wound through subsequent bacteremia which can progress to sepsis. The mortality rate in such cases is very high. In general, the patients most affected are those with a ventricular assist device (VAD), tunneled or non-tunneled atrial dialysis catheter (ADC), or peritoneal dialysis catheter (PDC). It is common that such devices are vital for the survival of these patients and, often, alternative options for therapy do not exist.

Fifty percent of all infections for hemodialysis patients are generated through the catheter [1]; 1.6–5.5% infections during 1000 tunneled-catheter days and a surprisingly high 3.8–6.6% through non-tunneled [2, 3]. It is reported that in the 2000 AD decade, the relevant US population was treated for 100,000 catheter-induced bacteremia cases yearly at a cost of US\$ 22,000 per case. The total cost of these infections may approach \$1 billion [4, 5]. Although the bacteremia incidents are considerably lower for patients with a peritoneal dialysis catheter, the risk for peritonitis increases regardless [6].

Driveline infections (DI) occur for VAD patients in 14–48% of the cases [7]. According to the INTERMACS-Database, an infection rate of 19% was described for the years 2006–2010 within the first 12 months [8]. Next to gastrointestinal bleeding and stroke, DI are the most common reason for unplanned hospital stays for left ventricular assist device (LVAD) patients at an average cost of US\$ 7000 per case [9].

The most widely used LVADs are currently the HeartWare device (Co. *Medtronic*) and the Heartmate device (Co. *Abbott*). The power supply for its pump is provided through an electric cable, the so-called driveline, which is coated with polyurethane and partially covered by Teflon. The driveline, partially transmuscular or completely subcutaneous, exits the body to the left or right of the central abdomen (M. rectus abdominis). Due to the large surface area, the potential for infection is considerable as a result of the formation of biofilms [10]. Inadequately treated infection areas can rapidly lead to rising infection levels resulting in death.

The most commonly encountered pathogens are Staphylococcus aureus, coagulase-negative Staphylococcus, Corynebacterium, Pseudomonas aeruginosa und Enterobacteriaceae [11].

12.2 **Diagnosis**

Founded in 2019, the "Driveline Expert Staging and Care (DESTINE)" study group concluded with and defined six condition stages of driveline exit-points for LVAD patients, whereby stages 0–2 are subdivided into a and b stage. In short, stage 0 classifies the exit-point as being without pathological findings, whereas a positive medical smear test is verified at stage 0b.

Stage 1a displays irritation and redness of a dry wound, whereas 1b constitutes a non-reddened, yet secreting, wound. A stage 2 wound presents a local infection with redness and swelling without detection of bacteria, while local pus formation and a positive medical swab is found in 2b. Stage 3 is a systematic infection defined by pyrexia and a positive blood culture. Hypergranulation at the exit-point or, as the case may be, phlegmonous changes, are added to stage 4. Stage 5 indicates a verified ascending infection [12].

12.3 **Standard Treatment Principles**

Changing wound dressing regularly for LVAD patients is essential for the prevention of impairment to the wound-healing process. The patient and the closest caregiver (e.g., family member, health care professional) are instructed on how to change the dressing correctly. If the skin is irritated at the contact point, the wound dressing needs to be changed daily, whereas the dressing of inconspicuous wounds can be changed less frequently at 2–3 times per week. In general, this will entail wiping the wound centrifugally with chlorhexidine or octenidine. Subsequently, the driveline exit-site is wrapped ("sandwich technique") with sterile compresses and plasters, by which the driveline is fixed next to the exit wound using a special fixation plaster on the abdominal wall to avoid friction.

This is essential to relieve strain or pull of any kind on the driveline exit-site, including relieving any steady mechanical strain, as these are a substantial factor in the emergence of adverse events on superficial wound healing. The second factor, on which only the patient can influence, is the excessive alimentary body fat of the abdominal wall as this can generally lead to a funnel effect at the driveline exit-site. The edges of this area are at risk due to mechanical macerations caused by the driveline itself or subsequent superinfections caused by to skin microbiota.

Should a superficial driveline exit-point become infected showing serous inflammation or putrid secretion and redness around the edges, it is to be treated with antibiotics (initial swab test to determine the efficacy of chosen treatment in case of antibiotic resistance) and by changing the wound dressing daily. If no improvement is reached or, rather, the condition worsens, such as deepening of the wound infection, then local surgery is necessary to excise the affected skin followed, if necessary, by negative pressure wound therapy (NPWT) and closing the wound a second time. Such procedures often require long periods of hospitalization with, under certain conditions, reoccurring negative impact on wound healing. Further therapies could include exposing and relocating the driveline. As a last resort, it could lead to a complete replacement of the mechanical system or, even, for a patient displaying the preconditions, a highly urgent heart transplant with considerable surgical risks.

12.4 Treatment Rationale

Especially these patients have often built up antibiotic resistance, through oral antibiotic therapies with tissue-penetrating active substances. For this reason, the search for a new method for sustainable wound disinfection and speeding up the healing process has become a high priority in scientific medical research. Cold atmospheric pressure plasma (CAP) appears to be such a new option for severe wound infection therapies. Already established in the 1970s, atmospheric-pressure plasma has been applied to and on the human body for medicinal purposes.

12.5 Cold Atmospheric Plasma (CAP) Therapy

The antimicrobial and wound-healing effects of CAP plasma have already been proven. Until now, no adverse or serious side effects resulting from plasma treatment have been noted. Based on the current fields of application for promoting the healing process, especially for the treatment of chronic wounds and infectious skin ailments, the medically approved *"kINPen med"* (approved since 2013, a medical device from the company *neoplas tools*, Greifswald) presents itself as a particularly useful tool in hospital treatments of beginning DI, on the one hand due to its potent antimicrobial effect and on the other due to its ability to regulate, target, monitor, and modify the doses, so as not to create a lethal impact on the mammalian cells or tissues.

Another, similarly effective option is the medical device "plasma care" (company *terrasplasma MEDICAL*, Garching). This device, which is considerably smaller and is not bound to a carrier gas vessel, is of particular interest for outpatient treatment of red exit-points or skin areas displaying only early-stage superficial DLI. The modification of this device for plasma application, including the required exchangeable spacers for treating cable exit-point wounds, is still being evaluated (◘ Fig. 12.1).

Preliminary investigations in 2014 by the Leibniz Institute for Plasma Science and Technology (INP) in Greifswald initially focused on the effects of the *"kINPen med"* on the driveline casing. In the experimental setup, driveline samples were selectively treated with a CAP jet between 15 and 240 minutes, the results being documented photographically (◘ Fig. 12.2a–f).

After a treatment time of 60 minutes, the polyurethane coating of the driveline showed light discoloration without damage to the coating itself (◘ Fig. 12.2c). After 240 minutes of radiation, a noticeably intense discoloration had appeared without damaging the insulation (◘ Fig. 12.2f). To rule out variables in the results by electromagnetic influence on the pump or the controller, the plasma treatment on the driveline was carried out by a pump dummy. No evidence was found related to influence on the pump function or controller parameters.

◘ Fig. 12.1 Model of a modificated spacer for the plasma care device for plasma application in VAD, ADC, and PDC patients

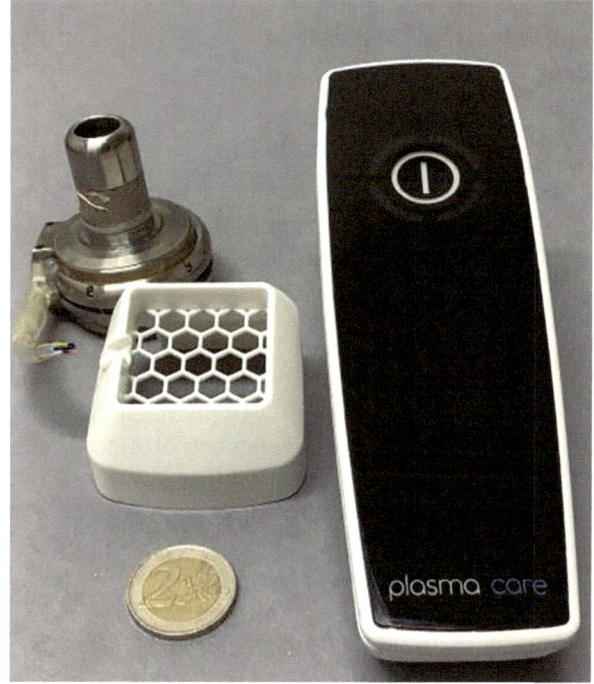

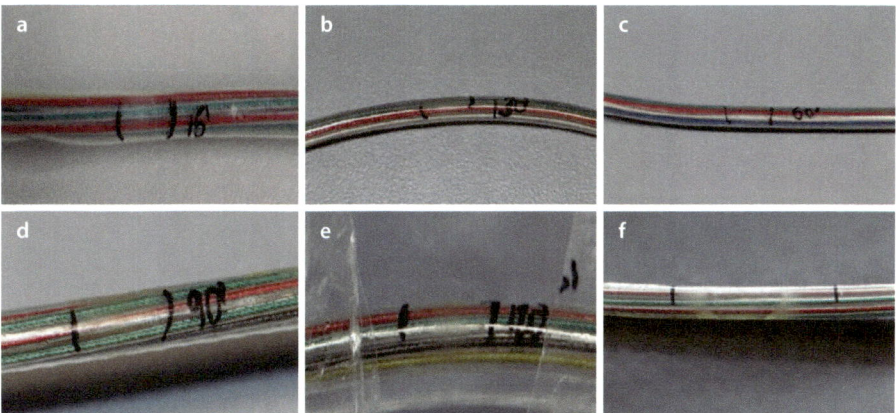

◘ Fig. 12.2 Effects of the continuous cold plasma application on the driveline isolation of the company *HeartWare/Medtronic*. **a–f**, After 15, 20, 60, 90, 120, and 240 minutes

12.5.1 Pretreatment Assessment

Preoperative diagnostics include a medical smear test, inflammation and antico-agulation laboratory parameters, ultrasonography of the ascending aorta, a thoraco-abdominal computer tomography to detect ascending DI, and in cases with suspected pump infection, a positron emission tomography computer tomography (PET-CT). Daily photo documentation of the driveline exit (DLE) has to be done.

12.5.2 Timing

The success of the treatment of DI depends on one side on its DESTINE stage and on the other side on an early and consequent treatment.

12.5.3 Diagnosis and Treatment Planning

The first implementation of CAP plasma in the Clinic for Cardiovascular Surgery, Clinic Karlsburg, was in September 2014, for a patient with a *HeartWare* pump implant who needed destination therapy after a fulminant myocardial infarction [13]. The *"kINPen med"* was continually applied at bedside. For this, the required cartridge of argon gas and the plasma generator were attached to a hand trolley, thereby making it mobile (◘ Fig. 12.3).

◘ **Fig. 12.3** Karlsburg plasma trolley for bedside plasma therapy

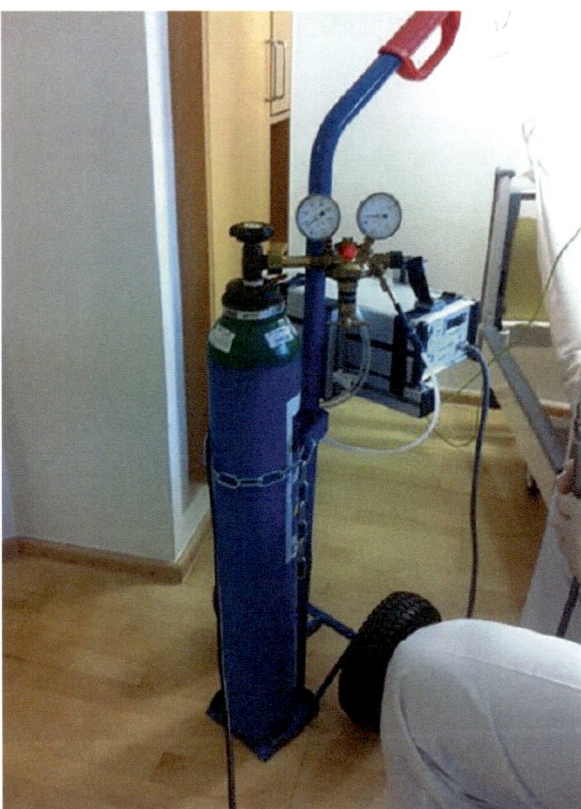

12

❶ Caution
> The hand-held nozzle with the plasma flame rotates at a distance of approximately 8 mm above the wound area to ensure that the application duration does not exceed 1 minute/cm^2.

The jet-like character of the device is greatly advantageous, optimal for radiation of fissures, canals, and wound cavities.

Clinical Tip

For surgical use, the handpiece and the gas-flow hose are packed in a sterile ultrasound cover, where a hole of approximately 1 cm diameter is cut at its end with a pair of sterile scissors. To ensure that only the capillary of the "*kinPen med*" perforates, the middle finger of a size-8 sterile glove, where the tip is pierced with an approximately 2 mm hole, is drawn through the hole in the sheath. Understandably, it is important to ensure that the capillary does not come into contact with the wound when operating the device. Before and after each operation, the capillary as well as the handpiece are swiped to prevent smear infections. In doing so, the disinfectant (liquid or drops) must not enter the capillary, as this will alter the quality of the plasma.

12.5.3.1 Superficial Driveline Infection (DESTINE-Stage 1a/b and 2a/b)

For these stages, along with increasing the frequency of changing the wound dressing to daily and 3-hour exposures of the DLE to air while at rest, a reasonable outpatient therapy is the CAP application at a rate of 2–3 times weekly over 3 weeks (■ Fig. 12.4). At the detection of pathogens, a suitable antibiotic treatment should accompany the CAP application. To improve the effectiveness of therapy in such cases, daily applications of plasma with the plasma care device provides a further option (■ Fig. 12.1).

12.5.3.2 Superficial Driveline Infection (DESTINE-Stage 3)

If positive blood cultures are verified, hospitalization and treatment of the patient with IV-antibiotics is inevitable. In such cases, the wound dressing is to be changed

■ **Fig. 12.4** Bedside treatment of a superficial DI (DESTINE-stage 2a)

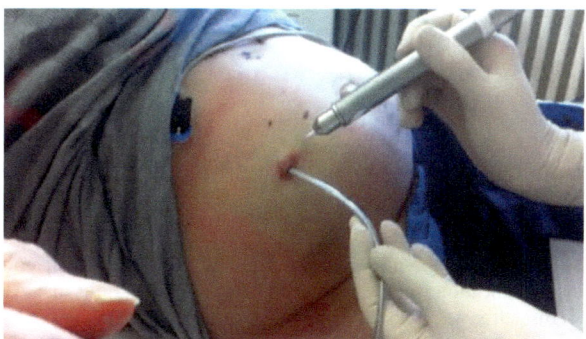

daily as in stage 1, and photographic documentation is necessary. Ten CAP treatments are recommended at first and doubled to twenty where necessary. These can be carried out on inpatient or outpatient basis. Furthermore, a computer tomography, as well as a TEE, shall follow to rule out an ascending DLI. Generally, the *"kINPen med"* can be used for the plasma therapy.

12.5.3.3 Superficial Driveline Infection (DESTINE-Stage 4)

Including the symptoms of stage 3, this stage further includes hemorrhagic hypergranulation in the sense of a fistula. At an early stage, often the same local treatment described in stage 2 is possible. The hypergranulation should, however, be treated with a silver nitrate stick to help it dissolve. Close attention is to be paid to ensure that silver nitrate remnants do not remain on the skin in the wound area, as this can lead to pronounced necroses. In principle, dissolving with silver nitrate removes the fistula tissue, making way for healing of the wound by CAP application.

A 68-year-old patient exhibited signs of an onset infection at the driveline exit-point 2 years after a *HeartWare* LVAD implant under cardiogenic shock due to a cardiac infarction. The initial intensely reddened and putrid secreting wound (pathogen: Clostridium difficile) worsened, despite a suitable antibiotic therapy using clindamycin. The wound developed circumscribed hypergranulation with continued infection. The antibiotic therapy had to be discontinued due to bacterial resistance.

After a singular application of silver nitrate, CAP was applied for over 1 minute each time on 12 consecutive days. Hypergranulation, secreting, and the redness declined sufficiently for the patient to be discharged. After four additional outpatient plasma treatments (once a week), the wound had completely healed [13]. Six months later, the patient returned to the clinic due to infectious complications at the driveline exit-point. The wound displayed hypergranulation and secretion at 7:00 (◘ Fig. 12.5a). The CAP therapy described above was subsequently repeated.

12

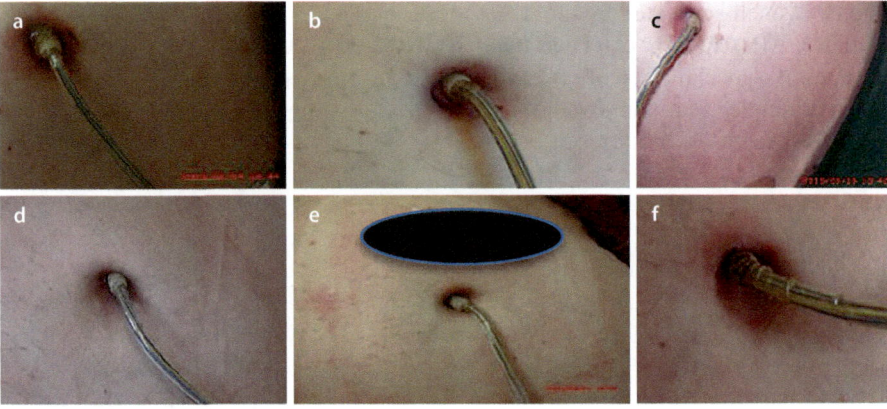

◘ **Fig. 12.5** Relapse of a superficial DI at the driveline exit-point at 8:00. **a** Original state, **b** Before local application of silver nitrate, **c** After 19 applications of CAP, **d** After 25 applications of CAP, **e** At discharge, **f** 2 years later

The wound healing improved as shown in ◘ Fig. 12.5. The patient remained without pathological findings for the duration of the following year (5f).

12.5.3.4 Ascending Driveline Infection (DESTINE-Stage 5) with Surgical Proximal Relocation Using Operative CAP Implementation and Primary Wound Closure

If an ascending infection occurs due to biofilm, an operative stabilization of this skin area is unavoidable and needs to be carried out promptly. Depending on the germ spectrum and anatomical conditions, a rise up to the pocket of the pump with the resulting consequences can develop within 14 days. The surgery should be conducted as follows: The incurred driveline canal is marked with methylene blue, the affected area excised, the biofilm and affected Teflon-felt area of the driveline is removed, and this skin area is closed after thorough disinfection using sodium hybrid solution and CAP treatments, using an inserted suction drain.

In the case of a 55-year-old patient suffering from nonischemic cardiomyopathy, the driveline was tugged after an LVAD implant (Company HeartWare/ Medtronic). This created micro-lesions of the skin which led to a rising DI (◘ Fig. 12.6b), triggered by the skin microbiota.

At first, the conservative approach described in case 1 patient was followed. Although improvement was seen soon after treatment, signs of a beginning/onset ascending DI appeared (◘ Fig. 12.6c). A surgical revision was required. After a spindle-shaped excision of the edges of the wound and flushing, the driveline was lateralized with intraoperative cold CAP application for 2 minutes (◘ Fig. 12.6d). The wound was closed using Prolene step-stitches and treated with CAP every alternative day. Although the driveline was tugged again after the stitches had been removed and a light prolapse occurred, the wound remained dry and non-irritated

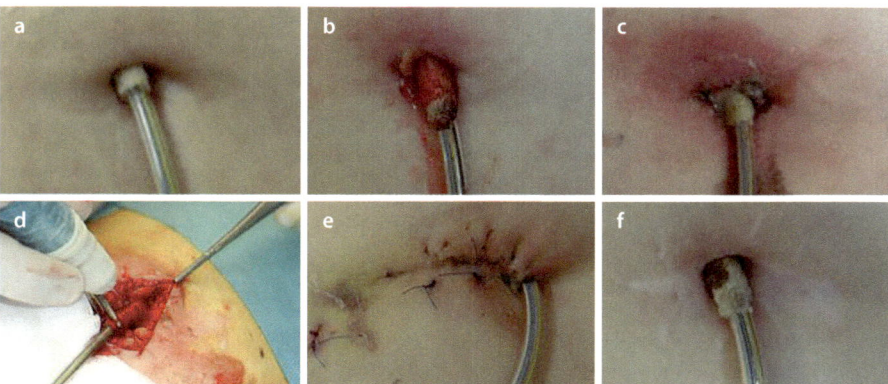

◘ **Fig. 12.6** Ascending DI with effective therapy and operative cold plasma treatments. **a** Original state, **b** Putrid secretion with hypergranulation at 11:00, **c** After a therapy trial using silver nitrate and cold plasma. The wound is dry, yet shows distinct signs of an ascending DI. **d** Surgical restoration by lateralization of the driveline exit-points and operative cold plasma treatment. **e** Status on postoperative day 13 after six superficial plasma applications. **f** Non-irritated status 1 year after surgical restoration as it was treated once again with 6 weeks of CAP therapy (■ Fig. 12.6e). Even after 12 months, no skin irritations or infections had appeared. The current condition is also non-irritated (■ Fig. 12.6f).

12.5.3.5 Ascending Driveline Infection (DESTINE-Stage 5) with Abscess Formation Near Exit-Points and Effective Subsequent Revisions Leading to Preservation of the Driveline Exit-Points; Use of NPWT with Intermediate CAP Therapy and Secondary Wound Closure

If through a CT scan or ultrasound an ascending abscess can be verified in the area where the initial superficial DI had been detected, an attempt at local stabilization can be made. This can be done through draining the abscess and subsequently treating the wound using 3-day NPWT therapy and local CAP application. In addition, the exit-points are treated with daily CAP applications.

An LVAD was implanted as destination therapy, in the case of a 55-year-old patient with ischemic cardiomyopathy. Half a year after implantation, a medical swab test showed Staphylococcus aureus at a superficial DI site. Because a conservative approach is unlikely to reduce such an infection, a surgical procedure was needed. Complete healing followed. At a planned checkup 6 months later, renewed wound secretion with verified Staphylococcus aureus (■ Fig. 12.7a) was observed. A CT showed light infiltration of the infection of the ascending driveline canal (■ Fig. 12.7b). As the patient displayed no or minimal infectious symptoms, the patient was treated on an outpatient basis with oral clindamycin. Four weeks later, a 2-dimensional planar redness of the skin appeared approximately 5 cm above the driveline exit-point.

12

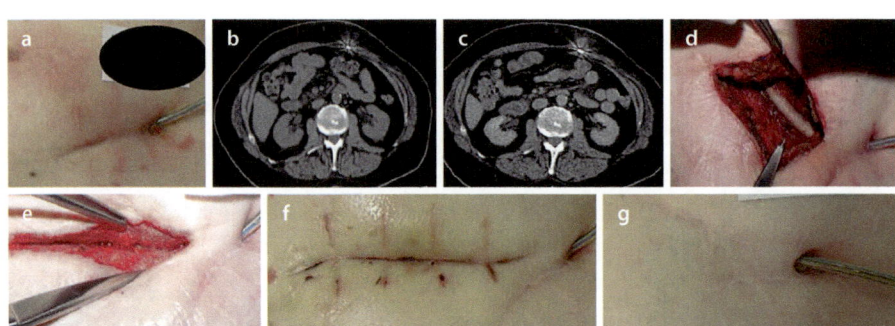

■ **Fig. 12.7** Abscess in region of the ascending driveline with surgical relief and following VAC plasma therapy. **a** Secreting driveline exit-point, distinct reddening in ascending driveline canal. **b** Mild tissue infiltration above the driveline exit-point in the abdominal CT scan. **c** Distinct increase in abscess formation. **d** Effective abscess relief. Felt cover of the exposed driveline visible. **e** Condition after 28 days of VAC plasma therapy, accompanied with dressing change every third day. The driveline is completely covered by granulation tissue, making a secondary closure of the wound possible. **f** Condition 24 days after secondary wound closure. **g** Condition 6 months after secondary wound closure

Both the CT and the ultrasound evidenced a 2×2 cm^2 abscess. A surgical stabilization was needed (■ Fig. 12.7c).

The operation confirmed the diagnostic findings. The medical swab test of the operation showed, again, a Staphylococcus infection. At the depths of the wound, the felt casing/covering of the exposed driveline was found (■ Fig. 12.7d). A canal leading to the driveline exit-point was found distally, and a further canal the length of approximately 2 cm, proximally. As an octenidine treatment of deep wound fistulas is not recommended due to its known cytotoxicity, the wound was rinsed with hydrogen peroxide and 5 minutes of cold plasma were applied. The procedure was concluded with additional rifampicin instilled in the canals. NPWT was applied postoperatively. Cold plasma was applied at each of the following dressing changes every 3 days. Complete granulation of the wound at the driveline exit-point followed (■ Fig. 12.7e). After inconspicuous medical swab tests at the wound site, the secondary wound closure could be applied after 28 days. The inserted Redon's (suction) drain was removed centimeter by centimeter on day 5 post surgery. Cold plasma therapy continued daily at the site of the stitches at the driveline exit-point. After another 11 days, the condition of the wound was completely free of irritation, so the patient could be discharged to continue outpatient therapy (■ Fig. 12.7f). A completely irritation-free driveline exit-point was still seen after another 6 months.

12.5.3.6 Ascending Driveline Infection (DESTINE-Stage 5) with Effective Driveline Revision; Negative Pressure Wound Therapy); Intermediate CAP Application and Secondary Wound Closure

If a surgical primary wound closure as depicted in case 4. is not an option based on the conditions given, one proceeds, at first, with the steps set forth under 5.; a combination of NPWT and intermediate CAP application (the so-called PlasVAC-therapy). This is to be done until a clean granulation of the wound floor is achieved. Based on our experience, for more extensive wounds it is advisable; in the case that no hypergranulation seems to be achievable; to remove the felt casing of the driveline completely. This lowers the high risk of reinfection after secondary wound closure (■ Fig. 12.8).

12.5.3.7 Severe, Secreting Ascending Pseudomonas Aeruginosa-Associated Driveline Infection with Surgical Plasma Therapy and Relocation of Driveline as Last Resort

The following example serves to illustrate a complicated development, which leads one to surmise that the success rate for the treatment of wounds associated to foreign bodies which are to be retained depends completely on the pathogen spectrum.

A 72-year-old patient suffering from dilated cardiomyopathy received an LVAD implantation (Co. *HeartWare/Medtronic*) as the destination therapy. Six months later a postoperative superficial DI appeared.

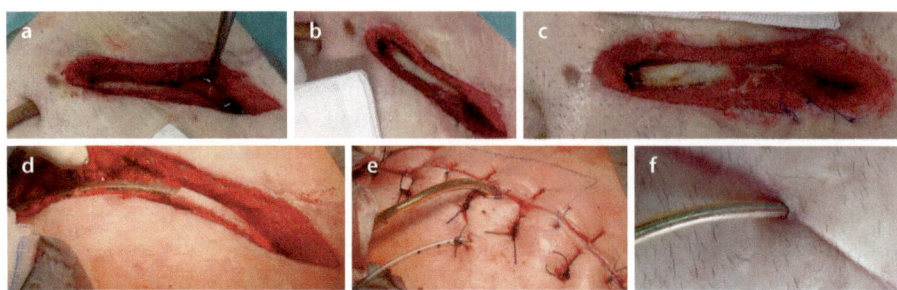

Fig. 12.8 Abscess in region of the ascending driveline with surgical relief and following VAC plasma therapy. **a** Secreting driveline exit-point, effective relief of the abscess in the ascending driveline canal. **b** Beginning hypergranulation. **c** Hypergranulation after three VAC therapy cycles. **d** Secondary wound closure with excision of the DLE, partial removal of the driveline felt and intraoperative CAP therapy. **e** Condition at the end of surgery. **f** Condition 30 days after secondary wound closure

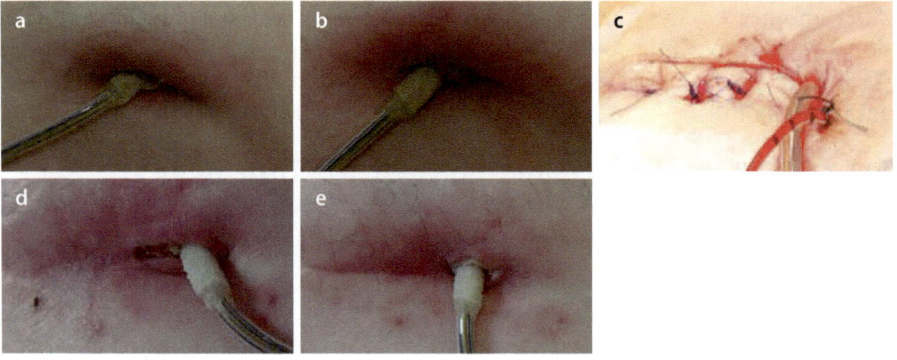

Fig. 12.9 Recurrence of superficial, onset ascending DI, colonized by Pseudomonas aeruginosa. **a** Original state with severe secretion; hypergranulation at 2:00. **b** After 30 days of conservative therapy no improvement. **c** After excision of driveline and lateral relocation. **d** Still postoperative wound dehiscence and redness after 3 weeks. **e** Wound also displays mild irritation 5 weeks post-operatively

It could be successfully treated as in case 1 patient. Four months later, an infection reoccurred (■ Fig. 12.9a); this time with Pseudomonas aeruginosa evidenced in the medical swab test. The conservative approach was repeated by way of plasma application and antibiotic-therapy; with tazobactam at first, uninterrupted use of ceftazidime later on. As this did not lead to improvement (■ Fig. 12.9b), a wound revision operation was indicated.

The intervention occurred as described in Patient case 2. Antibiotic therapy continued postoperatively and cold plasma was applied daily. The driveline exit-point remained conspicuously reddened, along with mild secretion evidencing Pseudomonas aeruginosa. The otherwise inconspicuous patient was discharged.

Four weeks later, the patient presented a still secreting, Pseudomonas-infected wound; a now hypertrophic driveline exit-point (■ Fig. 12.10a); latent rising CRP (C-reactive protein) values, and dot-like rash on the legs (■ Fig. 12.10b). Hospitalized once again, the patient received the required therapies; these being continuous ceftazidim and CAP applications. Intracavitary vegetation was ruled out by way of transoesophageal echocardiography. The condition of the wound improved (■ Fig. 12.10c) and the infection-associated rash largely disappeared (■ Fig. 12.10d). The patient was discharged.

An acute deterioration of the condition of the wound after 14 days led to renewed hospitalization. The indications of an ascending DI justified a surgical revision. Due to increasing wound infection, a total of 3 more revision surgeries spaced a month apart were necessary, despite cold plasma therapy. Subsequently, frequent resistance-modifications against the Pseudomonas bacteria eventually led to the development of a 3-MDRGN bacteria (Pseudomonas root). Nevertheless, cold plasma therapy continued, combined with dressing changes every third day. Although the wound closed, the skin remained red. Furthermore, the medical swab test of the wound verified a Pseudomonas species, making renewed wound revision necessary. This eventually led to exposing the entire driveline as far down as the subxiphoid region. A biofilm and the expanded polytetrafluorethylene (ePTFE) driveline casing had to be surgically removed. Finally, a gentamicin sponge was inserted and the wound was closed (■ Fig. 12.11f). Fourteen days later, hospital-

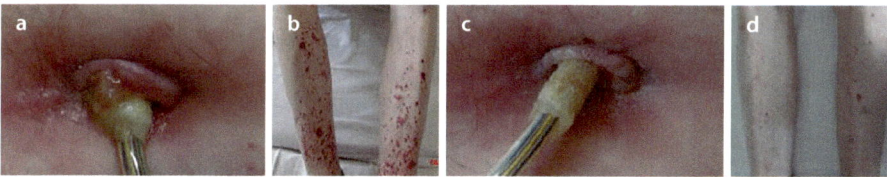

■ **Fig. 12.10** Secretion caused by Pseudomonas aeruginosa combines with infection-related rash on legs. **a** Pseudomonas infected secretion. **b** Infection-related splotch-shaped petechia on the lower legs. **c** Largely dry, hypertrophic driveline exit-points after antibiotic treatments and cold plasma therapy. **d** Reduction of rash on the lower legs

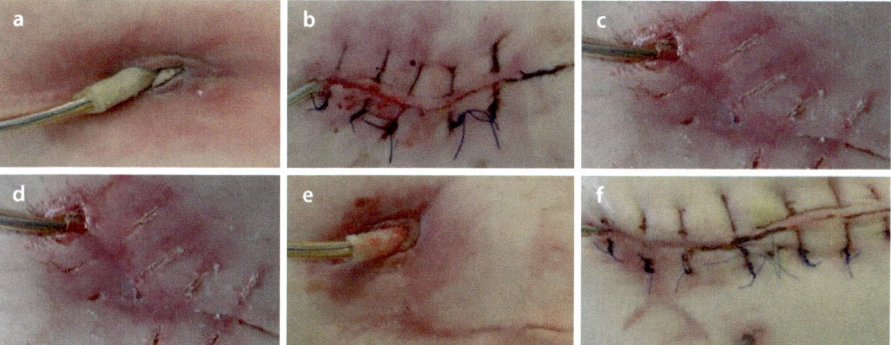

■ **Fig. 12.11** Repeated wound infections through Pseudomonas-related DI. **a** Repeated, increasing wound dehiscence and wound redness. **b** Renewed surgical lateral relocation with cold plasma application. **c** Persistent infection reaction despite cold plasma therapy. **d** Wound revision with NPWT. **e** Despite granulation using VAC and cold plasma therapy, persistent wound redness. **f** Renewed wound revision with exposure of the driveline as deep as the subxiphoidale region, insertion of gentamicin sponge and wound closure

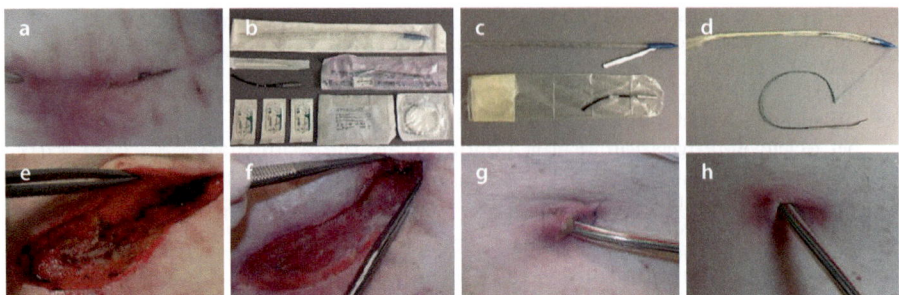

☐ **Fig. 12.12** Driveline-relocation therapy. **a** Renewed secretion with increasing splotchy redness. **b** Material required in order to tunnel the driveline. **c** Positioning the plug of the pump in the thorax chest tube. **d** Construction for sterile driveline relocation prepared by Hilker. **e** Former driveline bed. Remnant of driveline seen deep in the upper corner. **f** Granulation covering the driveline using VAC and cold plasma therapy. **g** Postoperative driveline neo-exit-point. **h** Driveline status after 12 months

ization was required once again due to the worsening condition of the wound (☐ Fig. 12.12a).

A driveline-relocation-therapy was necessary. The driveline was surgical mobilized subxiphoidally; disinfected; disconnected after applying 10,000 IU Heparin; packed into a sterile ultrasound-overcoat and thorax chest tube (☐ Fig. 12.11c); and finally tunneled into the opposite side, so that as little of the driveline as possible could be seen in the upper corner. Without delay, because an LVAD was involved, anesthesiological systems of supportive care; had to be in place prior to the procedure. The controller should be reconnected within 1 minute. The original driveline bed was treated with 3 days of alternating VAC and plasma applications; until the canal granulated over (☐ Fig. 12.9f). The neo-driveline-exit-point was treated daily with cold plasma (☐ Fig. 12.9g). The patient could be discharged soon after. Six months later, the wound was inconspicuous.

❯ Important to Know

> In summary, as illustrated by the patient's healing process, we can conclude that Pseudomonas aeruginosa colonized wound infections, as opposed to wound infections of other germ spectrums, pose a noticeable challenge, even for cold plasma therapy.

12.5.4 Anesthesia

Anesthetic management has to be organized as usual for LVAD patients with abdominal surgery. For the control of infusion and the catecholamine management a VAD-monitor is advantageous. The shock function of the defibrillator has to be interrupted during the operation. Perioperative antibiotic prophylaxis is indispensable. The interruption of anticoagulation has to be as short as possible.

12.5.5 **Posttreatment Care**

The posttreatment care depends on the surgical procedure. In cases with intraoperative NPWT a wound dressing change has to be done every 3 days. In these cases, the plasma application will be done during the dressing changes. After reaching a good granulation state, in the best case with granulation covered driveline a secondary wound closure should be done. After this dressing changes with concomitant CAP-application should be done daily. The enclosed Redon drainage should be left of this skin area for 3–7 days. Antibiotic treatment has to be continued for 10–21 days.

12.5.6 **Handling of Complications**

Most common complications are postoperative bleeding or wound reinfections, and has to be treated the usual way. Insufficient VAC dressings has to be changed immediately.

Conclusion

Meanwhile, CAP applications are established and routinely used for DI patients at the Clinic for Cardiovascular Surgery of the Clinic Karlsburg, despite the lack of reimbursement through health insurance. Other cardio surgery hospitals report the use of cold plasma applications [14]. With CAP therapy often potentially life-threatening, explanations could be prevented. In particular, using the simple and user-friendly bedside device with its jet-like character enabling application for deep fissures and canals has been of great advantage to patients. To date, the lack of side effects and displayed compatibility of the treatment is very good. Temporary pain-like paresthesia might be experienced only when the maceration wound is fresh.

To date, CAP has been used for greatly differing and complicated wound conditions and has repeatedly displayed its capability for accelerating the wound-healing process [15]. Experience gained when using cold plasma for beginning DI leads us to foresee that the use of cold plasma methods for prevention of catheter-associated infections for dialysis patients would be feasible in widespread, routine treatment. Catheter exit-points could even be treated with cold plasma during the dialysis therapy, to maximize efficiency of patient treatment time.

Further research is needed concerning the characteristics, capability, and application possibilities of varying forms of plasma, in order to determine how wounds in various regions of the human body, with varying pathogens, can be optimally treated. For this, the following fields of research are of particular value:
- Plasma modifications to optimize use for wounds of differing genesis in diverse regions of the human body and with the existence of diverse pathogens
- The possibility of sterilizing surgical instruments with plasma sterilization during surgical interventions
- Effects of plasma atmosphere during operations in visceral cavities
- Plasma wound disinfection for primary and secondary wound closures
- Plasma treatment of the closed wound in the early postoperative phase

- Plasma treatment of artificial fistula
- Activation of the plasma surfaces prior to implantations
- Plasma surface modifications to improve the biocompatibility of implants

Based on the very obvious benefits for the patients and the future social-economic advantages gained through plasma applications, we can hope and, according to our experience, expect that reasonable reimbursement will be instituted in due course and lead to wide recognition and acceptance of this method among the medical profession and patients.

References

1. Dittmer ID, Sharp D, McNulty CAM, et al. A prospective study of central venous haemodialysis catheter colonization and peripheral bacteraemia. Clin Nephrol. 1999;51:34–9.
2. Hannah EL, Stevenson KB, Lowder CA, et al. Outbreak of haemodialysis vascular access site infections related to malfunctioning permanent tunneled catheters: making the case for active infection surveillance. Infect Control Hosp Epidemiol. 2002;23:538–41.
3. Saxena AK, Panhorota BR, Al-Mulhim AS. Vascular access-related infections in haemodialysis patients. Saudi J Kidney Dis Transplant. 2005;16:46–71.
4. Engemann JJ, Friedman JY, Reed SD, et al. Clinical outcomes and costs due to Staphylococcus aureus bacteraemia among patients receiving long-term haemodialysis. Infect Control Hosp Epidemiol. 2005;26:534–9.
5. Manierski C, Besarab A. Antimicrobial locks: putting the lock on catheter infections. Adv Chronic Kidney Dis. 2006;13:245–58.
6. Williams VR, Quinn R, Callery S, Kiss A, Oliver MJ. The impact of treatment modality on infection-related hospitalization rates in peritoneal dialysis and hemodialysis patients. Perit Dial Int. 2011;31(4):440–9.
7. Pereda D, Conte JV. Left ventricular assist device driveline infections. Cardiol Clin. 2011;29: 515–27.
8. Goldstein DJ, Naftel D, Holman W, et al. Continuous-flow devices and percutaneous site infections: clinical outcomes. J Heart Lung Transplant. 2012;31:1151–7.
9. Akhter SA, Badami A, Murray M, et al. Hospital readmissions after continuous-flow left ventricular assist device implantation: incidence, causes, and cost analysis. Ann Thorac Surg. 2015;100:884–9.
10. Toba FA, Akashi H, Arrecubieta C, et al. Role of biofilm in staphylococcus aureus and staphylococcus epidermidis ventricular assist device driveline infections. J Thorac Cardiovasc Surg. 2011;141:1259–64.
11. Nienaber J, Wilhelm MP, Sohail MR. Current concepts in the diagnosis and management of left ventricular assist device infections. Expert Rev Anti-Infect Ther. 2013;11:201–10.
12. Bernhard AM, Schlöglhofer T, Lauenroth V, Mueller F, Mueller M, Schoede F, Klopsch C. Prevention and early treatment of driveline infections in ventricular assist device patients – the DESTINE staging proposal and the first standard of care protocol. J Crit Care. 2020;56: 106–12.
13. Hilker L, von Woedtke T, Weltmann KD, Wollert HG. Cold atmospheric plasma: a new tool for the treatment of superficial driveline *infections*. Eur J Cardiothorac Surg. 2017;51(1):186–7.
14. Rotering H, Hansen U, Welp H, DellÀquila AM. Kaltes atmosphärisches Plasma und "advanced negative pressure wound therapy". Z Herz-Thorax-Gefäßchir. 2020;34:52–61.
15. Hilker L, von Woedtke T, Titze R, Weltmann KD, Motz W, Wollert HG. The use of cold atmospheric pressure plasma (CAP) in Cardiac Surgery. In: Metelmann HR, von Woedtke T, Weltmann KD, Hrsg. Comprehensive clinical plasma medicine. Springer; 2018, p. 201–11.

12

Cold Plasma Treatment and Aesthetic Medicine

*Hans-Robert Metelmann, Kerstin Böttger,
and Thomas von Woedtke*

Contents

© Springer Nature Switzerland AG 2022
H.-R. Metelmann et al. (eds.), *Textbook of Good Clinical Practice in
Cold Plasma Therapy*, https://doi.org/10.1007/978-3-030-87857-3_13

🔘 **Core Messages**
- Aesthetic treatment is very likely the area with the most frequent applications of physical plasma in medicine.
- There are two different types of devices in use, generating either cold atmospheric pressure (CAP) or moderate thermal impact (MTI) plasma.
- CAP plasma is indicated for medical purposes, MTI plasma for cosmetic purposes.
- Typical diagnoses for CAP treatment are healing complications or risk of healing associated with aesthetic surgery, minimally invasive aesthetic medicine, and beauty treatment.
- Aesthetic disharmonies without causing disease and any pathological reason are no diagnosis for CAP plasma therapy, but MTI plasma application.
- The rationale of CAP plasma treatment concerning wound-healing complications is based upon randomized clinical trials and has been acknowledged by structured reviews.

13.1 Introduction

Aesthetic treatment is very likely the area with the most frequent applications today of physical plasma in medicine. In any case, plasma medicine is well established and plays an important role in aesthetic and cosmetic interventions.

However, it is important to distinguish between plasma medicine using devices generating cold physical plasma (below 40°C at target) and plasma medicine using devices generating physical plasma not so cold (below 70 °C at target).

The latter works by moderate thermal impact (MTI)-inducing shrinkage of soft tissue and skin [3, 13, 16, 27]. The MTI plasma is for cosmetic purposes like wrinkle removal, skin rejuvenation, or tightening of eyelids [6, 15]. MTI plasma devices are not approved for medical use.

Cold atmospheric pressure (CAP) plasma has no relevant thermal impact and is working by a completely different mechanism of action: It is not carbonizing and destructing cells and tissue by heat, but can selectively and therapeutically influence the redox balance and signal cascades in pathogenic and diseased cells.[1] CAP plasma is indicated for medical purposes like stimulation of insufficient wound healing and inhibition of surgical site infections. The first CAP plasma devices approved for medical use appeared in 2013.

13.2 Diagnosis

According to the present state of clinical research, CAP plasma is offering a rescue option in the event of specific complications caused by standard aesthetic interventions. Currently, typical diagnoses for CAP plasma treatment are healing complica-

---

1   See Part I.

tions or risk of healing associated with aesthetic surgery, minimally invasive aesthetic medicine, and beauty treatment.

13.2.1 Complications Associated with Aesthetic Surgery

A typical diagnosis for CAP plasma treatment is wound-healing complications following aesthetic surgery.

Aesthetic surgery is mostly a major intervention. It shares the operative procedures of reconstructive surgery and plastic surgery, but differs in goals and aims. For explanation only, reconstructive surgery is restoring the deep tissues and skin surface (e.g., after trauma or cancer) and plastic surgery is sculpting previously nonexistent structures (e.g., in cleft lip and palate). Aesthetic surgery, however, is doing both, for example, restoring the prematurely aged face and/or sculpting the unpleasant body contour. Even extensive surgical interventions are normally not based upon medical indication, but the strong desire of the patient. Without doubt, wound-healing complications resulting in unpleasant scars are the exact opposite to the intention of the patient: to look better after the surgical intervention (◘ Fig. 13.1).

13.2.2 Complications Associated with Minimally Invasive Aesthetic Medicine

Another typical diagnosis for CAP treatment is small local inflammations caused by minor penetration of skin and risk of infection in ablated or irritated skin areas.

Minimally invasive aesthetic medicine interventions in contrast to surgery are relatively smooth. The variety of treatment methods includes lasers and flash

13

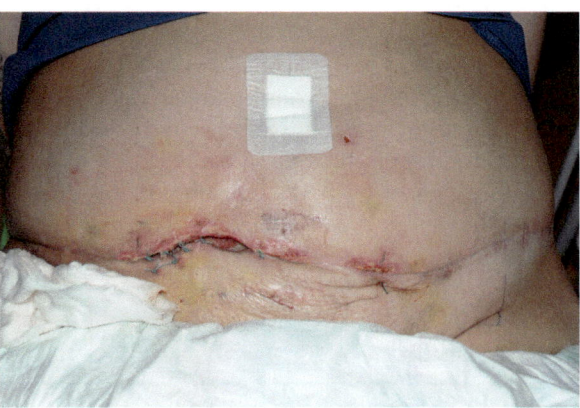

◘ **Fig. 13.1**   Clinical example of a severe complication caused by major aesthetic surgery: A classical abdominoplasty with extended removal of surplus fat and skin tissue and tightening of the abdominal wall muscles is being complicated postoperatively by a surgical site infection. The suture came loose, the opening measures several centimeters, the wound is suppurative and painful. The aim of CAP therapy is to eliminate the infection and stimulate secondary wound healing

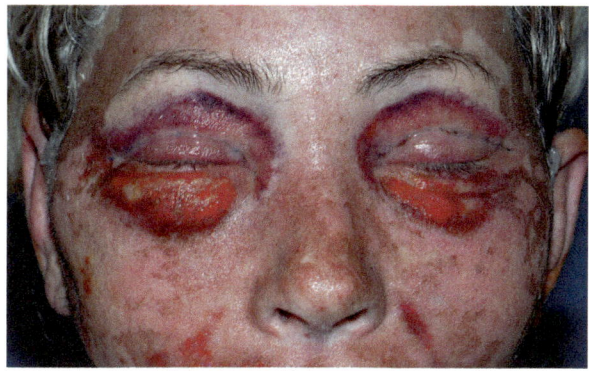

◘ Fig. 13.2   Clinical example of status after laser skin resurfacing. The laser procedure is minimally invasive, but treated area is large and extended which means a high risk of contamination and infection with pathogens. The aim of CAP therapy is to prevent infection and support closure of the epithelial cover as fast as possible

lamps, injections of botulinum toxin and fillers, thread lifts, dermabrasion, chemical peeling or needling, and low-heat plasma. The intention in general is rejuvenation, in detail to remove age spots, wrinkles, and blood vessel abnormalities in aesthetically relevant areas. A small local inflammation caused by the penetration or irritation of the skin is a major nuisance if this happens in the face. A superficial ablation of the epithelial layer puts the patient always at risk of surgical site infections (◘ Fig. 13.2).

13.2.3   Complications Caused by Beauty Treatment

An occasional diagnosis for CAP plasma treatment is small skin infections as misfortunes of a cosmetic procedure.

Cosmetics are "intended to be rubbed, poured, sprinkled, or sprayed on, introduced into, or otherwise applied to the human body...for cleansing, beautifying, promoting attractiveness, or altering the appearance" [8]. The cosmetic procedures to promote attractiveness or alter the appearance sometimes turn into a medical problem (◘ Fig. 13.3).

13.2.4   Beauty Flaws and Blemishes

Aesthetic disharmonies without causing disease and without any pathological reason are no diagnosis for CAP plasma therapy.

13.2.4.1   The Preserve of MTI Plasma Treatment

Beauty flaws and blemishes are the main indication for MTI plasma [11, 17, 31], and the typical field for nonmedical specialists working with nonmedical plasma

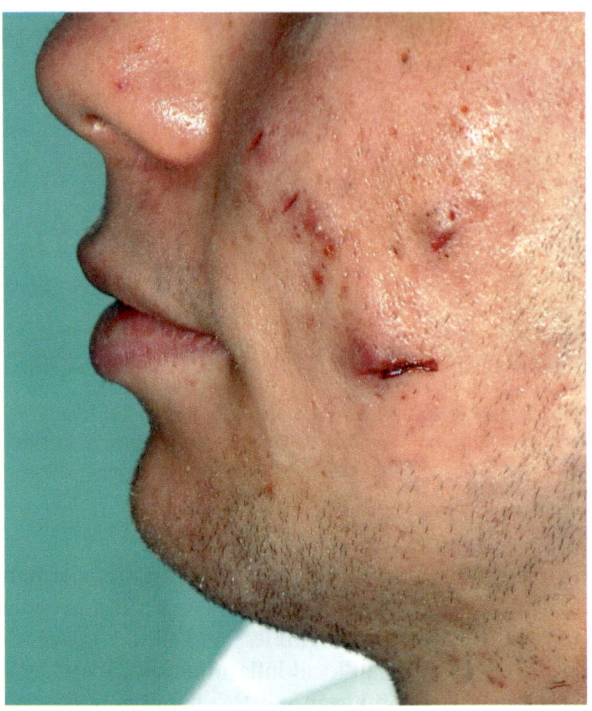

◘ Fig. 13.3 Clinical example of different appearances of skin infection as a result of failed cosmetic standard treatment. The aim of CAP therapy is to eliminate the infection and support discreet scaring

devices. R. Crofford, a cosmetic nurse specialist, is listing skin tags, lines of upper and lower face, milia, warts, stretch marks, verrucae, periumbilical laxity, tattoos, papuloma nigra, xanthelasma, scars, and permanent makeup, but she is mentioning skin shrinkage procedures like nonsurgical blepharoplasty and mini face lift as well, to be performed with MTI plasma [6].

13.2.4.2   A Future Role for CAP Plasma Treatment?

A number of studies is addressing the potential of CAP plasma application in terms of direct aesthetic effects. The issues are skin improvement, conditioning discreet scaring, and facilitating penetration of cosmetically relevant drugs.

The repetitive use of CAP plasma by dielectric barrier discharge devices boosts microcirculatory effects and blood perfusion of the skin [4, 7, 12, 18, 19, 28]. CAP plasma application is conditioning discreet scaring of CO_2 laser skin lesions [24]. Application of CAP plasma enhances skin permeability and might henceforth support the incorporation of cosmetically active substances [10, 14, 21–23].

These preliminary research results attract the attention of the laboratories of the cosmetic industry to CAP plasma [1, 29, 33].

> **❶ Caution**
> Sometimes apparent beauty flaws are side effects of diseases or medication, which may need rational medical therapy instead of beauty treatment. Seemingly harmless beauty flaws like dark skin spots may be of utmost medical importance as manifestation of, for example, a malignant melanoma, requiring immediate dermatological attention.

13.3 Physiology and Pathology

There is a flowing transition in wounds and wound healing from physiology to pathology.

13.3.1 No Pathology

Surgical wounds, ablated and penetrated skin, and irritations of skin are not pathologies right from the outset. Well-handled surgical wounds do not need additional targeted treatment because they are healing on their own under normal conditions. The same is true for skin defects by minimally invasive aesthetic medicine like injection, dermabrasion, chemical impact, or needling. In fact, loss of tenseness and progressing flaccidity of skin and soft tissues resulting in an undesired appearance are due to the physiological effects of aging.

13.3.2 Risk of Pathology

However, aging on its own is prone to retarded wound healing, complications, and pathologies. Unhealthy habits, eating, and lifestyle contribute their share. Patients with rapidly progressive aging or diseases altering the appearance suffer from special pathologies and demand a targeted medical treatment. There are always patients with generally weak healing conditions, some suffer especially from immediate or late rejection reaction to fillers, and invasive interventions are always connected with the risk of surgical site infections.

13.3.3 Pathology

Postoperative wound infections are mainly occurring from the resident flora of the skin [20]. Ablative laser skin resurfacing for facial rejuvenation, for example, is leaving behind the treatment area as a large superficial second-degree burn. Infection rates after use of non-fractionated laser are reported between 1.1% and 7.6%. With fractionated laser, the rate of surgical site infections is reduced to 0.3%–2.0%. Predominant pathogens are Herpes simplex-1, P. aeruginosa, S. aureus, and S. epidermidis. Postoperatively, risk of infection is increased when closed dressings are used excessively.

13.4   Standard Treatment Principles

Good clinical practice in aesthetic medicine is being aware of operating near the zone of nonmedical indications. Aesthetic medicine does "not impart any health benefits," since the only intention of interventions is "to improve appearance," according to the U.S. Federal Food, Drug, and Cosmetic Act [9]. This means heavy responsibility toward the patients benefit and attention to some out-of-standard treatment principles.

13.4.1   Integration of Nonmedical Specialists for Mutual Benefit

Teamwork in aesthetic medicine is based upon a structured cooperation within cosmetic nurse specialists and cosmeticians.

The main concern of the medical staff in terms of plasma medicine is rational CAP plasma treatment, based upon approved medical devices and procedures within the defined corridor of their medical indications.

The part of the cosmeticians within the team is beauty treatment by use of MTI plasma devices. Cosmeticians are not restricted to approved CAP medical devices and defined corridors of indications, since their treatment is purely cosmetically indicated.

13.4.2   Increased Attention to Aesthetic Indications

Nonmedical and especially aesthetic indications are challenging. To pick the winners is an important principle when the only reason for the patient to undergo a possibly invasive therapy is to look better afterward. The slightest imperfection caused by therapy could be considered as malpractice. Patients who passionately demand treatment might passionately strive for legal action in case of discontent.

13.4.3   Cross-Border Consideration of MTI Plasma Medicine

Aesthetic plasma medicine is not different from other plasma-related specialties when it comes to CAP. There are approved medical CAP devices available with a sound background of detailed preclinical and clinical investigations and with comprehensive physical and biological characterization: *kINPen MED* (neoplas tools GmbH, Greifswald, Germany), *PlasmaDerm Flex and Dress* (CINOGY GmbH, Duderstadt, Germany*), SteriPlas and PlasmaTact* (ADTEC, Hunslow, UK), and *Plasma care* (terraplasma medical GmbH, Garching, Germany).

Aesthetic plasma medicine from the cosmeticians' point of view is based upon other devices, generating MTI plasma, like *Plasma Elite, NanoPlasma, Plexr, Jett Plasma, Plasma IQ,* and *Plasma BT* to name a few [6, 15]. These devices are not approved for medical application, but permitted for cosmetic treatment only. They are effective in a different way and cause different side effects as surmised by non-medical practitioners:

"Plasma is produced when an electrical energy is charged or overheated, leading to a dissociation of molecular bonds and the production of a plasma arc. The arc delivers energy to the cell membrane, causing sublimation, changing a solid to a gas and bypassing the liquid phase which would potentially cause the skin to burn. The plasma arc hits the skin, creating an immediate contraction of the tissue and the stimulation of fibroblasts, initiating tissue regeneration and tightening of the skin" [15].

Thirty-seven medical practitioners completed a survey on Facebook, and a significant 64.9% answered "yes" to having witnessed side effects. The most common immediate (short-term) effects were swelling (83.3%) and erythema (62.2%). Longer-term side effects included mild hyperpigmentation (35.1%) hypopigmentation (10.8%) and erythema (24.3%) [6].

13.5 Treatment Rationale

At present, the rationale of CAP plasma treatment in aesthetic medicine is a rescue function by management of wound-healing complications and a prevention function by protecting jeopardized post-beauty-treatment areas. The rescue function concerning wound-healing complications is based upon randomized clinical trials by Brehmer et al. [5], Moelleken et al. [26], and Stratmann et al. [32]. The treatment rationale has been acknowledged in reviews by Sorg et al. [30], Kramer et al. [20], and Bernhardt et al. [2].

> **ℹ Cave**
> Research results addressing CAP plasma in terms of safety are not transferable to the treatment with MTI plasma, since the mode of action is totally different.

13.6 Therapy

CAP plasma-based therapy and MTI plasma application follow different treatment protocols.

13.6.1 CAP Plasma Treatment

13.6.1.1 Identifying Individual Risk Factors for Complications

Identification of risk factors comes too late in cases of obvious and apparent wound-healing complications. But it is important for taking a decision, whether irritated or ablated skin by beauty treatment in aesthetically relevant areas (Fig. 13.2) should be protected with CAP plasma for prevention of infection. There some general risk factors to be considered [25]:

Age over 60 years is an independent risk factor for retardation of wound closure, affecting about 15% of this group. The risk is attributable to hormone levels as well as the relatively longer exposition to influences such as sun or smoke. Concomitant diseases and malnutrition are relevant conditions as well.

Women after the menopause belong to the at-risk group of badly healing wounds. This is widely attributed to the decline of estrogen which is significant for the production of growth factors, cell migration, and proliferation.

Females in the age over 60 years are common patients in the aesthetic medicine practice. They should be considered in general for preventive plasma treatment of wound areas.

Concerning the rescue indication of CAP treatment, all wounds requiring more than 28 days of epithelial closure after aesthetic or cosmetic intervention raise suspicion to be on the way to chronic wounds and at risk of infection.

13.6.1.2 Informing the Patient

CAP plasma application as an innovative treatment requires extended information of the patient and written consent to undergo the treatment. Most patients for the time being are not familiar with CAP plasma medicine. They might have frequently asked questions.

▬ Is the clinical efficacy proved?

CAP plasma therapy of wound-healing complications is an aesthetic medicine based upon randomized clinical studies and approved medical plasma devices. Its application for treatment purposes is authorized by CE certification as a medical device Class IIa, according to the European Council Directive 93/42/EEC.

▬ No undesirable local or systemic side effects?

Approved plasma devices are in clinical use since 2013. There are no case observations or clinical studies known reporting severe side effects of any kind including carcinogenesis or genetic damage.

13.6.1.3 Obtain Written Consent

Written consent is self-evident in medical interventions but no normal practice in cosmetic and aesthetic procedures. However, even here written consent is seriously recommended: The patient understands the innovative application of cold plasma; there are no unwanted side effects known from standard medical applications of cold plasma; it cannot be guaranteed that the treatment result is fully satisfying the expectations of the patient since biological processes are not always predictable; and in cases of medical indication, costs of treatment are covered by health insurance.

> **⊘ Caution**
> An innovative treatment like CAP requires vitally extended information and written consent of the patient.

13.6.1.4 Treatment

CAP plasma will be applied without touch and is not causing pain in most of the patients. There is in principle no need for local anesthesia or cooling of the treatment area.

To prepare the field of application it might be useful to remove the biofilm; however, drying the area is not recommended because CAP Plasma is more active in wet surroundings.

There is no scientifically based standard how to apply CAP plasma. An exposure time of 1 minute per square centimeter is according to the clinical experience of most medical doctors. In correlation with hormesis, shorter exposure time will accelerate processes and longer exposure time will inhibit them. Therefore, treatment to stimulate wound healing will need in principle less CAP plasma applications per week (23 times) with longer treatment interruptions (2–3 weeks), mainly antiseptic treatment in principle might take place daily for 1 week.

Medical devices generating a jet plasma facilitate application under visual control, an accurately guiding of the plume, and they enable CAP application at deep tissue defects, extended fistula, undercut areas, and intra-oral findings. Medical devices generating a carpet-like CAP facilitate plasma application at large and plain areas.

Debridement of slough and necrotic tissue, wound cleansing procedures, and careful dressings will contribute to the healing success, and medical therapy of relevant comorbidities as well.

There is no special aftercare needed related to the use of CAP.

On principle, treatment can be delegated to a qualified nurse. However, an innovative treatment option like CAP and the very special relationship to patients in aesthetic medicine require at least careful supervision by the doctor.

13.6.2   MTI Plasma Treatment

Cosmetic treatment with devices generating moderate-temperature physical plasma is typically directed by nonmedical specialists. A. Kerr, as a nonmedical aesthetic practitioner, is describing this kind of plasma therapy presented by the example of a nonsurgical blepharoplasty [15]:

13.6.2.1   Patient Selection and Consultation

» Plasma is an ideal treatment for patients with skin laxity around the eye area, (although many other areas can also be treated). I personally use the Plasma Elite pen for this treatment. It is important to select patients based on the degree of laxity and to manage expectations. It is not possible to guarantee the shrinkage of the skin so therefore practitioners should be realistic regarding the outcome.

An in-depth medical history is taken before treatment including questions about immunosuppression or diabetes. Prolonged healing time is experienced in these patients, which can result in longer periods of isolation and time away from socialising or attending work. Assessment of the laxity of the skin using the 'snap test', consideration of the Fitzpatrick scale and any other skin conditions should be evaluated on consultation.

Although plasma does not affect the melanocytes, I would recommend avoiding treating patients with Fitzpatrick >3 unless a patch test is carried out to reduce risks of hyperpigmentation.

Keloid and hypertrophic scarring can be considered a contraindication; however, scarring such as stretch marks or pock marks can be treated [15].

13.6.2.2 Preparation

» The patient must not have had any other skin treatments (such as laser, skin needling or peels) in the three weeks prior to treatment, as this skin trauma could potentially interfere with natural skin healing.

A patch test is normally carried out on consultation a few days before the treatment is arranged. Cleaning the skin with a good skin disinfectant is imperative as I recommend dry healing for 7–10 days afterwards to allow for the carbon crusts to fall off naturally. This allows for less pitting of the skin if the crusts are knocked off or picked [15].

13.6.2.3 Treatment

» The carbon plume produced during the treatment is considered a biohazard therefore a plume extractor (recently launched by Plasma Elite) is essential in protecting both patient and practitioner.

After thoroughly cleaning the skin with a chlorhexadine solution and allowing to dry, a thin layer of local anaesthesia is applied. I find Emla® to be excellent in helping with the comfort of the procedure leaving it no longer than 15–20 minutes which can result in the anaesthesia wearing off and the patient becoming uncomfortable. Skin is cleansed again, and the plasma treatment is started.

Care should be taken on the thin, fragile skin of the eyelid; intervals of 1–2 mm between each dot respects the delicate structure of the orbital area.

I personally like to do a diced pattern on the upper eyelids as I feel it gives a tighter skin contraction on looser skin and good healing. A spray like pattern may also be used, which will give a subtle contraction and lift.

The plasma should not be held over the skin too long as this would result in a deeper penetration of the energy and can result in prolonged pitting of the skin after the carbon crusts have flaked off [15].

13.6.2.4 Aftercare

» The skin is cleaned of any carbon debris and I advise patients to dry heal for seven days. I also advise my patients that bilateral periorbital swelling is normal, can affect the whole eye, not just the area treated, and can last for a few days. Anti-inflammatory medication can be taken alongside antihistamines.

No makeup or creams should be applied and sunglasses with protection from UVA must be worn outside. When cleansing the newly treated area, lint free gauze with lukewarm water is advised and to pat dry immediately, no picking of the crusts as this can lead to scarring.

I recommend applying an SPF cream after the carbon crusts have flaked off, daily for up to three months post treatment. I personally recommend retinol cream in the evening after the crusts have fallen off; this acts as an antioxidant and can help encourage healthy new skin cells to develop.

Follow-up treatment can be offered at approximately six weeks to three months for optimal results [15].

Conclusion

Aesthetic treatment is very likely the area with the most frequent applications of physical plasma in medicine. There are two different types of devices in use, generating either cold atmospheric pressure (CAP) or moderate thermal impact (MTI) plasma. CAP plasma is indicated for medical purposes, MTI plasma for cosmetic purposes.

Currently, typical diagnoses for CAP plasma treatment are healing complications or risk of healing associated with aesthetic surgery, minimally invasive aesthetic medicine, and beauty treatment. Aesthetic disharmonies without causing disease and any pathological reason are no diagnosis for CAP plasma therapy, but for MTI plasma application.

At present, the rationale of CAP plasma treatment in aesthetic medicine is a rescue function by management of wound-healing complications and a prevention function by protecting jeopardized post-beauty-treatment areas. The rationale of the rescue function concerning wound-healing complications is based upon randomized clinical trials by Brehmer et al. [5], Moelleken et al. [26], and Stratmann et al. [32]. The treatment rationale has been acknowledged in structured reviews by Sorg et al. [30], Kramer et al. [20], and Bernhardt et al. [2].

To look ahead, CAP plasma has the potential to improve directly aesthetic appearance. Promising research projects are pointing at skin rejuvenation, conditioning of discreet scaring, and facilitating skin penetration of cosmetically relevant drugs. Preliminary research results are attracting at present the attention of the laboratories of the cosmetic industry to CAP plasma.

References

1. Baik KY. Application of atmospheric pressure plasma treated water for hair loss therapy. ISPB 2017, Jeju, Korea, 27 June 2017.
2. Bernhardt AM, Schlöglhofer T, Lauenroth V, Mueller F, Mueller M, Schoede A, Klopsch C, et al. Prevention and early treatment of driveline infections in ventricular assist device patients – the DESTINE staging proposal and the first standard of care protocol. Crit Care. 2020;56:106–12.
3. Bogle MA, Arndt KA, Dover JS. Evaluation of plasma skin regeneration technology in low-energy full-facial rejuvenation. Arch Dermatol. 2007;143:168–74. https://doi.org/10.1001/archderm.143.2.168.
4. Borchardt T, Ernst J, Helmke A, Tanyeli M, Schilling AF, Felmerer G, Viöl W. Effect of direct cold atmospheric plasma (di cap) on microcirculation of intact skin in a controlled mechanical environment. Microcirculation. 2017;24(8):e12399. https://doi.org/10.1111/micc.12399.
5. Brehmer F, Haenssle HA, Daeschlein G, Ahmed R, Pfeiffer S, Görlitz A, Simon D, Schön MP, Wandke D, Emmert S. Alleviation of chronic venous leg ulcers with a hand-held dielectric barrier discharge plasma generator (PlasmaDerm® VU-2010): results of a monocentric, two-armed, open, prospective, randomized and controlled trial (NCT01415622). Eur Acad Dermatol Venereol. 2015;29:148–55.
6. Crofford R. A review of plasma medicine. PMFA J. 2019;6(3):2–3
7. Daeschlein G, Rutkowski R, Lutze S, von Podewils S, Sicher C, Wild T, Metelmann HR, von Woedtke T, Jünger M. Hyperspectral imaging: innovative diagnostics to visualize hemodynamic effects of cold plasma in wound therapy. Biomed Eng/Biomed Technol. 2018;63(5):603–8. https://doi.org/10.1515/bmt-2017-0085.

8. FDA 2018a. https://www.fda.gov/cosmetics/cosmetics-laws-regulations/fda-authority-over-cosmetics-how-cosmetics-are-not-fda-approved-are-fda-regulated#What_kinds.

9. FDA 2018b. https://www.fda.gov/medical-devices/products-and-medical-procedures/cosmetic-devices.

10. Gelker M, Müller-Goymann CC, Viöl W. Permeabilization of human stratum corneum and full-thickness skin samples by a direct dielectric barrier discharge. Clin Plasma Med. 2018;9:34–40. https://doi.org/10.1016/j.cpme.2018.02.001.

11. Gloustianou G, Sifaki M, Tsioumas SG, Vlachodimitropoulos D, Scarano A. Presentation of old and new histological results after plasma exeresis (Plexr) application (regeneration of the skin tissue with collagen III). Pinnacle Med Sci. 2016;3:3. https://pjpub.org/pmms/pmms_241.pdf

12. Heuer K, Hoffmanns MA, Demir E, Baldus S, Volkmar CM, Röhle M, Fuchs PC, Awakowicz P, Suschek CV, Opländer C. The topical use of non-thermal dielectric barrier discharge (DBD): nitric oxide related effects on human skin. Nitric Oxide. 2015;44:52–60. https://doi.org/10.1016/j.niox.2014.11.015.

13. Holcomb JD, Kent KJ, Rousso DE. Nitrogen plasma skin regeneration and aesthetic facial surgery. Multicenter evaluation of concurrent treatment. Arch Facial Plast Surg. 2009;11:184–93. https://doi.org/10.1001/archfacial.2009.29.

14. Kalghatgi S, Tsai C, Gray R, Pappas D. Transdermal drug delivery using cold plasmas. 22nd International Symposium on Plasma Chemistry, 5–10 July 2015; Antwerp, Belgium; Conference Proceedings No. O-22-6, https://www.ispc-conference.org/ispcproc/ispc22/O-22-6.pdf.

15. Kerr A. How I do it – nonsurgical blepharoplasty using Plasma Elite® technology. PMFA J. 2020;8(1):2–3

16. Kilmer S, Semchyshyn N, Shah G, Fitzpatrick R. A pilot study on the use of a plasma skin regeneration device (Portrait® PSR3) in full facial rejuvenation procedures. Lasers Med Sci. 2007;22:101–9. https://doi.org/10.1007/s10103-006-0431-9.

17. King M. Focus on plasma: the application of plasma devices in aesthetic medicine. PMFA News 4 No 5; 2017. https://www.thepmfajournal.com/features/post/focus-on-plasma-the-application-of-plasma-devices-in-aesthetic-medicine.

18. Kisch T, Helmke A, Schleusser S, Song J, Liodaki E, Stang FH, Mailaender P, Kraemer R. Improvement of cutaneous microcirculation by cold atmospheric plasma (CAP): results of a controlled, prospective cohort study. Microvasc Res. 2016a;104:55–62. https://doi.org/10.1016/j.mvr.2015.12.002.

19. Kisch T, Schleusser S, Helmke A, Mauss KL, Wenzel ET, Hasemann B, Mailaender P, Kraemer R. The repetitive use of non-thermal dielectric barrier discharge plasma boosts cutaneous micro-circulatory effects. Microvasc Res. 2016b;106:8–13. https://doi.org/10.1016/j.mvr.2016.02.008.

20. Kramer A, Dissemond J, Willy C, Kim S, Mayer D, Papke R, Tuchmann R, Daeschlein G, Assadian O. Auswahl von Wundantiseptika – Aktualisierung des Expertenkonsensus 2018. WUNDmanagement. 2019;13:5–22.

21. Kristof J, Aoshima T, Blajan M, Shimizu K. Surface modification of stratum corneum for drug delivery and skin care by microplasma discharge treatment. Plasma Sci Technol. 2019;21:064001. https://doi.org/10.1088/2058-6272/aafde6.

22. Lademann O, Richter H, Meinke MC, Patzelt A, Kramer A, Hinz P, Weltmann KD, Hartmann B, Koch S. Drug delivery through the skin barrier enhanced by treatment with tissue-tolerable plasma. Exp Dermatol. 2011a;20:488–90. https://doi.org/10.1111/j.1600-0625.2010.01245.

23. Lademann O, Richter H, Kramer A, Patzelt A, Meinke MC, Graf C, Gao Q, Korotianskiy E, Rühl E, Weltmann KD, Lademann J, Koch S. Stimulation of the penetration of particles into the skin by plasma tissue interaction. Laser Phys Lett. 2011b;8:758–64. https://doi.org/10.1002/lapl.201110055.

24. Metelmann HR, von Woedtke T, Bussiahn R, Weltmann KD, Rieck M, Khalili R, Podmelle F, Waite PD. Experimental recovery of CO2-laser skin lesions by plasma stimulation. Am J Cosmetic Surg. 2012;29:52–6. https://doi.org/10.5992/AJCS-D-11-00042.1.

25. Metelmann I. Velocity of clinical wound healing without targeted treatment specified for age, gender, body weight, skin type, wound size and co-morbidities, Inaugural-Dissertation Greifswald University; 2018.

26. Moelleken M, Jockenhöfer F, Wiegand C, Buer J, Benson S, Dissemond J. Pilot study on the influence of cold atmospheric plasma on bacterial contamination and healing tendency of chronic wounds. Dt Dermatol Gesell. 2020; https://doi.org/10.1111/ddg.14294.

27. Pourazizi M, Abtahi-Naeini B. Plasma application in aesthetic medicine: clinical and physical aspects. J Surg Dermatol. 2017;2:113–4. https://doi.org/10.18282/jsd.v2.it1140.

28. Rutkowski R, Schuster M, Unger J, Seebauer C, Metelmann HR, Woedtke TV, Weltmann KD, Daeschlein G. Hyperspectral imaging for in vivo monitoring of cold atmospheric plasma effects on microcirculation in treatment of head and neck cancer. Clin Plasma Med. 2017;7:52–7. https://doi.org/10.1016/j.cpme.2017.09.002.

29. Robert E, Busco G, Grillon C, Pouvesle JM. Potential of low temperature atmospheric pressure plasma sources in cosmetic. COSMINNOV 2016, Orléans, France, 25 May 2016.

30. Sorg H, Tilkorn DJ, Hager S, Hauser J, Mirastschijski U. Skin wound healing: an update on the current knowledge and concepts. Eur Surg Res. 2017;58:81–94.

31. Sotiris TG, Nikolaos G, Irini G. Plexr: the revolution in blepharoplasty. Pinnacle Med Sci. 2014;1(5):2–3. https://pjpub.org/pmms/pmms_160.pdf.

32. Stratmann B, Costea TC, Nolte C, Hiller J, Schmidt J, Reindel J, Masur K, Motz W, Timm J, Kerner W, Tschoepe D. Effect of cold atmospheric plasma therapy vs standard therapy placebo on wound healing in patients with diabetic foot ulcers. A randomized clinical trial. JAMA Netw Open. 2020;3:e2010411.

33. von Woedtke T, Metelmann HR, Weltmann KD. Plasma in cosmetic applications: possibilities and boundary conditions. ISPB 2018. Incheon, Korea, 25 July 2018.

Cold Plasma Treatment for Dental Aesthetics

*Philine H. Doberschütz, Eun Ha Choi,
Jae-Sung Kwon, Gyoo-Cheon Kim, Seoul-
Hee Nam, and Hans-Robert Metelmann*

Contents

© Springer Nature Switzerland AG 2022
H.-R. Metelmann et al. (eds.), *Textbook of Good Clinical Practice in
Cold Plasma Therapy*, https://doi.org/10.1007/978-3-030-87857-3_14

Core Messages

- Approved cold atmospheric plasma medical devices are, on principle, qualified for application in dental medicine.
- Although a standardized technique of aesthetic plasma dentistry still needs to be developed, the practical use of cold atmospheric plasma as a beneficial treatment strategy is already on the doorstep of good dental practice.
- Current scientific investigations concerning bleaching mainly focus on approved argon-driven or helium-driven plasma jet devices in combination with low-dose hydrogen peroxide or carbamide peroxide or without chemicals, and a treatment time of 5–30 minutes.

14.1 Introduction

The clinical application of cold atmospheric plasma in dentistry is in line with the medical approval of certain well-established plasma devices. Basic and pre-clinical research in cold plasma dentistry significantly contributes to the physical and biological characterization of appropriate plasma sources [1]. Current research focuses on the treatment of caries and periodontitis, infections and wounds of the oral mucosa, the inactivation and removal of dental and implant biofilm, the disinfection of root canals, the surface conditioning for bone integration and bonding of restorations and orthodontic brackets, and the decontamination of dental prostheses [2–9].

And yet, cold atmospheric plasma treatment remains on the doorstep of clinical dentistry. "Although a standardized technique of cold plasma treatment still needs to be developed, with respect to standardization concerning the use of different plasma devices and treatment modalities, our results underline the practical use of cold plasma as a beneficial treatment strategy" [10]. This chapter is providing information for dentists willing to cross the doorstep, especially in dental aesthetics.

Dental aesthetics are an integral component of the oral health-related quality of life [11]. One of the most important factors that determine a patient's satisfaction with the own dental appearance is the tooth color [12–14]. Bleaching has therefore become the most commonly requested aesthetic dental treatment [12, 14].

14

14.1.1 Elective Indication

Interventions for aesthetic purposes are by definition never unavoidable or undeniable. They are justified only by a strong desire of the patient. The intention of the patient is to look better after the treatment. The slightest imperfection caused by the treatment could be considered as malpractice. Patients who passionately demand treatment might passionately strive for legal action. Picking the winners is an important principle of the highly elective indications in aesthetic plasma dentistry.

14.1.2 Not-Ideal Plasma Devices

Standard plasma medicine devices are approved for treating patients with chronic wounds and skin infections. Utilizing these devices for aesthetic procedures, such as tooth bleaching, is amounting to off-label use.

A huge number of cold plasma equipment is available on the market, not approved for medical purposes, but strictly intended for cosmetic application. Some of them are on sale as home devices for nonprofessional users. The performance of these devices is mostly too weak to deliver positive effects.

14.1.3 Competing with Conventional Methods

Application of cold atmospheric plasma has to compete with well-established standard methods of bleaching by teeth-whitening gel and light. Although it may not replace them, cold atmospheric plasma could improve established procedures by increasing their effectiveness or reducing their side effects. However, to receive a recommendation for use, cold atmospheric plasma has to be more effective and as safe as conventional methods.

14.2 Diagnosis

The tooth color is composed of a combination of extrinsic and intrinsic factors. Its perception is also influenced by the translucency and gloss of the tooth, as well as the color of the surrounding gingiva and lips [15].

Standardized color scales and electronic color measurement devices are used to determine the natural and desired tooth shade.

Teeth with a relatively uniform yellow color, age-related discolorations, endodontically treated teeth, and discolorations due to food and drink consumption respond well to bleaching procedures.

14.3 Physiology and Pathology

Substances absorbed on the enamel surface (extrinsic factors, e.g., tobacco, tea, red wine, chlorhexidine), as well as light scattering and the absorption capacity of enamel and dentin (intrinsic factors) both influence a patient's tooth color [16].

Additionally, the natural tooth color changes over the course of life and becomes darker and more yellow due to remodeling processes in the dentin and the physiological wear of the enamel.

The indication for bleaching is emotional, the outcome can be quantified using standardized color scales, but must be measured against the patient's perception of treatment success. Evidence-based medicine in aesthetic dentistry is not determinable by randomized clinical trials but at least by individual clinical expertise, according to the definition by Sacket: Evidence-based Medicine (EBM) is "(…) the conscientious, explicit and judicious use of current best evidence in making decisions about the care of individual patients. The practice of EBM means integrating individual clinical expertise with the best available external clinical evidence from scientific research" [17]. External clinical evidence is based upon randomized clinical trials comparing innovative treatment with standard treatment. Clinical trials are searching for improvement of pathologies, precisely definable, for example, by biopsies, lab data, and radiographs. Tooth bleaching is not a matter of improving pathologies but enhancing the healthy, youthful appearance of teeth.

> **Important to Know**
   Aesthetic dentistry cannot be assessed by the benchmarks of evidence-based medicine.

14.4   Standard Treatment Principles

The bleaching process is based on the oxidizing effects of peroxide, which is applied to the enamel in an aqueous solution and reacts with organic, colored materials after diffusion into the tooth. Apart from the type and etiology of the discoloration, the application time and the concentration of active ingredients are the main factors that influence the success of bleaching. Cold atmospheric plasma is used to increase the effectiveness of the bleaching materials while minimizing unwanted side effects, such as thermal damage to the pulp tissue, that may occur when using conventional light sources that heat up the peroxide.

There are no standard bleaching principles of cold atmospheric plasma application available at present. However, some research data provide insights concerning the main settings.

Several plasma devices with technologies based on helium [18, 19], argon [20, 21], ionized air [22], compressed air [23], and air enriched by oxygen [24] have demonstrated their effectiveness in tooth bleaching in interaction with hydrogen peroxide (5–40%) and carbamide peroxide (15–37%) or without the use of bleaching gels. Treatment times vary from 5 to 30 minutes. ■ Figure 14.1 shows an example of an experiment in which different cold atmospheric plasma compositions with or without the addition of carbamide peroxide exerted a whitening effect on tooth enamel.

The advantages over conventional methods are described as accelerated and enhanced tooth whitening [18] with 2–3 times more brightness [19, 23] and overall greater capability than conventional light sources like diode laser and plasma arc lamp [20, 25]. The use of cold atmospheric plasma showed positive effects not only for external enamel bleaching, but also for intracoronal bleaching of nonvital teeth [22].

All mentioned studies are identical in nature: they are based on extracted human teeth (except [24]). Having regard to the limited applicability of EBM in

14

before   after

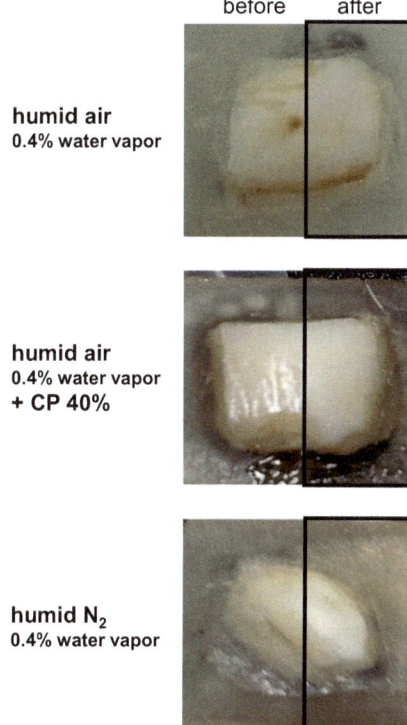

humid air
0.4% water vapor

humid air
0.4% water vapor
+ CP 40%

humid N$_2$
0.4% water vapor

◘ **Fig. 14.1** Exposure of bovine teeth to different cold atmospheric plasma compositions. The experiment was conducted using a plasma jet developed by Kwangwoon University and conducted in Yonsei University College of Dentistry. Extracted bovine teeth were stained with coffee solution overnight, half of the surface area was then exposed to various compositions of cold atmospheric plasma (20 minutes, 1 l/minute): humid air plasma jet (air with 0.4% of water vapor), humid air plasma jet combined with carbamide peroxide (CP, 40%), and humid nitrogen plasma jet (nitrogen with 0.4% of water vapor). The results show significant whitening on all three compositions, as can be seen when comparing the before photos (left) with the after photos (right, framed)

aesthetic indications, cold atmospheric plasma for tooth whitening comes close to level IV, meaning consent of scientific experts and practitioners in the dental office.

14.5 Treatment Rationale

The application of cold atmospheric plasma increases the production of free hydroxyl radicals that exert the bleaching effect on stained teeth. Thereby, the concentration of bleaching gel and the treatment time can be reduced. Cold atmospheric plasma-enhanced bleaching protocols are therefore less destructive on the enamel surface. Compared to conventional light sources, cold atmospheric plasma also reduces thermal damage.

14.6   Cold Plasma Therapy

The state of scientific knowledge in aesthetic plasma dentistry permits bleaching by approved plasma medical devices with aforementioned reservations. Generally, cold atmospheric plasma treatment can be delegated to a dental nurse. However, an innovative treatment option like cold atmospheric plasma, which is still under rapid development, should be carefully supervised by the dental doctor.

> **Tip**
>
> Delegation of the treatment to the dental nurse is only possible when supervision by the dental doctor is guaranteed.

14.6.1   Pretreatment Assessment

14.6.1.1   Indication

Tooth whitening is not a medical indication but is fully based on the patient's desire for treatment. Cold atmospheric plasma is particularly suitable when conventional methods of tooth whitening alone do not result in patient's satisfaction, or when negative side effects are to be reduced.

The general contraindications for conventional bleaching (e.g., insufficient fillings, poor oral hygiene, intolerances to ingredients of the bleaching material) also apply to the cold atmospheric plasma-enhanced bleaching procedures.

14.6.1.2   Informing the Patient

Cold atmospheric plasma bleaching as an innovative treatment requires extended information of the patient and written consent to undergo the treatment. Most patients for the time being are not familiar with plasma medicine. They might have some frequently asked questions.

- Is the clinical efficacy proved?

Bleaching is not the standard use of approved medical plasma devices like the plasma jet kINPen MED, particularly suitable for intraoral areas, but its application for treatment purposes is authorized by CE certification as medical devices Class IIa, according to the European Council Directive 93/42/EEC. The efficacy of plasma bleaching has been scientifically investigated. Additional application studies are underway.

- No undesirable local or systemic side effects?

Approved plasma devices are in clinical use since 2013. There are no case observations or clinical studies known reporting severe side effects of any kind including carcinogenesis or genetic damage.
- Bleaching effect reliable?

A certain bleaching effect is reliable. Nevertheless, since the indication is fully emotional, the individual evaluation of the result is emotional as well.
- Quick effect and lasting result?

Bleaching effects may occur quite fast. A lasting result depends mainly upon personal dental hygiene and life style.
- No inhibitory effect on normal flora of the mouth?

Cold atmospheric plasma has an antibacterial effect, therapeutically used in medicine for decontamination of infected wounds. Jet plasma devices recommended for bleaching direct the plume precisely to the surface of the tooth and do not significantly touch mucosa. There are no case reports or clinical studies of, for example, oral plasma surgery mentioning pathological changes of oral flora by cold atmospheric plasma application.
- Cost-effective?

Clinical experience shows that material consumption does not cost much. However, the purchase price of the plasma device and staff costs are noteworthy because treatment might be time-consuming.
- No alternative solution (could it be done easier)?

Patients in the dental chair usually have experience with a lot of alternative and easy-to-use solutions. They do not ask whether it could be done easier. The question is can it be done effectively.

14.6.1.3 Consent of Patient

Written consent is recommended. The patient understands that bleaching is an innovative application of cold atmospheric plasma, but there are no unwanted side effects known from standard medical applications of cold atmospheric plasma. It cannot be guaranteed that the treatment result is fully satisfying the expectations of the patient since biological processes are not always predictable. Costs of treatment are usually not covered by health insurance.

⚠ Caution
An innovative bleaching treatment like cold atmospheric plasma requires extended information and written consent of the patient.

14.6.2 Timing

Application of cold atmospheric plasma in combination with hydrogen peroxide and carbamide peroxide is subject to the precautions of chemical bleaching and should not happen more than twice a year. Cold atmospheric plasma alone or with deionized water replacing common bleaching agents is less destructive and not causing structural or morphological changes in enamel; so it can be applied more often in consultation with the dentist.

14.6.3 Diagnosis and Treatment Planning

In general, preparation and treatment planning of cold atmospheric plasma-enhanced bleaching are similar to those of a conventional bleaching procedure. The patient should be interviewed regarding existing allergies, known problems with tooth hypersensitivity, and possible reasons for tooth staining. Before starting the treatment, a careful dental examination and professional tooth cleaning should be performed.

Jet plasma technology is recommended for precise intraoral cold atmospheric plasma application. The current scientific data base speaks for an approved argon-driven or helium-driven HF plasma jet device, a combination with low-dose hydrogen peroxide or carbamide peroxide or without chemicals, and a treatment time of 5–30 minutes. Since the plasma jet directs an airflow onto the tooth surface, bleaching gels have to be reapplied repeatedly during the treatment time and gingival tissues should be protected by rubber dam. Pre- and Post-op documentation should include a scale of color and brightness and the date of treatment, and should follow the very basic requirements of scientific medical photography.

14.6.4 Anesthesia

Anesthesia is not needed in general. Slight local effects have to be considered like a minor pinprick or irritation of hypersensitive areas related to the tip of the plume of plasma jets.

14

14.6.5 Posttreatment Care

According to dental experience, there is no special posttreatment care needed with respect to cold atmospheric plasma.

14.6.6 Handling of Complications

As for clinical plasma medicine, there are most likely no complications to be expected in aesthetic plasma dentistry. All known side effects of bleaching are either of temporary nature or can be treated by simple dental procedures (e.g., fluoridation).

Conclusion

Although a standardized technique of aesthetic plasma dentistry still needs to be developed, the practical use of cold atmospheric plasma as a beneficial treatment strategy is already on the doorstep of good dental practice.

References

1. Jablonowski L, Kocher T, Schindler A, Müller K, Dombrowski F, von Woedtke T, et al. Side effects by oral application of atmospheric pressure plasma on the mucosa in mice. PLoS One. 2019;14(4):e0215099.

2. Rupf S, Idlibi AN, Marrawi FA, Hannig M, Schubert A, von Mueller L, et al. Removing biofilms from microstructured titanium Ex Vivo: a novel approach using atmospheric plasma technology. PLoS One. 2011;6(10): e25893.

3. Idlibi AN, Al-Marrawi F, Hannig M, Lehmann A, Rueppell A, Schindler A, et al. Destruction of oral biofilms formed in situ on machined titanium (Ti) surfaces by cold atmospheric plasma. Biofouling. 2013;29(4):369–79.

4. Kim GC, Lee HW, Byun JH, Chung J, Jeon YC, Lee JK. Dental applications of low-temperature nonthermal plasmas. Plasma Process Polym. 2013;10(3):199–206.

5. Kwon JS, Kim YH, Choi EH, Kim KN. Development of ultra-hydrophilic and non-cytotoxic dental vinyl polysiloxane impression materials using a non-thermal atmospheric-pressure plasma jet. J Phys Appl Phys. 2013;46(19):195201.

6. Cha S, Park YS. Plasma in dentistry. Clin Plasma Med. 2014;2(1):4–10.

7. Metelmann PH, Quooß A, von Woedtke T, Krey KF. First insights on plasma orthodontics – application of cold atmospheric pressure plasma to enhance the bond strength of orthodontic brackets. Clin Plasma Med. 2016;4(2):46–9.

8. Kwon JS, Kim YH, Choi EH, Kim CK, Kim KN, Kim KM. Non-thermal atmospheric pressure plasma increased mRNA expression of growth factors in human gingival fibroblasts. Clin Oral Investig. 2016;20(7):1801–8.

9. Gherardi M, Tonini R, Colombo V. Plasma in dentistry: brief history and current status. Trends Biotechnol. 2018;36(6):583–5.

10. Kleineidam B, Nokhbehsaim M, Deschner J, Wahl G. Effect of cold plasma on periodontal wound healing—an in vitro study. Clin Oral Investig. 2019;23(4):1941–50.

11. Sierwald I, John MT, Schierz O, Jost-Brinkmann PG, Reissmann DR. Zusammenhang von Overjet und Overbite mit ästhetischen Beeinträchtigungen der mundgesundheitsbezogenen Lebensqualität. J Orofac Orthop. 2015;76(5):405–20.

12. Samorodnitzky-Naveh GR, Geiger SB, Levin L. Patients' satisfaction with dental esthetics. J Am Dent Assoc. 2007;138(6):805–8.

13. Van Der Geld P, Oosterveld P, Van Heck G, Kuijpers-Jagtman AM. Smile attractiveness: self-perception and influence on personality. Angle Orthod. 2007;77(5):759–65.

14. Tin-Oo MM, Saddki N, Hassan N. Factors influencing patient satisfaction with dental appearance and treatments they desire to improve aesthetics. BMC Oral Health. 2011;11(1):6.

15. Reno E, Sunberg R, Block R, Bush R. The influence of lip/gum color on subject perception of tooth color. J Dent Res. 2000;79:381.

16. Joiner A. Tooth colour: a review of the literature. J Dent. 2004;32(Suppl):3–12.

17. Sackett DL. Evidence-based medicine. Semin Perinatol. 1997;21:3–5.

18. Claiborne D, Mccombs G, Lemaster M, Akman MA, Laroussi M. Low-temperature atmospheric pressure plasma enhanced tooth whitening: the next-generation technology. Int J Dent Hyg. 2014;12(2):108–14.

19. Lee HW, Kim GJ, Kim JM, Park JK, Lee JK, Kim GC. Tooth bleaching with nonthermal atmospheric pressure plasma. J Endod. 2009;35(4):587–91.

20. Nam SH, Lee HJ, Hong JW, Kim GC. Efficacy of nonthermal atmospheric pressure plasma for tooth bleaching. Sci World J. 2015;2015:581731.

21. Nam SH, Ok SM, Kim GC. Tooth bleaching with low-temperature plasma lowers surface roughness and Streptococcus mutans adhesion. Int Endod J. 2018;51(4):479–88.
22. Çelik B, Çapar İD, İbiş F, Erdilek N, Ercan UK. Deionized water can substitute common bleaching agents for nonvital tooth bleaching when treated with non-thermal atmospheric plasma. J Oral Sci. 2019;61(1):103–10.
23. Sun P, Pan J, Tian Y, Bai N, Wu H, Wang L, et al. Tooth whitening with hydrogen peroxide assisted by a direct-current cold atmospheric-pressure air plasma microjet. IEEE Transactions on Plasma Science. 2010;38:1892–6.
24. Choi HS, Kim KN, You EM, Choi EH, Kim YH, Kim KM. Tooth whitening effects by atmospheric pressure cold plasmas with different gases. Jpn J Appl Phys. 2013;52(11):11NF02-1-4.
25. Nam SH, Lee HW, Cho SH, Lee JK, Jeon YC, Kim GC. High-efficiency tooth bleaching using nonthermal atmospheric pressure plasma with low concentration of hydrogen peroxide. J Appl Oral Sci. 2013;21(3):265–70.

14

Devices

Contents

Basic Principles and Future Developments in Cold Plasma Therapy

Torsten Gerling, Robert Bansemer,
Eric Timmermann,
and Klaus-Dieter Weltmann

Contents

© Springer Nature Switzerland AG 2022
H.-R. Metelmann et al. (eds.), *Textbook of Good Clinical Practice in Cold Plasma Therapy*, https://doi.org/10.1007/978-3-030-87857-3_15

😊 Core Messages

- Plasma as the fourth state of matter has a rather long history in medicine and an even longer application in the decontamination of surfaces.
- The available commercial devices differ by ignition concept and generated plasma "cocktail", making them comparable in general, and unique in the details.
- Plasma medical devices are technically pioneered for the future in dentistry, endoscopy, cancer treatment and for large-scale treatments like burn wounds.
- Industrial trends of industry 4.0 are on the verge of implementation into plasma medicine, either by ambulant sensory supported treatment or artificial intelligence.
- Technological advances on plasma medical devices elevate related fields like medical hygiene and trigger new fields of investigation such as plasma agriculture.
- Joint approaches by medical experts, research experts, and companies are necessary to further explore and benefit from the high potential of CAP.

15.1 Introduction

Plasma technology is unique for its wide antimicrobial and antiviral efficacy even against multi-resistant germs and therefore attracts widespread attention [1–4]. This technology finds itself involved in various research fields and applications in medicine, out of which chronic wound treatment and cancer research are presently the most dominant ones [5].

Further areas under investigation are the treatment of skin donor samples, cardiac surgery, cleaning of surgical sites, dental medicine, aesthetic medicine, treatment of pigmentation disorders, immunology, ophthalmology, cancer treatment and even veterinary medicine [5]. In addition, the application of cold atmospheric pressure plasma is of high interest for clinical environments. In fact, its capacity for decontamination and hygiene improvement could be used in order to fight infection sources, for example, on surfaces.

However, with each advancement toward a new field, cold atmospheric plasma (CAP) development and characterization are essential steps. Presently four companies supply devices based on CAP technology for medical application as presented in the ▶ Chaps. 16, 17, 18 and 19. They all generate CAP with a range of reactive oxygen and nitrogen species (RONS), an electrical field, a certain temperature and irradiation from the ultraviolet until the infrared spectral range. However, the devices differ by ignition concept and the generated plasma cocktail.

❯ Important to Know

Each CAP device presently on the market differs by ignition concept and generated plasma cocktail.

This chapter introduces basic knowledge of the plasma state and the different types of devices in application. Furthermore, it presents an overview of conceivable future fields of medical CAP application and associated technological challenges. Moreover, several fields for CAP technologies strongly influenced by plasma medical applications are outlined.

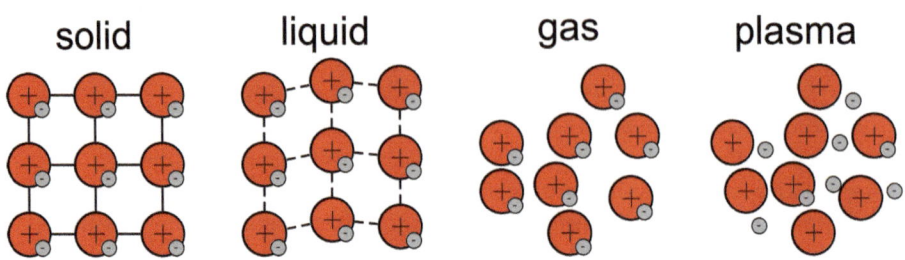

15.2 Plasma as Fourth State of Matter

Both from daily experiences as well as from general education, the appearance of substances or – to make use of a vocabulary more common in physics – of matter in different states is well-known. The most obvious example is water, which exists in a solid form below 0 °C (at normal pressure). Temperature is a macroscopically measurable state variable of matter and represents the mean internal energy stored in the random motion of its atoms and molecules.[1] Consequently, increasing the temperature means increasing the internal energy. At a certain threshold, the energy of the atoms and molecules is so high that they change the structure in which they arrange. This is depicted in a schematic and simplified form in Fig. 15.1.

If the internal energy of the solid ice is increased to such an extent that its temperature exceeds 0 °C, it changes to a liquid state (melting). This phase transition gives the molecules more degrees of freedom: while in the solid state they are fixed apart from an oscillatory movement, the liquid state allows them to move slightly toward one another. Macroscopically, this difference becomes visible in the lack of dimensional stability of water; it adapts to the shape of its (solid) environment. A further increase in temperature above 100 °C leads to boiling, with water changing into a gaseous state. The molecules now have even more energy and move freely from one to another at a large distance. The same amount of water molecules in the gaseous state takes up about 1000 times the volume compared to the liquid.

Beyond these classical states of matter, it is possible to achieve another state, which is characterized by an exceptional particle structure. With sufficient (i.e., a lot of) energy input into a gas, negatively charged electrons can be released from atoms or molecules, with the consequence that these remain now as ions. This state of matter is called plasma. The preferred technological way to transfer a gas into a cold (nonthermal) plasma state is exposing it to a very strong electric field, which forms between metal parts on which a very high electric voltage is applied.

---

1   Which is why there is the absolute zero at a temperature of 0 K or −273.15 °C: The particles are at rest then, so there is no way to cool down further!

15

Since there are electrically charged electrons and ions in the plasma, and not only electrically neutral atoms and molecules as in gases, plasmas are electrically conductive. Electrons and ions can induce chemical reactions which would not take place in a neutral gas, and they emit radiation. This allows a wide range of application fields, especially because it is possible to couple the very high energy – and hence the very high temperature – almost exclusively to the electrons. Since the electrons have about 1000–10,000 times lower mass than atoms and molecules, the conservation of momentum concludes a 1000–10,000 times reduced energy transmission. Atoms, molecules, and ions have a different, much lower temperature then. They can even remain at room temperature, which is the key aspect of CAP. Due to their unique physical and chemical properties, CAP is a versatile tool for working on technological problems, but also for interaction with biological and heat-sensitive systems.

❯ **Important to Know**
CAP is characterized by very hot electrons, but cold neutral particles and ions. This makes it suitable for heat-sensitive processes, but can still initiate chemical reaction networks that would either take place at much higher temperatures only, or are even unique to cold plasmas.

15.3 History of Plasma Application in Medicine

The first usage of plasmas for an indirect interaction with biological systems was the decontamination of water by ozone, for which plasma reactors were already investigated in 1857 by Ernst Werner Siemens (now known as Werner von Siemens) [6]. After the application on water, the decontaminating effect of ozone was also successfully used on technical surfaces and containers starting with a patent of 1968 [7]. With the first mention of so-called violet ray machines in the 1920s and the electro-therapeutic Zeileis method, medically intended applications without a scientific basis were performed early on as well [8]. However, with an advanced understanding and control of technological plasma devices, their application further extended into medicine.

One such example is the contactless surgical tool – the argon plasma coagulator (APC) [9]. It utilizes an arc discharge to create a localized plasma with a distinctive discharge current. Therefore, the temperature rises much higher than in CAP described in this book, which leads to controlled hemostasis, devitalization, and coagulation.

❯ **Important to Know**
Argon plasma coagulation is also applied in medicine; however, it is to be clearly distinguished from CAP devices, since it denatures the tissue surface through the action of heat.

Only in the early twentieth century, plasma technology was able to generate cold plasma at atmospheric pressure due to an enhanced understanding of nonthermal plasma together with an enhanced availability of new technical tools for manufacturing [10].

15.4 Basic Principles of CAP Generation

The ▶ Sect. 15.2 already explained electron-neutral collisions to be inefficient energy exchange processes. Of course, a more frequent supply of electrons caused by a high electrical current ("amperage") can enhance the number of such collisions and allow an alignment of electron temperature and gas temperature. This means that high current, as it is observed within lightning, usually leads to a hot plasma. However, for CAP, this can be inhibited by either a resistive or dielectric barrier that is placed between the high voltage electrode and the grounded electrode. Such a barrier could be a ceramic cover sheet, a glass plate, or even the skin of the patient.

The different technological solutions to generate CAPs are classified as follows. Dielectric barrier discharges (DBDs) are one player within the field. A dielectric covers the powered or the grounded electrode. This dielectric barrier limits the current and prevents the discharge from conversion into sparks or leaders, which are plasma discharges as parts within a lightning. ◘ Figure 15.2 shows two settings of DBDs. The first is the volume DBD, which can be used with a patient as the target electrode. The second setting shows a surface DBD, where the discharge is limited to the surface of the dielectric, and the generated reactive species are emitted into the surrounding toward the patient. For both types of discharges, there are implementations certified for medical application and presented in more detail in the upcoming chapters.

Another type of discharge arrangement used for application are the plasma jet arrangement (see ◘ Fig. 15.2 bottom). Plasma jets generate a high electrical field between a powered electrode and a grounded electrode around or inside a capillary. The capillary can act as a dielectric barrier and thus inhibit intense discharge formation. Due to the geometric setting, the discharge develops also outside of the device toward the patient. Optionally, this arrangement is supplied with a desired working gas like synthetic air, helium, or argon. A medical device of this setup will be presented in an upcoming chapter as well.

Each of the geometries in ◘ Fig. 15.2 is favorable for the generation of a different composition of cocktail components of CAP. Even within the same device, changes of operating parameters like voltage and gas selection can change the composition. Each component is already associated with respective contributions to medicine in individual fields and was until now partially proven to contribute similarly in plasma medicine as well:

(a) Electrons and ions
  - They are the essential building blocks of a plasma and relate to all subsequent generation of further components.
  - CAPs can generate exceptional ions like molecular argon ions, that can contribute by mechanical impact.
  - Ions are used in radiotherapy [12].
  - Negative ions were investigated in a series of animal studies to possibly prove their benefit in multiple ways; however, no consistent results were found [13].

15

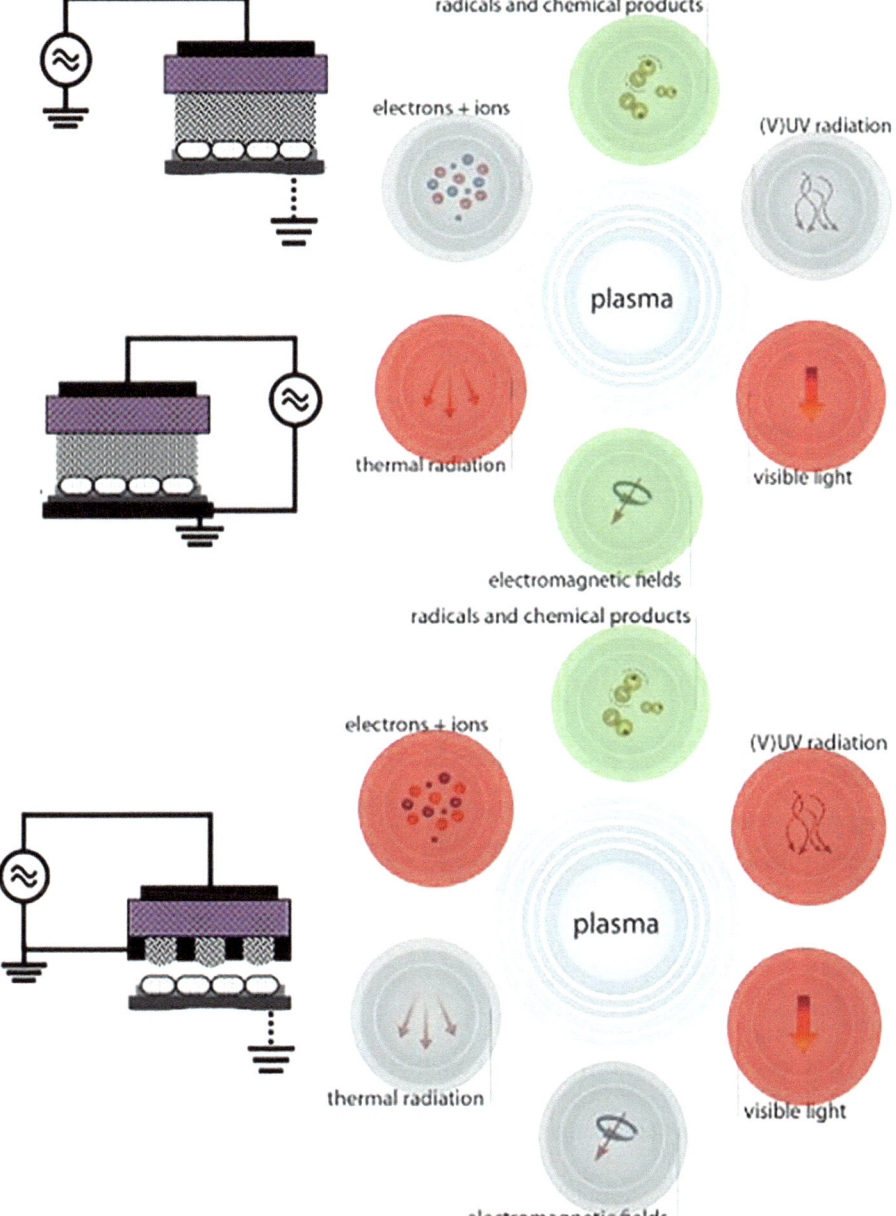

■ **Fig. 15.2** Geometry of common CAP arrangements. Top: two volume dielectric barrier discharges (DBDs), middle: surface DBD, bottom: plasma jet. For each type of CAP arrangement, typical characteristic contributions to the plasma cocktail are evaluated based on presumably dominant contribution of a component ("enhanced," green), rather indifferent contribution of the component ("indifferent," gray) or rather a nonsignificant contribution or generation of the respective component ("reduced," red). (Device pictures taken with permission from [11])

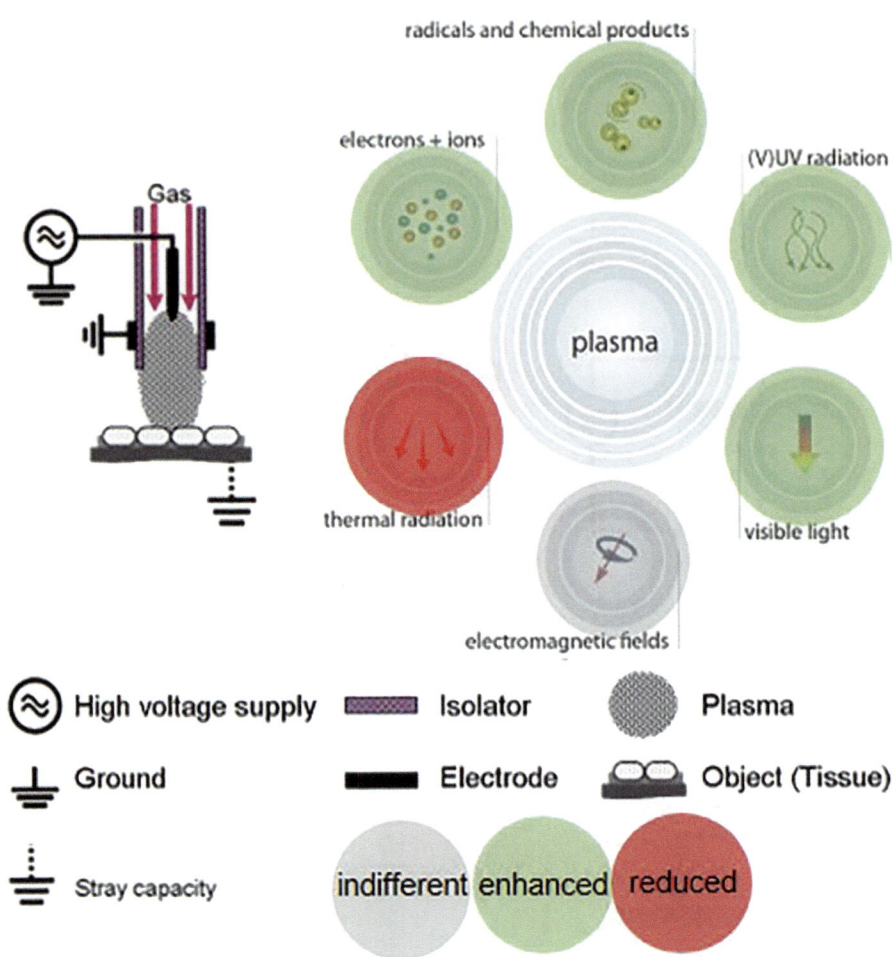

radicals and chemical products

electrons + ions

(V)UV radiation

Gas

plasma

thermal radiation

visible light

electromagnetic fields

High voltage supply   Isolator   Plasma

Ground   Electrode   Object (Tissue)

Stray capacity   indifferent enhanced reduced

■ **Fig. 15.2** (continued)

(b) Temperature
  - Closure of surgical wounds is sometimes supported by heat, as in coagulation applications.
(c) Radiation from the (vacuum) ultraviolet ((V)UV) to the near-infrared range (NIR)
  - UV radiation is applied in phototherapy of skin diseases [14].
  - UV radiation is recently applied for air or surface disinfection.
(d) Reactive species
  - RONS are known for their deleterious and beneficial effects in medicine [15, 16].
(e) Electrical fields
  - Pulsed electrical fields are investigated for cancer therapy [17].
  - Further medical applications are, for example, electrical muscle stimulation (EMS) and transcutaneous electrical nerve stimulation (TENS) [18, 19].

The overall understanding for tuning such devices in relation to intended indications and required set of components is not yet achieved, but rather represents a current research objective. However, an overall separation has been established in recent years and summarized in ◘ Fig. 15.2. Meanwhile, the balance of effectivity and harm has to be considered, for some cocktail components the effect changes based on concentration (e.g., ozone).

> ❯ **Important to Know**
> CAP generates a cocktail of components. However, the individual threshold for cocktail consumptions differ between targets.

One more system for medical application is based on a torch discharge arrangement with a hot and thermal plasma technology. The key part of this technology is the generation of an intense plasma between two electrodes at a distance of around 30 cm away from the patient and to have the generated radiation and reactive species being directed toward the intended spot. This results in a rather global treatment of the desired spot.

The transition cascade for CAP treatment of biological samples, crossing four states of matter, is depicted in ◘ Fig. 15.3. Within timescales of up to microseconds, CAP generates simple excited and reactive species, electrons and ions, electrical fields as well as UV and VUV radiation. The movement of especially the reactive and excited species through the gas phase takes a timeframe of up to milliseconds to reach the surface. There they interact on a timescale of up to minutes with the humid environment of the biological target and excite a solution chemistry before finally reaching the intended target – the cells, tissue, or bacteria. At the interface between each of the named phases in ◘ Fig. 15.3, complex chemical reaction networks are initiated, yet not fully understood to date. In addition, the desired individual treatment option available with CAP strongly depends on the composition and control of the cocktail of components (◘ Fig. 15.2). Ideally, each cocktail component should be assigned to a defined dose depending on the indication. However, that still needs more research to be conducted even for present medical application. A long-term result might also be a universal tunable device with an all-in-one doses variety.

15.5 New Fields for Medical Application of Cold Atmospheric Plasma Technology

The future of plasma medicine is closely linked to fundamental understanding and development of new CAP technologies, either by adjusting geometries, tuning operation parameters, or developing fundamentally new device concepts. Adjusting the geometries as performed for dimension and ergonometric adaptation for dental application, for example [21], proves to be a fundamental step, requiring a careful adaptation of especially the electrical safety concept.

Parameter tuning [22] is an effective approach to provide a composition of biologically active agents optimized for application requirements and conditions.

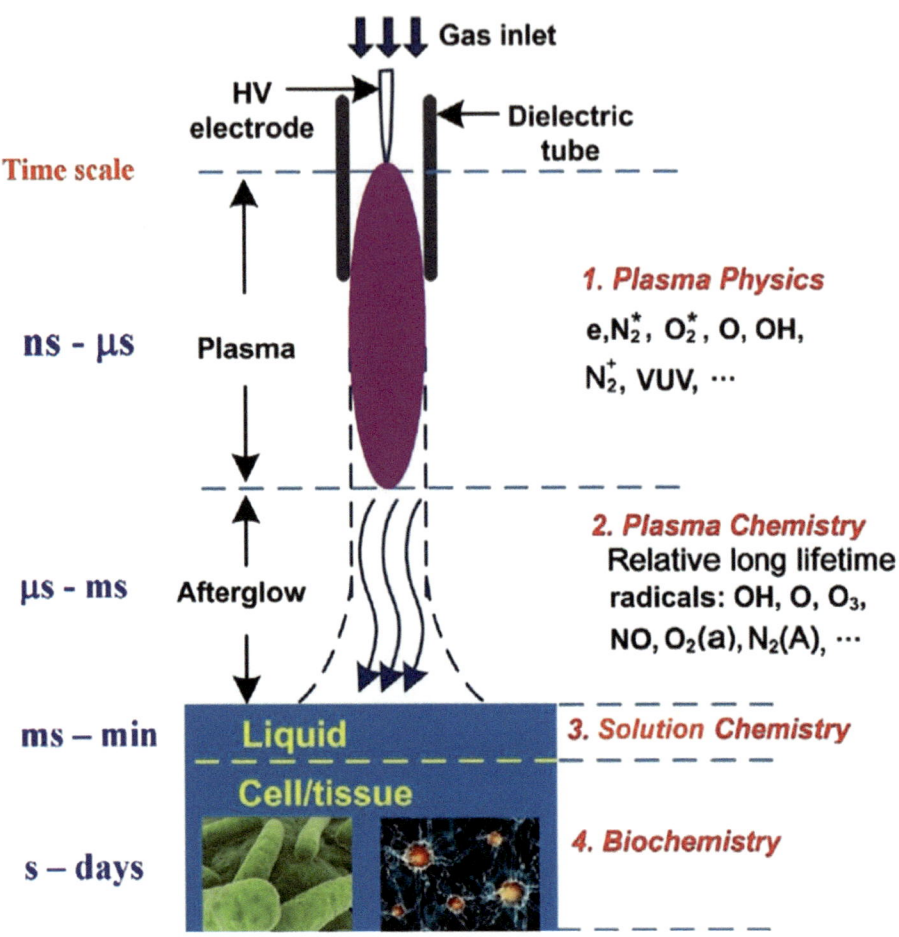

Fig. 15.3 Relevant timescale behind the treatment with CAP for the example of the plasma jet. (Taken with permission from [20])

However, it requires complex diagnostics and a careful scientific approach to understand correlations between device output and operating parameters.

Fundamental new CAP technologies are developed frequently, "plasma treated media", for example, crop posttreatment being one of the promising examples from recent years [23]. They greatly expand the possibilities of plasma therapy (compared to direct application), but also broaden the number of open and interdisciplinary research questions. Other approaches, like the piezoelectric-driven plasma generation promise more compact and safer devices [24].

In this section, an overview of the most recent and most innovative approaches for future plasma therapies in medicine is given. These topics will be differentiated by

1. Expanding CAP technologies to further medical fields
2. Trends, opportunities, and challenges of CAP in medicine
3. Emerging synergies to nonmedical topics

This chapter will give the reader an overview of the most interesting current technical developments and their current stage, while some of them are examined in more detail. Moreover, contemporary social demands and technological trends, which give CAP therapies opportunities for further development, are highlighted in the following section. It also explains the challenges that CAP therapy will face in the years to come. Finally, some promising synergies with related, but nonmedical topics are presented.

15.5.1 Expanding Application of Present CAP Technologies to Further Medical Fields

CAP technology provides a powerful and highly adaptable method to inactivate unwanted microorganisms, but also to excite and support the wound healing. Both features are uniquely suited for a broad range of medical fields, as two superior requirements for patient care are performed: reducing the number of present or hospital-acquired pathogens and increasing wound healing rates. Furthermore, CAP can be applied very precisely locally and has hardly any side effects [5]. In addition, promising results in cancer research are motivating new fields of application.

These results could only be achieved with pioneering devices, which opened up new fields of application, which in turn can be opened up with adapted devices and so on. Current research in plasma medicine is therefore an iterative process that is driven alternately by new devices and new scientific findings.

Some selected current and emerging fields for medical CAP treatment are depicted in ◘ Fig. 15.4. Current approved devices were developed for dermatologic wound treatment, but were also tested in other – always superficial – use cases (e.g., in ophthalmology). A more recent technical development in this area is shown in ◘ Fig. 15.5 – the plasma patch and the jet array, which aim to enable wounds to be treated easily over a large area. However, many other potential fields of application can only be tapped if the CAP can be applied inside the body (◘ Fig. 15.4). Therefore, two relevant developments are presented below.

15.5.1.1 CAP in Endoscopy

Modern, flexible endoscopes are operated via bowden controls and come with a powerful light source and a camera attached at their tip. While their diameter is being reduced further and further, there is still a working channel through which a variety of tools can be introduced. It was the logical conclusion to use this working channel to create access for plasma jets inside the body and thus open up many other areas of medical application.

The safe and reliable operation of such extremely miniaturized and flexible devices is the result of a large range of recent innovations in engineering and technology. In order to allow an ignition at the jet tip while avoiding parasitic plasma discharges in other parts of the system, specialized concepts to ensure a suitable electric field distribution in the complete assembly are necessary. Moreover, all

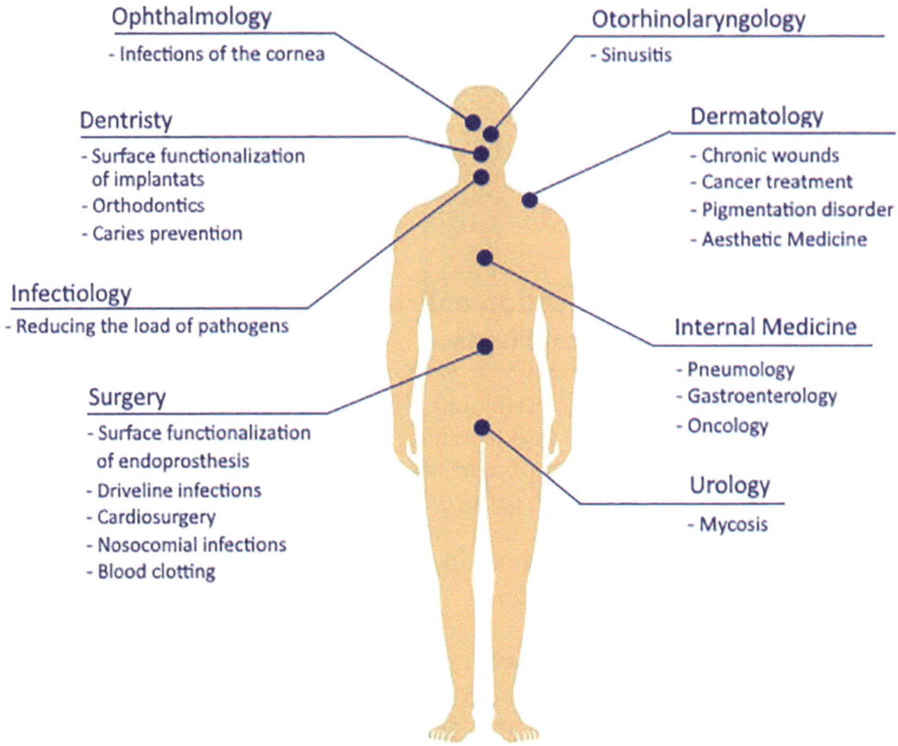

Ophthalmology
- Infections of the cornea

Otorhinolaryngology
- Sinusitis

Dentristy
- Surface functionalization
  of implantats
- Orthodontics
- Caries prevention

Dermatology
- Chronic wounds
- Cancer treatment
- Pigmentation disorder
- Aesthetic Medicine

Infectiology
- Reducing the load of pathogens

Surgery
- Surface functionalization
  of endoprosthesis
- Driveline infections
- Cardiosurgery
- Nosocomial infections
- Blood clotting

Internal Medicine
- Pneumology
- Gastroenterology
- Oncology

Urology
- Mycosis

Fig. 15.4   Selected current and emerging medical fields for CAP treatment

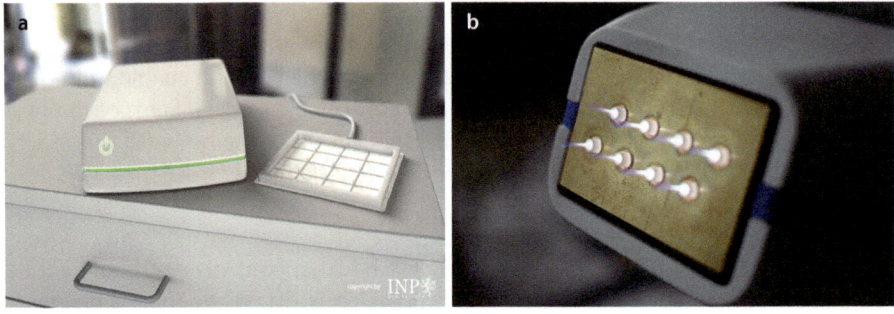

Fig. 15.5 **a** plasma patch for a large-scale DBD application for wound treatment; **b** upscaled plasma jet concept for a large-scale jet application in plasma medicine

materials used need to fulfill a variety of different, sometimes conflictive requirements to ensure flexibility, electrical safety, negligible erosion, robustness, and conformity with legal regulations. Despite all constructive challenges also with regard
to the electrical design, an uncompromising minimization of the patient leakage
current is inevitable in this application.

15

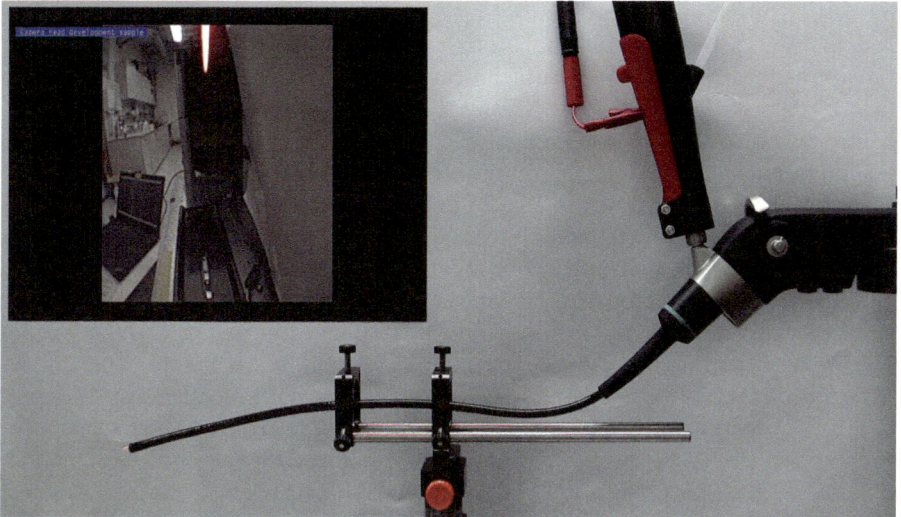

☐ Fig. 15.6 CAP jet at the tip of a prototype endoscope. Its gas and electric supply are inside the working channel. The perspective of the endoscope camera is depicted in the up*per left corner*

A notable prototype of a CAP jet for endoscopic applications with promising bactericidal effects in vitro is presented by Winter et al. [25, 26] (see ☐ Fig. 15.6). This device has an outer diameter of only 1.8 mm, and it can be used as a tool inside the working channel of an endoscope. Despite the high voltage necessary for the plasma and the low distances between system components, electromagnetic compatibility to the endoscope camera is given. Neon is used as the preferred feed gas, while carbon dioxide is needed as a shielding gas to ensure proper working inside cavities. This prototype was developed together with industrial and clinical partners in a public-founded project ("Plasmaskop"[2]). Preparations are currently being made to conduct animal experiments. Their aim is to show the relieving effect on acute sinusitis.

Examples of other approaches are the so-called plasma gun for the generation of pulsed plasma streams in a long, small-diameter tube [27] and the combination of a larger-volume plasma with a long, narrow tube with a plasma effluent at its downstream end [28].

15.5.1.2 Dental Application
The application of CAP in dentistry picked up interest early on when plasma medicine started. Already during the first big project on plasma medicine, the "Campus PlasmaMed,"[3] two fields for dental application were investigated using different

2   Funded by Federal Ministry of Education and Research via grant number 13GW0052C between 2015 and 2018

3   Funded by Federal Ministry of Education and Research via grant number 13N9779 and 13N11188, from 2008 until 2013

properties of plasma: functionalization of implants and reduction of microbial load [8, 28–31]. The target of implant treatment focused on coating with antibacterial agents to prevent bacterial attachment as well as the hydrophilicity of the surface for osseointegration [32]. Meanwhile, the reduction of microbial load in dentistry was focused on the implant surface as well as in the tooth root channel [33]. In recent years, the application toward oral tumor treatment has been of interest as well and was already investigated in the clinical environment [34, 35].

One major focus with a perspective for future medical application became the treatment of periimplantitis. Due to inflammation around the implant combined with the growth of microorganisms on the implant, the supporting bone structure is degenerated and a long-term implant failure might follow. Presently, this event has two negative outcomes. While the infected implant has to be replaced, generating additional costs for the patient, the bone structure itself mostly cannot support another implant. Hence, a new spot to mount the replacement implant has to be found or, in the worst case, to be generated. The present phenomenon of periimplantitis is just starting to emerge, since it can take several years to develop. However, the present observations only cover the situation of up to 10 years in the past. The fact that the number of implant usage is steadily increasing might indicate a potential rise of periimplantitis in the future.

One research project addressing periimplantitis is hosted at the University Medicine in Greifswald by Prof. T. Kocher and Dr. L. Jablonowski in collaboration with the industry ("PeriPLas"[4]). Their approach combines a mechanical cleaning to remove the biofilm, a laser application to inhibit the remaining bacteria, and a consecutive plasma application to improve the hydrophilicity of the surface. The project is expected to perform a clinical trial within the project timeframe.

15.5.2 Trends, Opportunities, and Challenges for CAP Technologies in Medicine

The main challenge for CAP treatment in the near future is to gain a detailed understanding of the mechanisms behind the observed biological effects (❏ Fig. 15.7). These efforts are complicated by the large number of possible variables during CAP treatment (plasma parameters, environmental, and target conditions). Breaking these down and examining them systematically remains the ambitious task of applied basic research - the creation of controlled field tests in the area of wound care being already difficult [36]. This knowledge would be the basis for CAP treatment optimized for the respective indication and surrounding conditions, but it would also facilitate the approval of devices.

On the device side, there are many published plasma sources that differ in terms of their different types of application, carrier gases as well as high voltage and plasma generation types, including those whose operating modes can change completely

4   Funded by Federal Ministry of Education and Research via grant number 13N14479 from 2017 until 2021

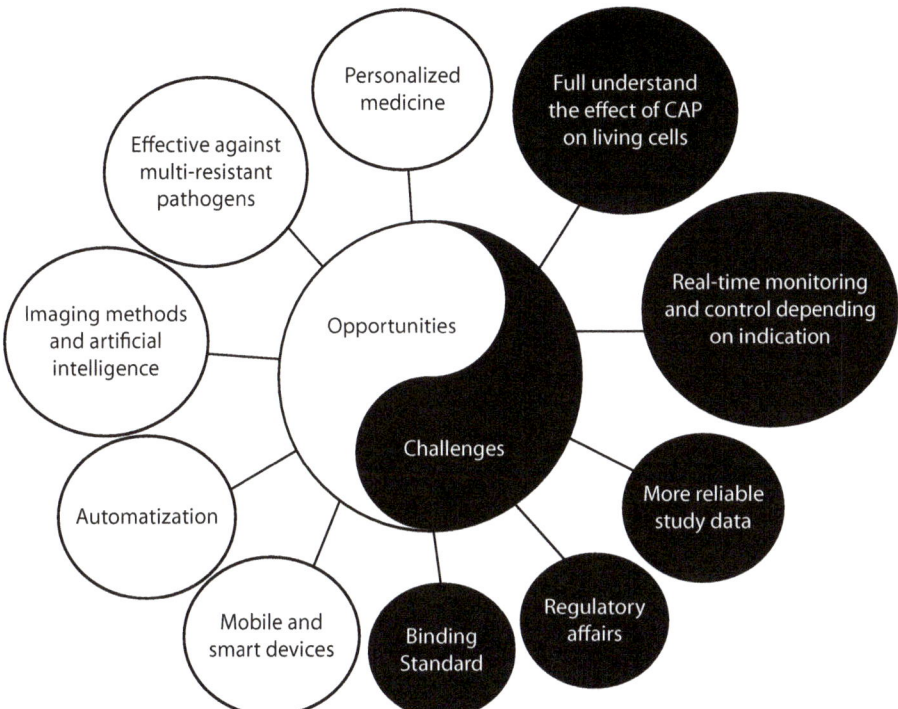

■ **Fig. 15.7** Opportunities and challenges associated with CAP technologies now and in the future

[22]. However, a standardized data set of each device applied in the research environment is not available. Establishing a systemization and storage opportunity here is the goal of the "INPTDat" data platform [37]. Moreover, a binding Standard for medical plasma devices must be developed to unify the elicitation of respective data. The first step in this direction is the DIN SPEC 91315, which is a collection of safety and efficacy-related tests (see 5.2.1). It allows medical plasma devices to be compared with one another, but does not impose any minimum requirements or limit values.

However, this adaptability and scalability of CAP devices also offer a number of attractive opportunities, which are driven by current social and technological trends. For example, plasma sources provide easy access to personalized medicine. The prerequisite here, however, is that real-time monitoring of the wound situation and the plasma parameters takes place. A possible technical approach is the combination with hyperspectral imaging, which allows conclusions to be drawn about tissue oxygenation and microbial contamination [38]. In addition, the size and shape of the wound can be determined from images using computer algorithms. Both would be a prerequisite for automated and optimized treatment. Moreover, comparative field tests would benefit from this. A further technical trend is the increasing mobility of equipment, made possible by ever-cheaper and more available battery technology.

15.5.2.1 Tracing Ambulant Treatment Conditions

The biggest success in application with plasma medicine was achieved in chronic wound treatment. However, the average patient with chronic wounds is not mobile and hence a mobile treatment solution should be considered. While a mobile treatment proves an opportunity for the patient, the risk prevails of rapidly changing ambulant conditions in patient homes compared to a clinic or medical practice.

To investigate this risk and to intensify the opportunity, a consortium with Prof. S. Emmert from the University Medicine Rostock, the Leibniz Institute for Plasma Science and Technology Greifswald and the OTaktiv GmbH Greifswald started a joint project on ambulant wound care and for the detection of ambient conditions ("AmbuPlas"). Different medical plasma devices (e.g., kINPen MED, neoplas med GmbH, and Plasma Derm, Cinogy GmbH) are used in a combination of ambulant and stationary settings. A mobile sensory unit is be applied to detect ambient conditions (e.g., temperature, humidity) as well as plasma operation time based on audio detection. In combination with this, a commercial wound camera is applied to trace the wound volume development in correlation with the respective sensory data.

For further motivation of plasma application in medicine, it is necessary to perform randomized clinical studies with a tracing of the wound healing process [39]. From a scientific viewpoint, the qualification of the wound properties like area, volume, and also the germ concentration and combination are of interest. However, to date, despite all progress in medical technology, the precise determination of wound dimensions is widely performed with a ruler placed on a wound and the consecutive evaluation of the wound based on a square or elliptic fit. However, wound healing is not just a matter of area but also the wound healing in the volume has to be considered.

One innovation addressing the shortage of wound data for detailed wound healing progress determination is based on artificial intelligence (AI). Under the slogan "KI Wound," a consortium of Prof. Steffen Emmert (University Medicine Rostock), Dr. Torsten Gerling, Dr. Kai Masur (both INP Greifswald), Ihda Chaerony Siffa (University Lübeck and INP Greifswald) and Christian Eschenburg (OTaktiv GmbH) initiated an approach combining AI with a sensor system to detect the wound volume without touching the surface. The approach shall require only a mobile phone and an attachable sensory unit. In the future, such easy access shall enable quick, convenient, and cheap options to document wound development and enable a database for further wound healing science, even outside the field of plasma medicine.

15.5.2.2 Further Development of DIN SPEC 91315

Defining a standard for technical products is very important in order to achieve the best possible benefits for the society, to increase transparency and safety for the user, but also to identify unsuitable devices on the market. In 2014, the first steps were taken to create a binding standard for medical plasma devices (intended for dermatologic use) in the very young discipline of plasma medicine. The result was the so-called DIN-SPEC 91315 [40] with the title "General requirements for medical plasma sources," which is regarded as the nonbinding forerunner of a DIN standard.

◻ **Table 15.1** Test procedures of the DIN SPEC 91315

Physical	Chemical	Biological
Temperature	Gas emissions	Inhibition zone tests
Thermal output	pH in liquid	Microbial suspensions
Optical emissions (UV)	H_2O_2 in liquid	Cytotoxicity
Leakage current	NO_2^- and NO_3^- in liquid	

The DIN-SPEC 91315 contains a set of generally applicable physical, biological and chemical test procedures, defining information to be obtained about performance characteristics as well as efficacy and safety of the plasma source (◻ Table 15.1). The measurement results are not evaluated or only by reference to standards that are already in force. When choosing the tests, it was also taken into account that they can be carried out with simple laboratory equipment. Furthermore, the description is deliberately kept general so that it can be adapted to the different plasma sources [40].

During the past few years, the DIN SPEC has been used frequently by manufacturers to test the general suitability of their (sometimes completely different) plasma sources for medical use. The individual tests of the DIN SPEC are described shortly below. With this insight, the authors would also like to encourage medical users to provide feedback.

The patient leakage current is measured using a defined circuit that is intended to reflect the sensitivity of the human body to alternating electrical currents of different frequencies [41]. The measurements can be carried out quickly and easily, as there are commercial measuring devices and defined limit values [41]. The temperature of the plasma source is another key parameter. A small increase in temperature (38.5 °C) is associated with stimulation of wound healing, while temperatures above 45 °C lead to burns. A maximum temperature of 40 °C is typically given as a guide. Both measurements are conducted in dependence on the distance between target and the CAP device. A safe distance can be easily maintained in the finished medical product using spacers.

Optical emission spectroscopy and measurements of the position-dependent gas emissions complement the physical safety tests. From the measured optical spectrum, an effective UV radiation and maximum daily dose on the human skin are calculated [42]. Ozone and nitrogen oxides are typical long-living and potentially lung damaging species for which strict thresholds exist. Furthermore, the effect of time-dependent CAP treatment on a human cell vitality assay accounts for the identification of the cytotoxicity.

In contrast, the time-dependent antimicrobial efficacy of the CAP device is determined by inhibition zone assays and via treatment of microbial suspensions. Moreover, RONS are generated by complex plasma-liquid interactions. They play a major role in the biological effects of plasma treatment, as living cells and microorganisms usually are surrounded by liquid environments. Thus, a decrease of the pH and the production of nitrite (NO_2^-), nitrate (NO_3^-), and hydrogen peroxide (H_2O_2) in plasma-treated liquids enable the determination of the potential biological activity of the CAP device.

> **❶ Caution**
> New devices should always be subjected to thorough estimations of potential risks prior to application on patients. Therefore, the DIN SPEC 91315 should be applied and conformity declared.
>   ! Safety first

15.5.3   Emerging Synergies to Nonmedical Topics

The research but also the development in the field of plasma medicine generated and still generates enhanced plasma technological solutions. These solutions are not limited to plasma medicine and rather boost other existing fields or even initiate new fields of research (■ Fig. 15.8).

Along these existing fields, the application of CAP technology for surface treatments, in the context of this book for disinfection purposes or the use in air or water purification are just examples. New fields recently discussed are along veterinary medicine, and plasma agriculture and beauty applications.

Most of these fields even have lower legal restrictions on the device performance; however, this results in these fields also being overcrowded with many nonplasma technological solutions with potentially less efficacy investigation prior to

15

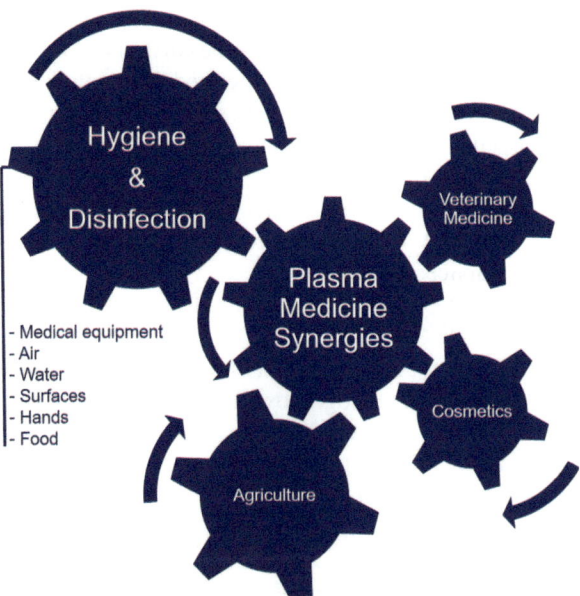

■ **Fig. 15.8**   Synergies between plasma medicine and selected, related topics

application. A clear statement to improve performance is hence harder to achieve. With the synergy input from plasma medicine, the device control can be enhanced, and thus an easier statement concerning cost-benefit is more accessible.

15.5.3.1 CAP in Clinical Hygiene

The antimicrobial properties of CAP treatment clearly suggest an application within clinical hygiene measures. The most advanced applications are plasma sterilizers, which dissociate hydrogen peroxide into highly effective free radicals. These devices are commercially available since 1993 and mainly used when steam sterilization is not possible, for example, with thermolabile materials (e.g. plastics), such as flexible endoscopes.

Although CAP is also able to disinfect or purify water and indoor air, such systems still play a minor role in clinical practice. On the one hand, this is because existing technologies are sophisticated and economically more attractive, but also because CAP applications sometimes have undesirable side effects that request higher effort of development and permission in this particular field. For example, the plasma treatment of indoor air is always accompanied by the production of ozone, the concentration of which is strictly limited (MAK value) due to its effect as a lung poison. Appropriate ozone filters could nullify the advantages of plasma treatment over other technologies like filters. An alternative application could be the disinfection of empty rooms, for example, overnight. In clinical wastewater treatment, plasmas can contribute to the destruction of stubborn compounds such as pharmaceutical residues (e.g., Diclofenac) or radiocontrast media (Diatrizoat). The promising usability of CAP for food processing and decontamination as well as reducing the chemical treatment of plants should be mentioned too.

In recent years, CAP-based water treatment has been investigated as a possible surface and volume disinfectant. It is characterized by a broad spectrum of antimicrobial activity, which can be traced back to a synergistic interaction of the RONS as well as in combination with electric fields. Peroxynitric acid in particular appears to have an important role. The biocidal effect wears off after a while, leaving only the original water. This could make it a greener alternative to conventional disinfectants, although there are still unanswered questions about upscaling, applicability, outgassing, and the detailed mechanism of action [43].

Infections with clostridium difficile play a special role, as they are extremely resistant in the form of spores (e.g., to alcohol-based disinfectants) and contribute to many nosocomial infections. They are mainly transmitted through frequently used surfaces (handles, touchscreens, …) – that is, through indirect contact. Although there are also promising approaches with antimicrobial copper coatings [44], self-cleaning with the help of CAP technologies is at least worth investigating, as it has been proven that they can inactivate clostridium difficile [45] and other spores [46].

In general, however, the inanimate environment plays a rather subordinate role as the origin of nosocomial infections [47]. Many, if not most, of the 2.6 million cases in Europe per year [48] can be traced back to endogenous pathogens [47]. This means that the microorganism moves from one place of the patient's body, where it does no harm, to another, where it causes infection. This is usually provoked by foreign bodies penetrating, for example, in catheter-associated urinary tract infections [49]. Nosocomial pneumonia as well as bloodstream, driveline, and surgical site infections also belong to this category. Unfortunately, this kind of hospital-acquired infections cannot be avoided by basic hygiene measures and often occur in connection with antibiotic-resistant microorganisms [50]. In this case, CAP technologies could make an important contribution, in particular, because they are effective against antibiotic-resistant microorganisms [1]. Moreover, they are applicable in the smallest gaps and they could in principle be operated in vivo as a built-in function of the medical product. This possibility could be demonstrated for the inside of endoscopes, for example, whereby the occurring material erosion was still problematic and has to be solved in future [51].

The application of CAP measures to avoid nosocomial infections by endogenous microorganisms can certainly be assigned a high potential. Especially in this area between hygienic and medical applications, to which wound therapy can also be counted, CAP technologies can still make a major contribution due to their advantageous properties compared to alternatives [3].

15.5.3.2 CAP Liquid Interaction for Agriculture

In plasma medical applications, CAP devices are required to operate reliably and to provide biologically active agents also under conditions involving certain amounts of humidity. Working in these humid environments is a challenge, but also accompanied with opportunities to purposefully extend mechanisms of interaction with biological systems provided by the influence of humidity. This is immediately relevant for plasma medicine [52–54], but also for application fields in decontamination and agriculture [55, 56]. The latter two can benefit from a plasma treatment of water, in which then short-living species as well as nitrite and nitrate accumulates and, in some circumstances, acidification occurs. The resulting liquid has an antimicrobial effect, and due to the nitrite and nitrate content, the usage as a fertilizer with an additional disinfecting effect could be feasible [57].

Beyond the mentioned examples, the field of plasma-liquid interactions took over an important place in basic research in recent years, driven by its importance for a large variety of applications. Due to the complex nature of plasma-liquid interactions, research in this topic is inherently multidisciplinary and holds out the prospect of advances for plasma medicine and environmental sciences as well as for topics with a weaker relation to plasma medicine, such as material synthesis [58].

15.6 How Can We Transfer the Ideas of the Future to the World of Today

One major experience leading to a later advantage of plasma medicine is the strict interdisciplinary approach followed for all different indications and topics. However, of course each participator needs to gain a benefit to motivate the self-involvement into such a project. Even more, for a certain effort, especially public-funded entities need a funding source to be able to place a certain amount of workforce onto such projects. Due to the high risk at the very beginning of new fields of investigation, companies are also often struggling with limited development capacities. This is something that all sites need to be aware of. In a similar way, a company will and can only participate, if a business case comes into view. The medical participators are driven by an inner impulse to reduce the distress of patients encountered in daily work.

While every stakeholder needs to take into account individual interests, they also depend on everyone else involved in the innovation process in order to make it successful. Here the joint approach is formulated and innovation opens up. Researchers need to request feedback from application specialists as a basis for a demand-driven advancement of ideas and technologies in a joint approach together with industry partners. Companies, on the other hand, need the feedback and the research impulse to expand and secure new business fields, while medical doctors are involved in technological innovations by collaborating with R&D partners, which transform their ideas into prototypes for clinical evaluation.

For the development, testing, and implementation, the research community of plasma medicine requires funding, clinical partners, and companies. To coordinate and support this, the "Nationales Zentrum für Plasmamedizin e.V." (national center for plasma medicine, ▶ http://www.plasma-medizin.de/) was founded. Several companies presently providing medical devices for plasma medicine are part of it as well. So in order to not miss our chance, new ideas should grow, be approached, tested in a clinical environment and the future may show more ideas for plasma medical applications than mentioned here.

❯ Important to Know

To coordinate the development, testing, and implementation of plasma medicine, the "Nationales Zentrum für Plasmamedizin e.V." (national center for plasma medicine, ▶ http://www.plasma-medizin.de/) was founded in 2013 in Germany.

Take-Home-Messages

Plasma as the fourth state of matter is well-known from the sun, the initiator of life on earth. Now, CAP is used to sustain life and to improve quality of life for some patients. Despite a long history of plasma technology in medicine like in argon plasma coagulation, the invention of CAP enabled wound healing approaches. Simultaneously, several different technical solutions were developed toward medical products to supply a cocktail of active components onto the wound with individual compositions.

Subsequent to the now established field of chronic wound care, future fields of plasma application in medicine are under investigation like endoscopic or dental access or for large-scale applications and the very new field of cancer treatment by CAP. The global trends of industry 4.0 can enhance the benefits of plasma medical therapies, especially as quality control in ambulant settings. Further elevation of future topics in medical hygiene is observed and impulses toward new fields of CAP application such as plasma agriculture are described.

In order to utilize further potential of CAP technology in various scopes of treatments, a joint approach of medical experts, research experts, and companies is required and encouraged.

References

1. Daeschlein G, Napp M, von Podewils S, Lutze S, Emmert S, Lange A, Klare I, Haase H, Gümbel D, von Woedtke T, Jünger M. In vitro susceptibility of multidrug resistant skin and wound pathogens against low temperature atmospheric pressure plasma jet (APPJ) and dielectric barrier discharge plasma (DBD). Plasma Process Polym. 2014;11(2):175–83.
2. Zimmermann JL, Dumler K, Shimizu T, Morfill GE, Wolf A, Boxhammer V, Schlegel J, Gansbacher B, Anton M. Effects of cold atmospheric plasmas on adenoviruses in solution. J Phys D Appl Phys. 2011;44:505201.
3. O'Connor N, Cahill O, Daniels S, Galvin S, Humphreys H. Cold atmospheric pressure plasma and decontamination. Can it con-tribute to preventing hospital-acquired infections? J Hosp Infect. 2014;88(2):59–65.
4. Xia T, Kleinheksel A, Lee EM, Qiao Z, Wigginton KR, Clack HL. Inactivation of airborne viruses using a packed bed non-thermal plasma reactor. J Phys D Appl Phys. 2019;52:255201.
5. Metelmann H-R, von Woedtke T, Weltmann K-D. Comprehensive clinical plasma medicine. Cham: Springer; 2018.
6. Siemens EW. Ueber die elektrostatische Induction, die Verzögerung des Stroms in Flaschendrähten. Ann Phys. 1857;178:66–122.
7. Menashi WP. Treatment of surfaces. USA Patent 3,383,163, May 1968.
8. Weltmann K-D, Polak M, Masur K, von Woedtke T, Winter J, Reuter S. Plasma processes and plasma sources in medicine. Coontribut Plasma Phys. 2012;52(7):644–54.
9. Raiser J, Zenker M. Argon plasma coagulation for open surgical and endoscopic applications: state of the art. J Phys D Appl Phys. 2006;39(16):3520.
10. Foest R, Kindel E, Ohl A, Stieber M, Weltmann K-D. Non-thermal atmospheric pressure discharges for surface modification. Plasma Phys Control Fusion. 2005;12B:B525.
11. Weltmann K-D, Kindel E, von Woedtke T, Hähnel M, Stieber M, Brandenburg R. Atmospheric-pressure plasma sources: prospective tools for plasma medicine. Pure Appl Chem. 2010;82(6):1223.
12. Muramatsu M, Kitagawa A. A review of ion sources for medical accelerators. Rev Sci Instrum. 2012;83(2):02B909.
13. Bailey WH, Williams AL, Leonhard MJ. Exposure of laboratory animals to small air ions: a systematic review of biological and behavioral studies. Biomed Eng Online. 2018;17(1):1–32.
14. Grundmann-Kollmann M, Ludwig R, Zollner TM, Ochsendorf F, Thaci D, Boehncke W-H, Krutmann J, Kaufmann R, Podda M. Narrowband UVB and cream psoralen-UVA combination therapy for plaque-type psoriasis. J Am Acad Dermatol. 2004;50(5):734–9.
15. Valko M, Leibfritz D, Moncol J, Cronin MTD, Mazur M, Telser J. Free radicals and antioxidants in normal physiological functions and human disease. Int J Biochem Cell Biol. 2007;39(1):44–84.
16. Martínez-Sánchez G, Al-Dalain SM, Menéndez S, Re L, Giuliani A, Candelario-Jalil E, Álvarez H, Fernández-Montequín JI, León OS. Therapeutic efficacy of ozone in patients with diabetic foo. Eur J Pharmacol. 2005;523(1.3):151–61.
17. Nuccitelli R, Pliquett U, Chen X, Ford W, Swanson RJ, Beebe SJ, Kolb JF, Schoenbach KH. Nanosecond pulsed electric fields cause melanomas to self-destruct. Biochem Biophys Res Commun. 2006;343(2):351–60.
18. Maffiuletti NA, Minetto MA, Farina D, Bottinelli R. Electrical stimulation for neuromuscular testing and training: state-of-the art and unresolved issues. Eur J Appl Physiol. 2011;111:2391.
19. Kara M, Özcakar L, Didem G, Özcelik E, Yörübulut M, Güneri S, Kaymak B, Akinci A, Cetin A. Quantification of the effects of transcutaneous electrical nerve stimulation with functional magnetic resonance imaging: a double-blind randomized placebo-controlled study. Arch Phys Med Rehabil. 2010;91:1160–5.
20. Lu X, Naidis GV, Laroussi M, Reuter S, Graves DB, Ostrikov K. Reactive species in non-equilibrium atmospheric-pressure plasmas: generation, transport, and biological effects. Phys Rep. 2016;630:1–84.
21. Jablonowski L, Kocher T, Schindler A, Müller K, Dombrowski F, von Woedtke T, Arnold T, Lehmann A, Rupf S, Evert M, Evert K. Side effects by oral application of atmospheric pressure plasma on the mucosa in mice. PLoS One. 2019;14(4):e0215099.

15

22. Bansemer R. Computer assisted development and optimization of a variable dielectric barrier discharge (Diss.). Rostock: Universität Rostock; 2020.
23. Schnabel U, Handorf O, Yarova K, Zessin B, Zechlin S, Sydow D, Zellmer E, Stachowiak J, Andrasch M, Below H, Ehlbeck J. Plasma-treated air and water—assessment of synergistic anti-microbial effects for sanitation of food processing surfaces and environment. Foods. 2019;8(2):55.
24. Timmermann E, Bansemer R, Gerling T, Hahn V, Weltmann K-D, Nettesheim S, Puff M. Piezo-electric-driven plasma pen with multiple nozzles used as a medical device: risk estimation and antimicrobial efficacy. J Phys D Appl Phys. 2020;54:025201.
25. Winter J, Nishime TMC, Glitsch S, Lühder H, Weltmann K-D. On the development of a deploy-able cold plasma endoscope. Contrib Plasma Physics. 2018;58(5):404–14.
26. Winter J, Nishime TMC, Bansemer R, Balazinski M, Wende K, Weltmann K-D. Enhanced atmo-spheric pressure plasma jet setup for endoscopic applications. J Phys D Appl Phys. 2018;52(2):024005.
27. Robert E, Vandamme M, Brullé L, Lerondel S, Le Pape A, Sarron V, Riès D, Darny T, Dozias S, Collet G, Kieda C, Pouvesle JM. Perspectives of endoscopic plasma applications. Clin Plasma Med. 2013;1(2):8–16.
28. Kostov KG, Nishime TMC, Machida M, Borges AC, Prysiazhnyi V, Koga-Ito CY. Study of cold atmospheric plasma jet at the end of flexible plastic tube for microbial decontamination. Plasma Process Polym. 2015;12(12):1383–91.
29. von Woedtke T, Metelmann H-R, Weltmann K-D. Clinical plasma medicine: state and perspec-tives of in vivo application of cold atmospheric plasma. Contrib Plasma Physics. 2014;54(2):104–17.
30. Kerlikowski A, Matthes R, Pink C, Steffen H, Schlüter R, Holtfreter B, Weltmann K-D, von Woedtke T, Kocher T, Jablonowski L. Effects of cold atmospheric pressure plasma and disinfect-ing agents on Candida albicans in root canals of extracted human teeth. J Biophotonics. 2020;13:e202000221.
31. Hertel M, Schwill-Engelhardt J, Gerling T, Weltmann K-D, Imiolczyk SM, Hartwig S, Preissner S. Antibacterial efficacy of plasma jet, dielectric barrier discharge, chlorhexidine, and silver diamine fluoride varnishes in caries lesions. Plasma Med. 2018;8(1):73–82.
32. Matthes R, Jablonowski L, Holtfreter B, Gerling T, von Woedtke T, Kocher T. Fibroblast growth on zirconia ceramic and titanium disks after application with cold atmospheric pressure plasma devices or with antiseptics. Int J Oral Maxillofac Implants. 2019;34(4):809–818a.
33. Bussiahn R, Brandenburg R, Gerling T, Kindel E, Lange H, Lembke N, Weltmann K-D, von Woedtke T, Kocher T. The hairline plasma: an intermittent negative dc-corona discharge at atmo-spheric pressure for plasma medical applications. Appl Phys Lett. 2010;96:143701.
34. Semmler ML, Bekeschus S, Schäfer M, Bernhardt T, Fischer T, Wizke K, Seebauer C, Rebi H, Grambow E, Vollmar B, Nebe JB, Metelmann H-R, von Woedtke T, Emmert S, Boeckmann L. Molecular mechanisms of the efficacy of cold atmospheric pressure plasma (CAP) in cancer treatment. Cancers. 2020;12(2):269.
35. Metelmann H-R, Seebauer C, Miller V, Fridman A, Bauer G, Graves DB, Pouvesle J-M, Rut-kowski R, Schuster M, Bekeschus S, Wende K, Masur K, Hasse S, Gerling T, Hori M, Tanaka H, Choi EH, Weltmann K-D, Metelmann PH, Von Hoff DD, von Woedtke T. Clinical experience with cold plasma in the treatment of locally advanced head and neck cancer. Clin Plasma Med. 2018;9:6–13.
36. Cutting KF. Evidence and practical wound care: an all-inclusive approach. Wound Med. 2017;16:40–5.
37. INPTDAT – The Data Platform for Plasma Technology, Leibniz Institute for Plasma Science and Technology, 2020. [Online]. Available: https://www.inptdat.de/. [Zugriff am 11 12 2020].
38. Hornberger C, Herrmann BH, Daeschlein G, von Podewils S, Sicher C, Kuhn J, Masur K, Meis-ter M, Wahl P. Detecting bacteria on wounds with hyperspectral imaging in fluorescence mode. Curr Direct Biomed Eng. 2020;6(3):264–7.
39. Stratmann B, Costea T-C, Nolte C, Hiller J, Schmidt J, Reindel J, Masur K, Motz W, Timm J, Kerner W, Tschoepe D. Effect of cold atmospheric plasma therapy vs standard therapy placebo on wound healing in patients with diabetic foot ulcers. JAMA Netw Open. 2020;3(7):e2010411.

40. DIN Deutsches Institut für Normung e.V., DIN SPEC 91315. General requirements for plasma sources in medicine. Berlin: Beuth; 2014.
41. DIN EN 60601-1. Medical electrical equipment - part 1–6: general requirements for basic safety and essential performance. Berlin: Beuth; 2010.
42. ICNIRP. Guidelines on limits of exposure to ultraviolet radiation of wavelengths between 180 nm and 400 nm (incoherent optical radiation). Health Phys. 2004;87(2):171–86.
43. Zhou R, Zhou R, Prasad K, Fang Z, Speight R, Bazaka K, Ostrikov K. Cold atmospheric plasma activated water as a prospective disinfectant: the crucial role of peroxynitrite. Green Chem. 2018;20(23):5276–84.
44. Weaver L, Michels HT, Keever CW. Survival of Clostridium difficile on copper and steel: futuristic options for hospital hygiene. J Hosp Infect. 2008;68(2):145–51.
45. Tseng S, Abramzon N, Jackson JO, Lin W-J. Gas discharge plasmas are effective in inactivating bacillus and clostridium spores. Appl Microb Cell Physiol. 2012;93(6):2563–70.
46. Ehlbeck J, Schnabel U, Polak M, Winter J, von Woedtke T, Brandenburg R, von dem Hagen T, Weltmann K-D. Low temperature atmospheric pressure plasma sources for microbial decontamination. J Phys D Appl Phys. 2010;44(1):013002.
47. Schulze-Röbbecke R. Schulze-Röbbecke, Roland. Übertragung nosokomialer Infektionen und Prinzipien der Transmissionsprävention. (german). Krankenhaushygiene Up2date. 2014;9(4):281–300.
48. Cassini A, Plachouras D, Eckmanns T, Sin MA, Blank H-P, Ducomble T, Haller S, Harder T, Klingeberg A, Sixtensson M, Velasco E, Weiß B, Kramarz P, Monnet DL, Kretzschmar ME, Suetens C. Burden of six healthcare-associated infections on European population health: estimating incidence-based disability-adjusted life years through a population prevalence-based modelling study. PLoS Med. 2016;10:e1002150.
49. Tambyah PA. Catheter-associated urinary tract infection. Curr Opin Infect Dis. 2012;25(4):365–70.
50. Xia J, Gao J, Tang W. Nosocomial infection and its molecular mechanisms of antibiotic resistance. Biosci Trends. 2016;10(1):14–21.
51. Polak M, Winter J, Schnabel U, Ehlbeck J, Weltmann K-D. Innovative plasma generation in flexible biopsy channels for inner-tube decontamination and medical applications. Plasma Process Polym. 2012;9(1):67–76.
52. Hansen L, Schmidt-Bleker A, Bansemer R. Influence of a liquid surface on the NOx production of a cold atmospheric pressure plasma jet. J Phys D Appl Phys. 2018;51(47):474002.
53. Jablonowski H, Sousa JS, Weltmann K-D, Wende K, Reuter S. Quantification of the ozone and singlet delta oxygen produced in gas and liquid phases by a non-thermal atmospheric plasma with relevance for medical treatment. Sci Rep. 2018;8(1):12195.
54. Jablonowski H, Schmidt-Bleker A, Weltmann K-D, von Woedtke T, Wende K. Non-touching plasma–liquid interaction – where is aqueous nitric oxide generated? Phys Chem Chem Phys. 2018;20(39):25387–98.
55. Wannicke N, Wagner R, Stachowiak J, Nishime TMC, Ehlbeck J, Weltmann K-D, Brust H. Efficiency of plasma-processed air for biological decontamination of crop seeds on the premise of unimpaired seed germination. Plasma Process Polym. 2020;18:e2000207.
56. Nishime TMC, Wannicke N, Horn S, Weltmann K-D, Brust H. A coaxial dielectric barrier discharge reactor for treatment of winter wheat seeds. Appl Sci. 2020;10(20):7133.
57. Schmidt M, Hahn V, Altrock B, Gerling T, Gerber IC, Weltmann K-D, von Woedtke T. Plasma-activation of larger liquid volumes by an inductively-limited discharge for antimicrobial purposes. Appl Sci. 2019;9(10):2150.
58. Bruggeman PJ, Kushner MJ, Locke BR, Gardeniers JGE, Graham WG, Graves DB, Hofman-Caris RCHM, Maric D, Reid JP, Ceriani E, Fernandez RD. Plasma–liquid interactions: a review and roadmap. Plasma Sources Sci Technol. 2016;25(5):053002.

15

kINPen® MED – The Precise Cold Plasma Jet

Ulrike Sailer

Contents

© Springer Nature Switzerland AG 2022
H.-R. Metelmann et al. (eds.), *Textbook of Good Clinical Practice in Cold Plasma Therapy*, https://doi.org/10.1007/978-3-030-87857-3_16

🎓 **Core Messages**

- The kINPen® MED is a CE-certified medical device class IIa used for the precise treatment of infected wounds and pathogen-caused skin diseases.
- The utmost fine jet of cold physical plasma facilitates high-precision handling in anatomically and pathologically demanding areas under visual control and without touch, which is unfeasible for other physical treatment methods like negative pressure, ultrasound-assisted, laser-based or DBD-plasma wound therapy.
- Benefits of cold plasma therapy with the CAP argon-based jet include the effective inactivation of microorganisms (including multi-resistant germs), stimulation of cell proliferation and microcirculation resulting in the regeneration of destroyed tissue, acceleration of wound healing without evidence of side effects and development of resistance.
- Overall clinical and pre-clinical data available up to date provide an evidence for safe use in human subjects.
- First placebo-controlled clinical trial proves the successful application of the CAP argon-based jet kINPen® MED in diabetic foot ulcers reactivation and acceleration of wound healing [1].

16.1 Introduction

The kINPen® MED is an atmospheric pressure argon plasma jet, manufactured by neoplas med GmbH, Greifswald, Germany which is used for the treatment of infected wounds and pathogen-caused skin diseases. It is a CE-certified medical device class IIa, which was introduced on the European market in 2013.

The first prototype (kINPen01) was developed in 2005 at the Leibniz Institute for Plasma Science and Technology, INP, in Greifswald, Germany – the largest non-university institute in the field of low-temperature plasmas in Europe. The prototype was developed throughout an interdisciplinary research project including partners from medicine and industry. The device was investigated as plasma jet for biological, technical and sensitive surface treatment. The design history of the CAP jet kINPen® product family is presented in ◘ Fig. 16.1 [2].

The spin-off company neoplas med GmbH participated in prototype development as well as the following further development and manufacturing leading to the current version of the atmospheric pressure argon plasma jet. It was the first of its kind to obtain a medical device approval for the treatment of chronic wounds and pathogen-induced skin diseases.

16.2 About the Device

16.2.1 Basic Principles/Technology

The cold atmospheric plasma (CAP) devices can be generally classified into three different types: direct, indirect and hybrid plasma sources [3, 4]. The kINPen® MED is an argon-based CAP jet device intended for indirect plasma

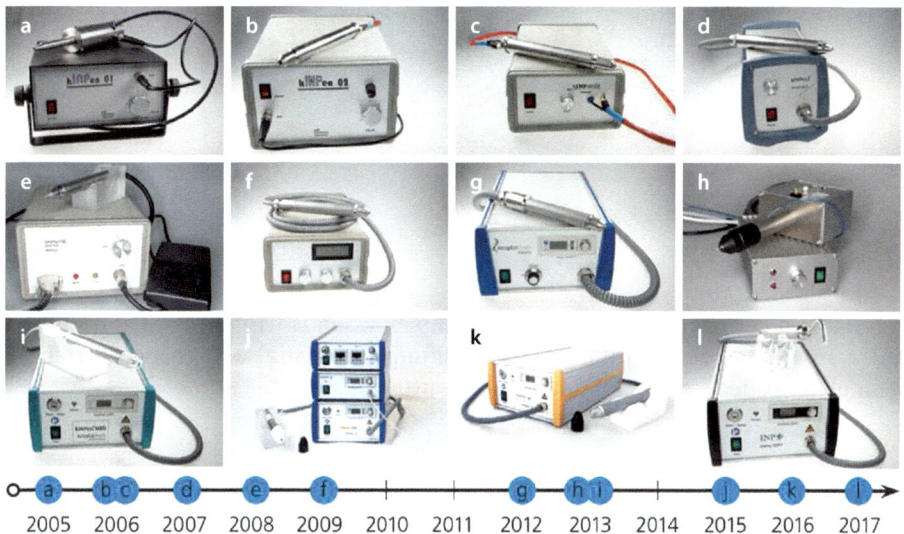

Fig. 16.1 kINPen design history: **a** kINPen01, **b** kINPen02, **c** kINPen04, **d** kINPen07, **e** kIN-Pen08, **f** kINPen09, **g** kINPen 10/11, **h** kINPenSci, **i** kINPen® MED with distance piece, **j** kINPen IND, **k** kINPen VET, **l** kINPen Dent prototype [2]

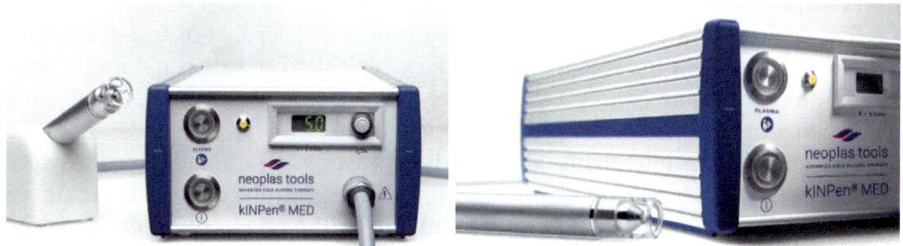

Fig. 16.2 Picture of kINPen® MED. (©neoplas med GmbH)

treatment and consists of a base unit and a permanently connected handpiece (■ Fig. 16.2).

The base unit is connected to the external power supply with a power cable and to an external argon supply with a pressure tube. At the head of the handpiece, the plasma jet or also called effluent is set up/ formed (see also ▶ Sect. 16.2.2).

The effluent is composed of reactive species and excited photons (■ Fig. 16.3). During indirect treatment, only long-lived species can reach the targeted surface. It is due to recombination events that take place inside the effluent in which most metastable species and ions react to neutral species [5].

The therapeutic effects of cold plasma are induced by reactive oxygen and nitrogen species, an irradiation in the UV light range, and a topical short-term increase in temperature. It provides a consistently stable atmosphere around the plasma beam – and thus, a controlled plasma composition with a consistent quality, both

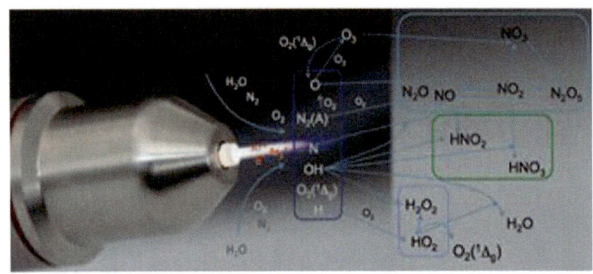

☐ **Fig. 16.3** Reactive species generated by plasma jet [2]

on flat and complex surfaces even on complex wounds with recesses and cavities. As a result, there are antimicrobial, antifungal, antiviral and cell proliferation-stimulating effects on the plasma-treated surface.

16.2.2 General Parameter (Electrical/Mechanical/Physical/ Chemical/Biological Characteristics)

The cold plasma of the kINPen® MED, with a temperature below 40 °C, is generated by a high frequency generator (1 MHz). The system power is at about 50 VA. The electrical safety of the device was validated by certified laboratories and complies with EU standards (certificate number 609.003.1).

The device operates only with argon, emitting the plasma jet of 6, 5–8 mm long visible 'effluent' (☐ Fig. 16.4a). The gas flow typically lies between 4 and 6 standard litres per minute (slm) [2]. The power and gas supply units are connected to the handpiece via a flexible tube of 1, 5 m in length.

The device has interchangeable heads consisting of an outer cone-shaped grounded electrode, a gas diffusor system, a dielectric tube and an inner driven electrode (☐ Fig. 16.4c) [2]. The shape and size of the handpiece connected with the head reminds a pen. The concentric, light-weighted and pen-like design allows precise and adjustable 3D movements and is therefore well suited for the individual treatment of complex surface structures. A replaceable spacer (sterile single use) was designed to support the maintenance of hygiene and the predefined distance during the treatment (☐ Fig. 16.4b) [6]. The intensity of the treatment is determined by its duration. When the start/stop button is triggered or the main switch is operated, both the voltage and the gas flow can be immediately cut off allowing, in consequence, a very precise and easy control of treatment exposure time.

☐ Table 16.1 summarizes the technical specifications of the kINPen® MED plasma jet.

16.2.3 Risk Assessment and Product Safety

Several parameters need to be considered when designing a plasma jet device for safe medical applications. Therefore, during the development phase of the kINPen® MED an explicit risk assessment followed by appropriate mitigation measures was carried out to ensure that the use of the device in human subjects

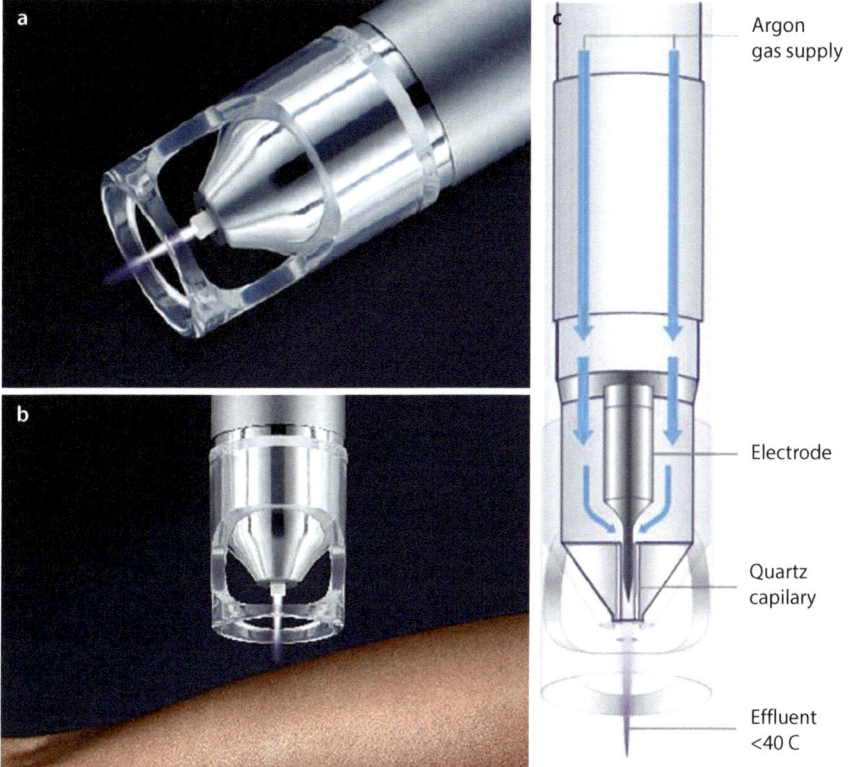

Argon gas supply

Electrode

Quartz capilary

Effluent <40 C

◘ **Fig. 16.4** **a** Picture of the kINPen® MED plasma jet; **b** Treatment of skin with the plasma jet (application with spacer); **c** Schematic set up of the plasma jet. (©neoplas med GmbH)

is safe and the therapeutic window defined for the application – supporting treatment of chronic wounds and inflammatory diseases of skin- is appropriate.

In order to establish general requirements for plasma sources in medicine, a DIN SPEC 91315 standard has been published by Mann et al. in 2014 [7, 8]. Performance, effectiveness and safety of medical CAP devices depend on certain physical and biological characteristics that need to be evaluated during the V&V activities. Physical performances include temperature, optical emission spectrometry (OES), UV irradiance, gas emission, leakage current. Biological performances include antimicrobial activity, cytotoxicity and chemical composition of the liquid. The CAP argon-based jet kINPen® MED was a subject of extensive pre-clinical testing, conducted as a part of V&V activities. The device meets all the relevant requirements of applicable standards, including the DIN SPEC 91315 [8–10]. According to the available literature, the cold atmospheric plasma jet does not pose any health risks in humans with regard to UV exposure, thermal damage, tissue toxicity or mutagenicity [10, 11]. The summary of risk assessment for this device was presented in a review article, published by Bekeschus et al. [11] in 2016. Overall, it was demonstrated that all the physico-chemical parameters (i.e., temperature, UV radiation, generation of ozone and reactive species) and biological parameters

■ Table 16.1   Cold atmospheric plasma jet kINPen® MED

Total weight		4.0kg
Power supply	Supply voltage frequency	230VAC, 50/60 Hz
	Mains fuses	T 1A E 250V
	Maximum power input	50VA
Gas supply	Gas Type	Argon
	Purity	Min 4.8 (specification according to pharmacopeia)
	Gas flow rate	5 ± 1 slm (standard litre per minute)
	Supply Pressure	2–3 bar (2–3 × 10^5 Pa)
	Fed gas flow control	Yes (integrated)
Supply unit (main unit)	Dimensions (L × W × H)	330 × 180 × 105 (mm)
Plasma generator (applicator)	Dimensions (Ø × L)	20 × 180 mm
	Feed line length	1.50 m
Other parameters	Mode of operation	Pulsed
	Duty cycle	Plasma on/off 1:1
	Typical effluent length	6.5–8 mm
	Temperature at the recommended working distance	Below 40 ºC
	UV-irradiation at working distance (free jet)	UVA: 5–15 µW/cm^2 UVB: 5–15 µW/cm^2
	Phase stabilization during plasma generation	Automatic PLL-circuit

(i.e., mutagenicity, penetration depth into the skin, subjective sensation, cytotoxicity and histocompatibility) of the cold plasma jet are well within the specifications and pose no safety-related concerns (see also ▶ Chap. 5).

Schmidt et al. performed a 1-year follow-up study on mice exposed to 14-day plasma treatment in an ear wound model. Histological, biochemical and imaging analysis were used to assess long-term side effects of repetitive treatment with the argon-based plasma jet on using a total of 84 study animals [12]. None of the plasma-treated animals differed from control groups in health state, nutrition or behaviour and displayed no chronic wound inflammation or other side effects while wound healing progressed physiologically.

In addition, the safety of the cold plasma jet is also substantiated through the manufacturer's PMS data and PMCF activities (i.e., the extended clinical literature research and the review of relevant safety report databases). Since the market launch in 2013, neither incidents nor serious adverse events have been reported for the cold plasma jet resulting in the highest possible safety ratio of the product.

In total, 17 clinical articles (for more detail refer to ▶ Sect. 16.4) have been published up to date, where the plasma jet was used in human subjects. No serious adverse events were reported during the conducted clinical studies so far. In general, the treatment with the device was well tolerated by the patients and did not cause any safety-related issues. Investigations of the cold plasma jet on the skin of healthy human volunteers showed that plasma was well tolerated in terms of paraesthesia, pain and heat without causing damage to the skin barrier or resulting in skin dryness [13, 14]. In vivo risk assessments of temperature and UV exposure by plasma indicated that UV radiation of the plasma jet was an order of magnitude below the dose inducing sun burn, and that thermal damage of the tissue by cold plasma could be excluded [15]. No side effects or inflammation were registered in trials using the cold plasma jet for treatment of wounds such as chronic leg ulcers [16] or wound healing disorder [17] or when employed as an adjuvant anti-fungal treatment in oral applications [18].

In conclusion, the available pre-clinical and clinical data show that the application of the cold plasma jet kINPen® MED in humans is safe when it is used according to the manufacturer's instructions.

16.3 Indications

The most common and highly accepted health care professional's indication of CAP is its application in wound healing therapy (i.e., chronic and acute). This is achieved by its antimicrobial activity (i.e., anti-bacterial, anti-fungal and anti-viral). The kINPen® MED was developed for supporting the treatment of chronic wounds and inflammatory diseases of skin and skin appendices of the extremities and torso.

Wound healing is a complex process. It is defined by four continuous, overlapping and precisely programmed phases: haemostasis, inflammation, proliferation and remodelling (maturation) [11]. The healing process is only completed once all phases have been successfully run through. Its duration depends mostly on the severity of an injury but also on other factors such as the general health condition of the patient and underlying diseases (e.g., diabetes or age). A distinction should be made between acute wounds caused by external influences such as cuts, bruises or abrasions and chronic wounds that have an internal cause [19].

Complications in wound healing affect millions of people in the world and is considered a strong burden to patients and health care systems. Although many different wound therapies are available challenges remain in the treatment of problematic, chronic wounds. Chronic wounds are known to display an imbalance in redox processes and inflammation, ultimately disturbing the sequence of events necessary for healing [20]. Chronic wounds are often populated by microorganisms causing chronic infections, which decrease the wound healing processes. In addition, those types of wounds show a weak inflammatory profile that has a negative effect on the skin cell division and wound remodelling. Thus, many patients suffered years from chronic wounds with no therapeutic option. The cold atmospheric plasma jet and other CAP devices are a new therapeutic option for the treatment of chronic wounds. The effect of the cold atmospheric argon-based plasma jet kINPen® MED therapy is based on two levels, which have a synergistic effect on wound healing:

- Inactivation of microorganisms (bacteria, fungi) and viruses – including multi-resistant germs such as MRSA
- Stimulation of cell proliferation and microcirculation resulting in the regeneration of destroyed tissue

It should be stressed that the antimicrobial effect of the cold plasma jet has the potential to reduce the use of antibiotics in wound treatment and can contribute to the fight against antibiotic resistance [11].

In summary, the application of the cold plasma jet on chronic wounds enhances the wound healing process and leads to pain and itching relief. The effectiveness of the cold plasma jet was underlined in a first placebo-controlled, patient-blind prospective clinical trial on the use of cold plasma in diabetic foot syndrome, which was published in July 2020 and provides further relevant findings on cold plasma therapy with the cold plasma jet (see ▶ Sect. 16.4 *Clinical Trials*).

16.3.1   Use and Treatment Recommendations

The therapy with the cold plasma jet should be used as a supplement to standard wound management in wounds that do not respond to standard treatment methods (e.g., infectious and non-infectious skin disorders). The application may take place in 1–3-day intervals. The duration of cold plasma therapy depends on the individual wound condition and the frequency of treatment.

In general, wounds must be debrided before plasma treatment. Plasma treatment should be performed prior to topical medication to avoid undesirable interactions with any other substances.

During the treatment with the cold plasma jet, the hand unit is placed in such a way that it is perpendicular to the surface to be treated and a replaceable spacer is guided without contact at a distance of approx. 1 mm above the treatment area. The skin areas to be treated have to be covered meander-shaped and with a moderate speed of about 5 mm/s. The effective plasma area of the cold plasma jet covers about 1 cm^2 directly in front of the spacer.

The device is easy to use: It has a power switch and an on/off button to start the flow of gas. Both physicians and medical staff such as technicians or nurses can use the device safely and successfully.

16

The kINPen® MED was launched in 2013 and is commercially marketed since 2017. Before the cold atmospheric plasma jet was put on the market, extensive studies regarding antiseptic and antimicrobial effects as well as analyses of wound healing on artificial wound models were carried out and have been published.

The collective pre-clinical (i.e., in vivo animal models and in vitro studies) and clinical data provide a strong evidence of **antimicrobial performance** of the cold plasma jet and its **positive effect in wound healing processes**.

Antimicrobial performance   The kINPen® MED has been shown in series of in vitro studies to be effective against various bacteria (i.e. *Escherichia coli*, *Klebsiella* group (*K. pneumoniae*, *K. oxytoca*), *Staphylococcus aureus hemolysing*, *Lancefield Streptococci* (group A and B), *Proteus* group (*P. mirabilis*, *P. vulgaris*), *Acinetobacter spp.*, *Stenotrophomonas spp.*, *Enterococcus faecalis* and *Staphylococcus epidermidis*) [11], including highly resistant bacteria such as methicillin-resistant *Staphylococcus aureus* (MRSA), *Pseudomonas aeruginosa* or *Deinococcus radodurans* [5, 21]. The efficacy of CAP against bacteriophages, viruses and fungal species with some strains that are resistant to common antifungal treatments has also been demonstrated in vitro [5, 22–26]. This potent antimicrobial property of the cold atmospheric argon-based plasma jet application was confirmed in clinical studies, where a significant reduction of the bio-burden (bacterial contamination) of wounds or intact skin was achieved [14, 27, 28].

Positive effect in wound healing processes   In vitro studies provide further evidence that cold plasma treatment can affect wound healing not only by a reduction of bacterial colonization but also by direct effects on epidermal and dermal cells [4, 24, 29]. It has been observed that wound-relevant processes, including activation and/ or enhanced proliferation of fibroblasts, endothelial cells and keratinocytes are supported by CAP treatment [24, 29]. The potential of the cold plasma application in chronic wound healing was successfully evaluated by Schmidt et al. [20] Conducting an in vivo experiment the authors showed that the cold plasma jet accelerates re-epithelialization. Experiments with hyperspectral camera performed at Leibniz Institute for Plasma Science and Technology (INP) demonstrate that the haemoglobin level and the oxygen supply increase significantly in treated wounds after application of cold plasma with the kINPen® MED (◘ Fig. 16.5). The effect was observed not only on the surface area directly reached by the cold plasma but also in deeper skin layers (up to 8 mm in depth). This data indicates that perfusion and oxygen supply in wounds are increased after cold plasma therapy and support the healing process.

16.3.2 Successful Examples

There are many case studies presenting successful application of the kINPen® MED in wound healing. Härling [30] described a case of a 68-year-old male patient who sustained a third-degree open fracture of the interphalangeal joint with the destruction of the proximal joint surface of the thumb as part of a circular saw injury. After the third treatment session with the cold plasma jet there was a significant reduction in the local signs of infection, and he had an improvement in the pain symptoms. A microbial control smear after 14 days of treatment showed no

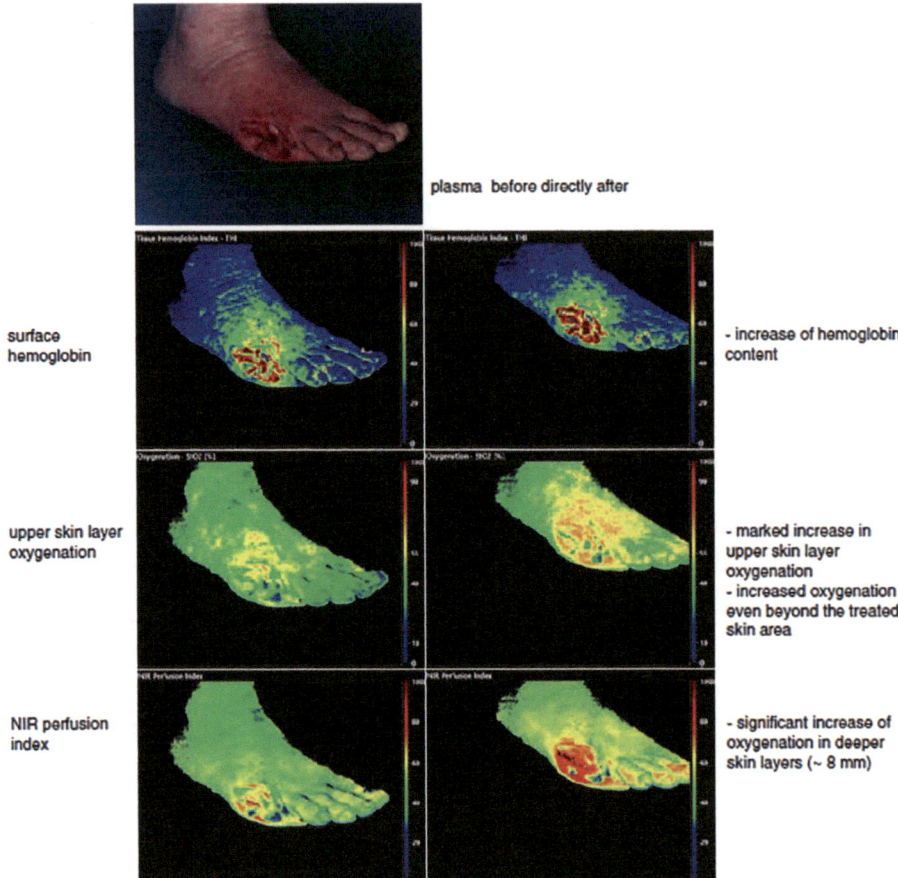

□ Fig. 16.5 Hyperspectral analysis image of microcirculation changes in a diabetic foot. (Printed with the kind permission of Kai Masur)

more germ growth. Hilker et al. [31] reported another successful cold plasma jet application where the device was used to treat driveline infection (DI) in a 66-year-old patient. After treatment, the local infection was completely regressed without any signs of exudation or recurrence. Barten et al. [32] reported a case of the cold plasma jet application in a postoperative sternum wound. After a few applications, the patient could be treated on an outpatient basis. After initial daily use, the interval could be expanded to three or two times a week. The patient returned to work 3 months after starting cold plasma therapy.

    □ Figure 16.6 presents examples of case studies registered at the Hospital of Thun in Switzerland. The aim of the study was to gain initial clinical experience in patients with chronic venous ulcer. Five patients were included. The duration of treatment was a maximum of 8 weeks with two to three applications per week per patient. Treatment with cold plasma was passed on all five patients in addition to an existing «best medical treatment» using optimized wound management and adequate compression. The evaluation was passed based on digital photographs. The primary parameter of success was the reduced wound area. The treatment was

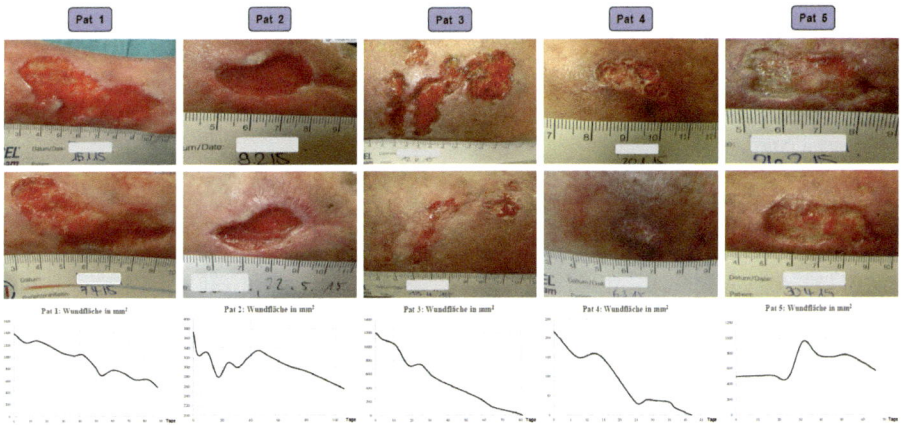

Fig. 16.6 Examples of case studies; kINPen® MED influence on chronic wounds. (Printed with the kind permission of Spital Thun, Switzerland)

reported as painless in all cases. There were no complications, that is, no clinical manifestation of infection and no need for antibiotics. In four of the five cases, a significant reduction of the size of the wound during treatment was reported and two of the five wounds were completely closed. One case (patient 5, **■** Fig. 16.6) did not respond to the treatment, possibly due to insufficient granulation.

Further successful cases of kINPen® MED applications in wound healing are provided in **■** Table 16.2

— In general, the overall clinical experience with the cold atmospheric plasma jet demonstrates high compliance and satisfaction of patients. The cold plasma treatment is safe and painless. In most cases after the first application of the cold plasma jet patients´ persistent wound pain decreases significantly or disappears completely. Effective pain relief motivates especially patients with chronic wounds. Patients with itchy skin conditions report a reduction or complete disappearance of their symptoms.

In summary, the benefits of CAP argon-based therapy with the kINPen® MED combine a safe and user-friendly treatment, the improvement of well-being of patients with chronic wounds and the prospect of convalescence. In addition, the utmost fine jet of cold physical plasma facilitates high-precision handling in anatomically and pathologically demanding areas under visual control and without touch, which is unfeasible for other physical treatment methods like negative pressure, ultrasound-assisted, laser-based or DBD-plasma wound therapy.

16.4 Clinical Trials

In total, 17 clinical articles (interventional and observational clinical studies) have been published up to date where the kINPen® MED was used in human subjects. The overview of clinical data and evidence summary are provided in **■** Table 16.3.

☐ **Table 16.2**   Case study examples of the kINPen® MED application in wound healing

Case study	Picture
Wound type: dog bite, acutely infected wound **Problem:** infected wound, pain VAS 5, irritated wound environment, increase in inflammation despite antibiotic treatment **Treatment:** inflamed area only **Result:** elimination of irritation, infection and inflammation, beginning of epithelization	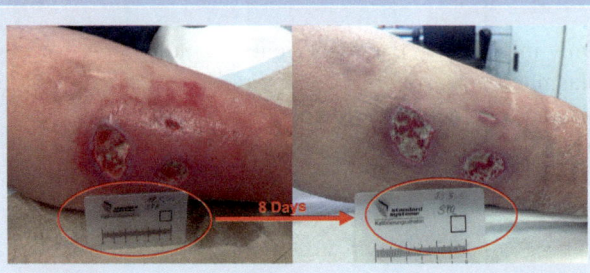
Wound type: diabetic ulcer **Problem:** continuous deterioration after 7 weeks of treatment, smell, onset of infection **Result:** granulation, significant reduction of the wound area, beginning of epithelization	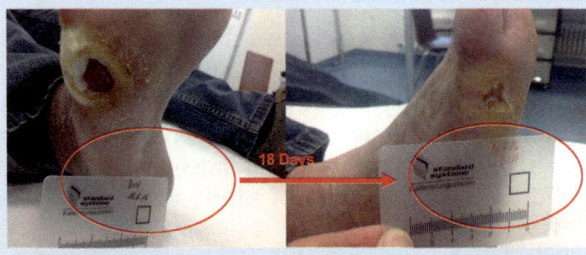
Wound type: age 80, venous leg ulcers, PAVK IV, resistant pseudomonas **Problem:** enlargement of the wound area and deterioration of wound healing **Result:** after amputation of the third toe, plasma treatments 24x + 40x, complete healing, elimination of resistant pathogens	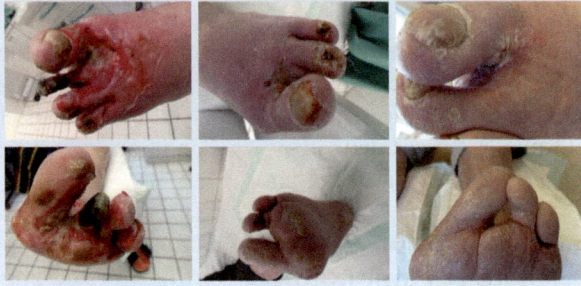
Type: accident at work with crushing and broken wreckage **Problem:** infected wound, resistant to therapy, pain, preparation for amputation **Result:** wounds completely healed after 42 days, complete elimination of the infection, start of physiotherapy	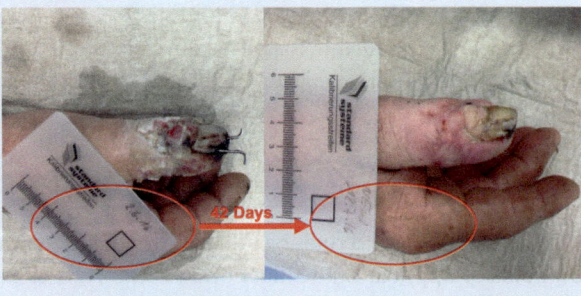

16

◘ **Table 16.2** (continued)

Case study	Picture
Type: venous leg ulcers + ischemic bacteria **Problem:** non-healing wound **Result:** the wound healed completely after 31 treatments with the kINPen® MED plasma jet	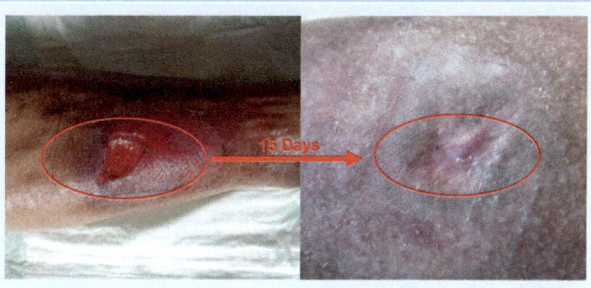

Printed with the kind permission of Gilbert Hämmerle, LKH Bregenz, Austria, and Dr. Birgit Schwetlick, Clinic Altenburger Land, Germany

◘ **Table 16.3** Overview of clinical studies with kINPen® MED

Studies with healthy volunteers

1	Reference	**Lademann et al. [28]**
	Study design	No randomized, case control study
	Study objective	Efficacy comparison of antiseptic solution (Octenisept) and the CAP (kINPen 09; the prototype of kINPen® MED) on healthy human skin.
	Patients no	10 healthy volunteers
	Performance outcome	Both antiseptic methods have been proved to be highly efficient and led to a significant reduction in the bacterial colonization ($p < 0.05$). Cutaneous treatment of the skin with Octenisept was significantly more efficient than treatment with kINPen 09 and lead to a 99% elimination of the bacteria. 74% elimination was achieved by CAP treatment. **Note:** Technical challenges with an early prototype kINPen 09 device could be held responsible for the slightly reduced antiseptic properties of CAP, compared to a standard antiseptic solution, since the manual treatment of the skin surface with a small beam of the CAP device might have led to an incomplete coverage of the treated area. This issue has been solved by the design of the new version of the device kINPen® MED
	Safety outcome	No signs of inflammation such as dilate blood vessels, leukocyte rolling or inflammatory infiltrate within the epidermis were observed before and after both treatments. In any of the volunteers' signs of skin damage could be observed.

(continued)

◘ Table 16.3 (continued)

2	Reference	**Vandersee et al. [33]**
	Study design	Case control study (4 armed) Arm A: no treatment Arm B: kINPen® MED Arm C: OCD Arm D: kINPen® MED + OCD
	Study objective	Analysis of wound healing parameters, that is, area decline and histomorphological characteristics of tissue repair in six healthy volunteers with vacuum-generated wounds on the forearm.
	Patients no	6 healthy volunteers with vacuum created wounds
	Performance outcome	kINPen® MED treatment led to a more rapid area decline that was statistically significant in comparison to other treatment groups. It is notable that statistically significant differences in favour of treatment arm B (kINPen® MED) existed, illustrating the potential of CAP to accelerate wound repair
	Safety outcome	Besides mild pain, all treatment types were well tolerated by study participants
3	Reference	**Daeschlein et al. [13]**
	Study design	Open label, pilot study
	Study objective	Investigation of cold plasma effects of three different plasma sources (pulsed, non-pulsed atmospheric pressure plasma jet (kINPen 09) and a dielectric barrier discharge (DBD)) on the trans-epidermal water loss (TEWL) and skin moisture after treating the fingertips of four healthy male volunteers
	Patients no	4 healthy volunteers
	Performance outcome	No performance endpoints were assessed during the study.
	Safety outcome	All cold plasma treatments were well tolerated and did not damage the skin barrier nor cause skin dryness. The study results confirm the safe use of CAP devices on human skin.

16

◻ Table 16.3 (continued)

4	Reference	**Daeschlein et al. [14]**
	Study design	Open label, pilot study
	Study objective	Investigation of decontamination power of two cold plasma sources: kINPen 09 and a dielectric barrier discharge (DBD)
	Patients no	9 healthy volunteers
	Performance outcome	The bacterial load was determined after counting and subject's treatment tolerance (i.e., paraesthesia, pain and heat) was measured using a numerical rating scale. Both plasma devices led to a significant reduction in physiological and artificially contaminated flora (*Staphylococcus epidermidis and Micrococcus luteus*). The study results demonstrated the effectiveness of both CAP devices in eradicating contaminated flora from the fingertips of healthy volunteers
	Safety outcome	Treatment with both devices was well tolerated.
5	Reference	**Fluhr et al. [34]**
	Study design	Open label, pilot study
	Study objective	Investigation of CAP (kINPen 09) influence on a carotenoid profile in relation to skin physiology parameters (epidermal barrier function, stratum corneum (SC) hydration, surface temperature and irritation parameters). The main study focus was the interaction of CAP and the antioxidative network, as well as the consequences for skin physiology parameters.
	Patients no	7 healthy volunteers
	Performance outcome	No performance endpoints were assessed during the study
	Safety outcome	It has been concluded that the induction of reactive oxygen species is probably the major contributor to CAP efficacy in skin disinfection. Skin physiology parameters were influenced without damaging the skin or skin functions, demonstrating the safe use of CAP in human subjects

(continued)

◘ Table 16.3 (continued)

6	Reference	**Metelmann et al. [35]**
	Study design	Experimental case series Each of 4 wounds per subject was allocated by randomization to: Arm A: 10 seconds of plasma stimulation, Arm B: 3 seconds of plasma stimulation Arm C: 10 seconds of plasma stimulation over the following 3 days Arm D: control (no treatment)
	Study objective	Generation of basic clinical data about the early wound healing phase treated with kINPen® MED.
	Patients no	5 healthy volunteers with experimental laser wounds created by CO2 laser in a single shot: 4 wounds per study subject
	Performance outcome	Short-term plasma stimulation, repeatedly applied for 3 days, showed the most effective results in wound treatment in terms of early aesthetic recovery. All blinded observers have voted this treatment pattern was more effective in comparison to other treatment protocols. The numeric aesthetic assessment scored twice the highest number of satisfaction ('10'), four times a '9' and seven times an '8'; all together standing for an outstanding cosmetic benefit at this very early time of healing
	Safety outcome	No safety-related outcomes were reported during the study
7	Reference	**Metelmann et al. [36]**
	Study design	Observational study (follow-up to previously described series of 5 cases, Metelmann et al. [35], 2012)
	Study objective	The assessment of scar formation during the 10 days, 6 months and 12 months follow-up.
	Patients no	5 healthy volunteers
	Performance outcome	The immediate reaction to wound setting differed from patient to patient, which made inter-individual comparisons of plasma treatment effects impossible; however, intra- individual comparison was performed. At day 10, the group of lesions without plasma treatment (Arm D) showed signs of acute inflammation (4 cases out of 5). It has been demonstrated that plasma treatment has no disturbing influence on healing inflammation and is possibly even supporting it at this early stage of wound healing.
	Safety outcome	The time span of controlling cancer risk was 12 months after plasma treatment. There was no observation of any precancerous lesion of the skin in 15 wounds set by laser and afterwards treated by non-thermal plasma.

16

◼ **Table 16.3** (continued)

Studies with patients with chronic wounds

8	Reference	**Hartwig et al. [17]**
	Study design	Prospective case series
	Study objective	Evaluation of the assisted effect of kINPen® MED in wound healing disorders in addition to routine wound care.
	Patients no	4 patients who had undergone radial forearm free flap procedures and developed wound healing disturbance leading to exposed flexor tendons
	Performance outcome	The primary outcome of wound closure was reached in all cases, but the courses were heterogeneous. As the size of the defect was different in all cases and the plasma initiation did not start at the same time post-surgery (5.9 weeks to 8.9 weeks;), a meantime for the wound closure was 10.1 weeks (range 4.9–16)
	Safety outcome	No undesirable side effects were observed and no inflammation or infection occurred
9	Reference	**Klebes et al. [27]**
	Study design	Non-randomized, 3 arms clinical trial Treatment arms: Arm A: only kINPen 09, Arm B: only ODC Arm C: combination of both;
	Study objective	Investigation of potential antimicrobial effects of sequential applications of CAP using kINPen 09 and the conventional liquid antiseptic octenidine dihydrochloride (ODC) compared to each treatment method alone.
	Patients no	34 patients with chronic leg ulcers
	Performance outcome	The reduction of bacterial growth due to all antiseptic procedures was significant in all study arms ($p < 0.05$). Arm C displayed the highest antimicrobial efficacy; suggesting that combined use of kINPen and conventional antiseptics might represent the most efficient strategy for antiseptic treatment of chronic wounds
	Safety outcome	No safety outcomes were reported in the study.

(continued)

□ Table 16.3 (continued)

10	Reference	**Ulrich et al. [16]**
	Study design	Monocentric pilot study Arm A: only kINPen® MED, Arm B: only ODC
	Study objective	Comparison of wound area and bacterial load in chronic wounds between two different treatment methods: octenidine (ODC) and CAP (KINPen® MED)
	Patients no	16 patients with chronic leg ulcers
	Performance outcome	Immediately after the treatment, wounds treated with ODC showed a significantly higher microbial reduction (64%) compared to wounds treated with kINPen® MED (47%). The wound area decreased from 14.1 ± 12.2 (mean ± standard deviation) cm^2 to 11.6 ± 10.2 cm^2 over the 2-week study period, by 12.5% in the ODC-treated group and by 39.0% in the CAP-treated group (4.4 ± 4.3 cm^2 to 2.9 ± 3.3 cm^2). It should be noted, however, that the initial volume of the APP-treated wounds were significantly smaller (4.4 cm^2) compared to the OCT-treated study group (14.1 cm^2).
	Safety outcome	Clinically, there were no signs of delayed wound healing observed in the two groups and both treatments were well tolerated.
11	Reference	**Blatti and Zehnder [37]**
	Study design	Pilot study, open label (no control arm)
	Study objective	Gaining initial clinical experience with the 'cold plasma' method in patients with chronic venous ulcer. The treatment with cold plasma was carried out in addition to an existing 'best medical treatment' using optimized wound management and adequate compression.
	Patients no	5 patients with chronic venous ulcer
	Performance outcome	The wounds lasted an average of 16.6 ± 12 months. On average, 19 ± 6.2 applications were carried out per patient, which took around 5–10 minutes in addition to standard therapy. In four of the five cases, there was a significant reduction in area during treatment and two of the five wounds were practically closed. The conclusions of this pilot study indicate that the CAP application is very simple and safe and painless for the patient.
	Safety outcome	The treatment was painless in all cases. There were no complications, in particular no clinically manifest infection occurred during therapy, and antibiotics were not used.

16

◻ Table 16.3 (continued)

12	Reference	Schwetlick [38]
	Study design	Observational study
	Study objective	To observe the effect of kINPen® MED adjustment therapy in chronic wound management.
	Patients no	61 patients with chronic wounds
	Performance outcome	Complete wound healing was achieved in 44.3%, reduction of wound area in 52.5%. No effect was observed in 3.2%. Multi-resistant bacteria were eradicated in all 18 cases.
	Safety outcome	CAP-related side effects were not observed

Studies with cancer patients (CAP decontamination of infected cancer ulcerations as a part of palliative care)

13	Reference	**Schuster et al. [39]**
	Study design	Descriptive evaluation of the clinically visible influence of the intervention in one group of patients together with a histological analysis of tissue effects in a comparable second group of patients
	Study objective	Evaluation of whether clinical application of CAP (kINPen® MED) can cause (i) visible tumour surface effects, (ii) apoptotic cell kill in squamous cell carcinoma and (iii) whether CAP-induced visible tumour surface response occurs as often as CAP-induced apoptotic cell kill.
	Patients no	21 patients with advanced squamous cell carcinoma were assigned to one of both groups due to their individual different clinical treatment plans. Group I ($n = 12$) was treated with CAP as part of their palliative program, not primarily intended to influence tumour growth but to reduce microbiological contamination of their infected ulcerations. Group II ($n = 9$) was treated by curatively intended surgery and received CAP before total tumour resection.
	Performance outcome	12 patients with head and neck cancer received superficial CAP followed by palliative treatment. 4 of them revealed tumour surface response appearing 2 weeks after intervention. The tumour surface response is expressed as a flat area with vascular stimulation (type 1) or a contraction of tumour ulceration rims forming recesses covered with scabs, in each case surrounded by tumour tissue in visible progress (type 2). In parallel, 9 patients with the same kind of cancer received CAP before radical tumour resection. Tissue specimens were analyzed for apoptotic cells. Apoptotic cells were detectable and occurred more frequently in tissue areas previously treated with CAP than in untreated areas. In case of cancer response, visible effects at the tumour surface became obvious 2 weeks after CAP application and appeared in 2 different types. There was no clinical observation of stimulated tumour growth in all the patients
	Safety outcome	There were no severe adverse effects or adverse effects to be reported in group I. CAP was safe and well tolerated, both treatment team and patients never considered effects of CAP to be a reason for discontinuation of procedure. However, patients complained about a stinging, but moderate pain.

(continued)

▣ Table 16.3 (continued)

14	Reference	**Schuster et al. [40]**
	Study design	Retrospective analysis
	Study objective	Assessment of safety and evaluation of side effects related to supportive CAP palliative treatment of patients with head and neck cancer.
	Patients no	20 patients with advanced head and neck cancer and contaminated ulcerations, who underwent palliative treatment with CAP for decontamination.
	Performance outcome	Performance was not assessed during the study
	Safety outcome	14 out of 20 patients reported discomfort, uneasiness or several side effects (i.e., bad taste, exhaustion, bleeding) while under CAP treatment, and 6 out of 20 did not report any side effects or discomfort. As a conclusion, no severe side effects were observed, mainly mild reactions, uneasiness and discomfort. It has been judged therefore, there is no risk of severe side effects when applying CAP in cancer patients for palliation.
15	Reference	**Metelmann et al. [41]**
	Study design	A retrospective cohort; (clinical follow-up of 12 patients afflicted with advanced squamous cell carcinoma of the head and neck)
	Study objective	(CAP) (kINPen® MED) was used to decontaminate infected cancer ulcerations as a part of palliative care. The aim of the study was to additionally evaluate anti-cancer effects.
	Patients no	12 patients with advanced squamous cell carcinoma of the head and neck
	Performance outcome	CAP had no immediately observable impact on the treated tissue. Visible changes in this study began after 2 weeks of CAP treatment, mainly expressed like a scar or as shrinking or flattening of a previously augmented tumour surface. While under treatment, tumour growth did not return. CAP did reduce contamination of cancer ulcerations; however, the decontaminated ulcers still had a higher microbial load than healthy tissues. Pathogenic species found in lesions prior to treatment could not be detected after CAP. Many patients receiving CAP had a reduction in pain as evaluated by a decrease in patient requests for medication; however, there are some confounders to be considered. The extent of pain reduction differs remarkably between patients receiving CAP
	Safety outcome	CAP treatment of cancer ulcerations was not free from side effects (i.e., extreme fatigue, small but sharp pain, bad taste, collateral oedema, superficial bleeding), but none of them were severe. 9 patients died within the period of investigation. Clinical and pathologic diagnoses determined that cancer progression was the cause of death.

16

◻ **Table 16.3** (continued)

16	Reference	**Metelmann et al. [42]**
	Study design	Prospective observational study
	Study objective	Evaluation of clinical CAP (kINPen® MED) treatment results in terms of survival time, course of disease, tumour remission and safety. The approved indication of CAP was antimicrobial control as part of a standard treatment protocol for palliation.
	Patients no	6 patients with locally advanced (pT4) squamous cell carcinoma of the oropharynx suffering from open infected ulcerations
	Performance outcome	CAP treatment resulted in a reduction in odour and pain medication requirements, in improvement in social function and a positive emotional affect. Further observance revealed partial remission in two patients for at least 9 months. Incisional biopsies at remission demonstrate a moderate amount of apoptotic tumour cells and a desmoplastic reaction of the connective tissue.
	Safety outcome	Four of the six patients enrolled in this observation considered CAP treatment as a noticeable palliation in terms of quality of life, in particular fatigue, social function and emotionality. Following their individual courses of tumour development, two patients were suffering from fast-growing carcinoma, another two from slow or during longer periods not growing tumours and two patients enjoyed a strong response to CAP, one still persistent, the other having experienced a sudden relapse.

Other application (denture stomatitis disease)

17	Reference	**Preissner et al. [18]**
	Study design	Randomized double-blinded, split-mouth pilot study Arm A: (control) nystatin, chlorhexidine and placebo treatment Arm B: (intervention arm) nystatin, chlorhexidine and kINPen® MED administered six times each 7 days
	Study objective	Investigation of antifungal efficacy of adjunctive administered CAP in denture stomatitis (DI) patients.
	Patients no	8 patients with denture stomatitis (DI) disease
	Performance outcome	The initially measured mean erythema surfaces (standard deviation) were 2.92 (1.52) cm^2 on the test side and 4.04 (2.84) cm^2 on the control side. After therapy initiation, the affected surface was reduced significantly more on the test sides compared to the control sides after 2, 3, 4, 5 and 6 weeks ($P \leq 0.05$). This result suggests that additional plasma irradiation provided a significantly accelerated and more extensive remission of the erythema. Visual analogue scale values and the frequency of moderate or heavy growth of Candida post-treatment did not differ significantly between both sides ($P > 0.05$)
	Safety outcome	No adverse events were recorded. Only one male patient reported a slight tingling sensation during the first plasma irradiation on the test site. Another male patient reported irritation of the oral mucosa after having used chlorhexidine for 3 weeks, which he felt was tolerable. Additionally, a brown stain was evident on the back of the tongue in this subject. No side effects of nystatin were observed.

In summary, clinical data show that the kINPen® MED application has a positive influence on:

- Reduction of wound size
- Reduction of pain
- Reduction of bioburden (bacterial contamination) of wounds or intact skin
- Improvement of wound healing
- Improvement of tissue perfusion
- Decontamination of infected cancer ulcerations as a part of palliative care. However, the number of clinical reports concerning CAP treatment of cancer areas is very limited, so this subject needs to be further investigated.

The data clearly demonstrate that there are no safety concerns related to the application of the cold plasma jet in human beings.

Although published clinical studies have shown a beneficial impact of the use of the kINPen® MED on the wound healing process, there is still a limited number of controlled randomized clinical trials reported up to date that assess the effectiveness of the cold atmospheric argon-based plasma jet and CAP in general. As presented in ◘ Table 16.3, most of the current clinical evidences come from the low sample size pilot studies, case reports and non-controlled settings. Well-designed randomized controlled trials are therefore required to confirm current clinical evidence.

Recently the Heart and Diabetes Centre, Bad Oeynhausen in cooperation with the Heart and Diabetes Centre Karlsburg in Germany conducted a prospective, placebo-controlled, single-blinded, randomized study using the kINPen® MED. The study has been completed and its results have been published [1] and will be made available in ► Chap. 9 of this compilation. The objective of this investigation was to demonstrate that the use of cold plasma in addition to standard care treatment compared to placebo combined with standard of care could accelerate wound healing in terms of more rapid and clinically meaningful wound surface regression. Wound closure progression and microbiological analysis were monitored over time to assess the effects. Further collected endpoints were patient's well-being and subjective perceptions during the treatment procedure. Sixty-five participants have been enrolled in total. The cold atmospheric argon-based plasma jet was applied on a group of patients eight times within 14 days; thus, CAP therapy was applied in the first week of treatment on a daily schedule, in the second week CAP was provided every second day. Most important outcomes measured were (a) the change in wound surface area and (b) changes in wound surface area within 14 days of treatment. The results provide relevant evidence to support the effectiveness of the cold plasma jet in chronic wound treatment. It has been demonstrated that avital chronic wounds can be 'activated' using the cold plasma therapy and transferred from the chronic stage to an active stage. Due to the simultaneous antiseptic effect, the germ pressure was successfully reduced in a resource-saving manner. This finding confirms that cold plasma therapy can reduce the duration of the wound and therapy time. For more detail on the results of this study please refer to ► Chap. 9.

16.5 Outlook and Further Developments

To provide additional clinical evidence for the cold atmospheric argon-based plasma jet effectiveness in wound healing, neoplas med GmbH is continuously collaborating with hospitals, universities and research institutions. Furthermore, the company is investigating new possible areas to extend the kINPen® MED applications. The preliminary results are promising. However, the evidence needs to be supported by case studies and well-designed clinical trials.

Conclusion

In conclusion, the safety and performance of the kINPen® MED medical device have been established. The overall clinical and pre-clinical data available up to date collectively demonstrate that the device has a positive influence on wound milieu in infected wounds and pathogen-caused skin diseases and is safe for use in humans. The advantages of cold plasma therapy with the kINPen® MED include the non-invasiveness of the application, high-precision handling in anatomically and pathologically demanding areas under visual control and without touch, pain and itching symptoms relief, lack of side effects, enhancement of wound healing process through the inactivation of a wide range of pathogens – including multi-resistant germs; stimulation of tissue regeneration and promotion of microcirculation.

The results of a new prospective, placebo-controlled, single-blinded, randomized study using the kINPen® MED, that has been conducted at the German Heart and Diabetes Center, Bad Oeynhausen in cooperation with the Heart and Diabetes Center Karlsburg in Germany, provide strong clinical evidence of kINPen® MED's effectiveness in supporting chronic wound management. Moreover, new potential applications of kINPen® MED in the areas of dentistry and ophthalmology are currently under investigation.

References

1. Stratmann B, Costea T-C, Nolte C, Hiller J, Schmidt J, Reindel J, Masur K, Motz W, Timm J, Kerner W, Tschoepe D. Effect of cold atmospheric plasma therapy vs standard therapy placebo on wound healing in patients with diabetic foot ulcers. A randomized clinical trial. JAMA Network Open. 2020;3(7):e2010411.
2. Reuter S, von Woedtke T, Weltmann K-D. The kINPen—a review on physics and chemistry of the atmospheric pressure plasma jet and its applications. J Phys D Appl Phys. 2018;51:233001.
3. Isbary G, et al. Cold atmospheric plasma devices for medical issues. Expert Rev Med Devices. 2013;10:367–77.
4. Heinlin J, et al. Plasma medicine: possible applications in dermatology. J Dtsch Dermatol Ges. 2010;8:968–76.
5. Lackmann J-W, Bandow JE. Inactivation of microbes and macromolecules by atmospheric-pressure plasma jets. Appl Microbiol Biotechnol. 2014;98:6205–13.
6. Schönebeck R. Comprehensive clinical plasma medicine. Springer; 2018.
7. Mann M, Tiede R, Ahmed R, et al. DIN SPEC 91315: general requirements for plasma sources in medicine. Beuth Verlag; 2014.

8. Bernhardt T, et al. Plasma medicine: applications of cold atmospheric pressure plasma in dermatology. Oxidative Med Cell Longev. 2019;2019:3873928.
9. Mann M, et al. Introduction to DIN-specification 91315 based on the characterization of the plasma jet kINPen® MED. Clin Plasma Med. 2016;4:35–45.
10. Lehmann A, Pietag F, Arnold T. Human health risk evaluation of a microwave-driven atmospheric plasma jet as medical device. Clin Plasma Med. 2017;7–8:16–23.
11. Bekeschus S, Schmidt A, Weltmann K-D, von Woedtke T. The plasma jet kINPen – a powerful tool for wound healing. Clin Plasma Med. 2016;4:19–28.
12. Schmidt A, et al. One year follow-up risk assessment in SKH-1 mice and wounds treated with an argon plasma jet. Int J Mol Sci. 2017;18:868.
13. Daeschlein G, et al. Cold plasma is well-tolerated and does not disturb skin barrier or reduce skin moisture. J Dtsch Dermatol Ges. 2012;10:509–15.
14. Daeschlein G, et al. Skin decontamination by low-temperature atmospheric pressure plasma jet and dielectric barrier discharge plasma. J Hosp Infect. 2012;81:177–83.
15. Lademann JM, et al. Risk assessment of the application of a plasma jet in dermatology. J Biomed Opt. 2009;14:1–6.
16. Ulrich C, et al. Clinical use of cold atmospheric pressure argon plasma in chronic leg ulcers: a pilot study. J Wound Care. 2015;24:196–203.
17. Hartwig S, et al. Treatment of wound healing disorders of radial forearm free flap donor sites using cold atmospheric plasma: a proof of concept. J Oral Maxillofac Surg. 2017;75:429–35.
18. Preissner S, et al. Adjuvant antifungal therapy using tissue tolerable plasma on oral mucosa and removable dentures in oral candidiasis patients: a randomised double-blinded split-mouth pilot study. Mycoses. 2016;59:467–75.
19. Schultz GS, Chin GA, Moldawer L, Diegelmann RF. Principles of wound healing. In: Fitridge R, Thompson ME, editors. Mechanisms of vascular disease: a reference book for vascular specialists. Cham: Springer; 2011.
20. Schmidt A, Bekeschus S, Wende K, Vollmar B, von Woedtke T. A cold plasma jet accelerates wound healing in a murine model of full-thickness skin wounds. Exp Dermatol. 2017;26: 156–62.
21. Daeschlein G, et al. In vitro susceptibility of important skin and wound pathogens against low temperature atmospheric pressure plasma jet (APPJ) and dielectric barrier discharge plasma (DBD). Plasma Process Polym. 2012;9:380–9.
22. Izadjoo M, Zack S, Kim H, Skiba J. Medical applications of cold atmospheric plasma: state of the science. J Wound Care. 2018;27:S4–S10.
23. Daeschlein G, et al. Skin and wound decontamination of multidrug-resistant bacteria by cold atmospheric plasma coagulation. J Dtsch Dermatol Ges. 2015;13:143–50.
24. Arndt S, Schmidt A, Karrer S, von Woedtke T. Comparing two different plasma devices kINPen and Adtec SteriPlas regarding their molecular and cellular effects on wound healing. Clin Plasma Med. 2018;9:24–33.
25. Koban I, et al. Treatment ofCandida albicansbiofilms with low-temperature plasma induced by dielectric barrier discharge and atmospheric pressure plasma jet. New J Phys. 2010;12:73039.
26. Daeschlein G, Scholz S, von Woedtke T, Niggemeier M, Kindel E, Brandenburg R, Weltmann K-D, Junger M. In vitro killing of clinical fungal strains by low-temperature atmospheric-pressure plasma jet. IEEE Trans Plasma Sci. 2011;39:815–21.
27. Klebes M, et al. Combined antibacterial effects of tissue-tolerable plasma and a modern conventional liquid antiseptic on chronic wound treatment. J Biophotonics. 2015;8:382–91.
28. Lademann J, et al. Comparison of the antiseptic efficacy of tissue-tolerable plasma and an octenidine hydrochloride-based wound antiseptic on human skin. Skin Pharmacol Physiol. 2012;25:100–6.
29. Gan L, et al. Medical applications of nonthermal atmospheric pressure plasma in dermatology. J Dtsch Dermatol Ges. 2018;16:7–13.
30. Häring NS. F. Behandlung einer superinfizierten Wunde mit Kaltplasma. JATROS Dermatologie Plast Chir. 2016;4:12–3.
31. Hilker L, von Woedtke T, Weltmann KD, Wollert H-G. Cold atmospheric plasma: a new tool for the treatment of superficial driveline infections. Eur J Cardio-thoracic Surg. 2017;51:186–7.

16

32. Barten MJ & Stratmann B. Kaltplasmatherapie zur Behandlung chronischer Wunden. Forum Sanitas – Das Inf Medizinmagazin. 2017;33–35.

33. Vandersee S, et al. Laser scanning microscopy as a means to assess the augmentation of tissue repair by exposition of wounds to tissue tolerable plasma. Laser Phys Lett. 2014;11:115701.

34. Fluhr JW, et al. In vivo skin treatment with tissue-tolerable plasma influences skin physiology and antioxidant profile in human stratum corneum. Exp Dermatol. 2012;21:130–4.

35. Metelmann H-R, et al. Experimental recovery of CO2-laser skin lesions by plasma stimulation. Am J Cosmet Surg. 2012;29:52–6.

36. Metelmann H-R, et al. Scar formation of laser skin lesions after cold atmospheric pressure plasma (CAP) treatment: a clinical long term observation. Clin Plasma Med. 2013;1:30–5.

37. Blatti M, Zehnder T. Anwendung von Kaltplasma bei Patienten mit einem chronisch venösen Ulcus cruris. WUNDmanagement. 2018;12:294–6.

38. Schwetlick B. Kaltplasmatherapie - ein vielversprechender Therapieansatz für die Behandlung peripherer Ulcerationen und multiresistenter Erreger. Spitzenforsch. der Dermatologie - Alpha Informations-Gesellschaft mbH; 2017.

39. Schuster M, et al. Visible tumor surface response to physical plasma and apoptotic cell kill in head and neck cancer. J Craniomaxillofac Surg. 2016;44:1445–52.

40. Schuster M, et al. Side effects in cold plasma treatment of advanced oral cancer—clinical data and biological interpretation. Clin Plasma Med. 2018;10:9–15.

41. Metelmann H-R, et al. Head and neck cancer treatment and physical plasma. Clin Plasma Med. 2015;3:17–23.

42. Metelmann H-R, et al. Clinical experience with cold plasma in the treatment of locally advanced head and neck cancer. Clin Plasma Med. 2018;9:6–13.

DBD-CAP PlasmaDerm® Flex and Dress

Dirk Wandke, Benedikt Busse, and Andreas Helmke

Contents

© Springer Nature Switzerland AG 2022
H.-R. Metelmann et al. (eds.), *Textbook of Good Clinical Practice in Cold Plasma Therapy*, https://doi.org/10.1007/978-3-030-87857-3_17

⊜ Core Messages

- PlasmaDerm® technology is based on the concept of dielectric barrier discharge
- Additional to CAP PlasmaDerm® utilizes pulsed electric fields in the treated tissue
- For medical applications, specific device and process engineering developments have been implemented
- Intended to use in treatment and management of chronic and acute wounds by germ reduction, increase of microcirculation and wound healing
- Effectiveness of PlasmaDerm® proven by clinical studies

17.1 Introduction

In principle, a physical plasma emerges as soon as the electric field strength in a gas exceeds a characteristic limit above which, among other effects, ionization of gas particles occurs as a result of energy transfer by collisions with energetic electrons. The avalanche-like charge separation into ions and electrons causes the gas to become increasingly conductive and thus able to conduct electric current. This current flow heats up the gas, just like with all other materials that are not ideal conductors. If sufficient time and energy are available, a thermodynamic equilibrium can be established in the gas (the plasma), which can reach gas temperatures well above the ambient temperature.

One of the central challenges in the technical utilization of the healing potentials of plasma technology is to minimize the transfer of (thermal) energy into the tissue. Only a few gas discharge concepts are particularly well suited for this purpose at atmospheric pressure conditions – among them the so-called *dielectric barrier discharge* (DBD), which is also referred to as *silent discharge* or *barrier discharge* (*shown in* ◘ Fig. 17.1). This chapter describes the implementation of this type of gas discharge in medical devices based on PlasmaDerm® technology. In addition to technical device characteristics and their influence on implementation in clinical workflows, selected indications are mentioned and results from clinical trials are presented.

◘ **Fig. 17.1** Typical discharge of a dielectric barrier discharge (DBD) operated in ambient air

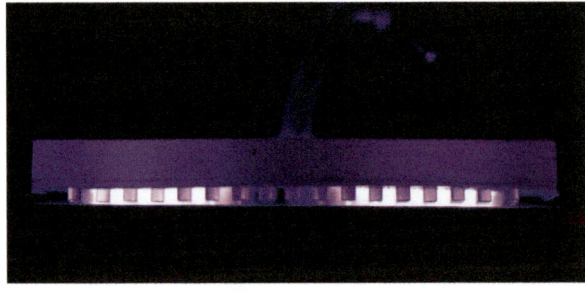

17

17.2 About the Device

17.2.1 Basic Principles/Technology

Just like in any other gas discharge configuration at atmospheric pressure, the electric field strength required to establish the physical plasma is of the order of some kV/mm. These comparatively strong fields are provided technically by generating an electrical potential of the order of kV between at least two electrodes at distances of only a few mm. The characteristic and eponymous feature of the DBD concept is the presence of at least one dielectric material in the electric field between the aforementioned electrodes. This arrangement bears slight technical challenges in terms of plasma generation, since the presence of the dielectric slightly reduces the electric field strength available in the gas. Yet, this issue can be easily addressed by utilizing a power supply that is matched to the properties of the electrode configuration. This minor technical challenge, however, is overcompensated by the spatial and temporal modifications of plasma-physical processes, which include in detail:

- The dielectric significantly reduces the conduction current between the electrodes, since it can only occur in the gas space with a limited amount of total charge.
- Gas discharge events usually occur stochastically distributed over the dielectric surface (microdischarges) thus limiting the local current density.
- Freely moving charge carriers accumulate on the dielectric surfaces and seal off the "external field" generated by the electrodes. As a result, the individual discharge events last only a few tens to hundreds of nanoseconds (10^{-9} s) – even if the applied alternating high voltage would allow a much longer current flow and thus energy transfer.

The sum of these properties prevents an effective heating of gas and tissue and thus supports the formation of a cold plasma at atmospheric pressure conditions. Together with the comparatively simple scalability and the large, technically feasible areas (from cm^2 up to a few 100 cm^2) compared to other gas discharge concepts, DBD has proven to be a versatile, flexible and powerful tool for a wide range of applications.

The PlasmaDerm® technology is also based on the concept of DBD and is referred to as DBD-CAP. For medical applications, specific device and process engineering developments have been implemented. These include:

- A power supply that provides specially shaped high-voltage pulses to generate a cold plasma for the nonthermal treatment of tissue
- The design of the device as a single-electrode (up to 27.5 cm^2) or double-electrode (up to 100 cm^2) system (◘ Fig. 17.2), thus utilizing the tissue itself as a second electrode
- A functional structure (spacer) on the electrode surfaces that ensures the presence of ambient air at the tissue surface interface at all times

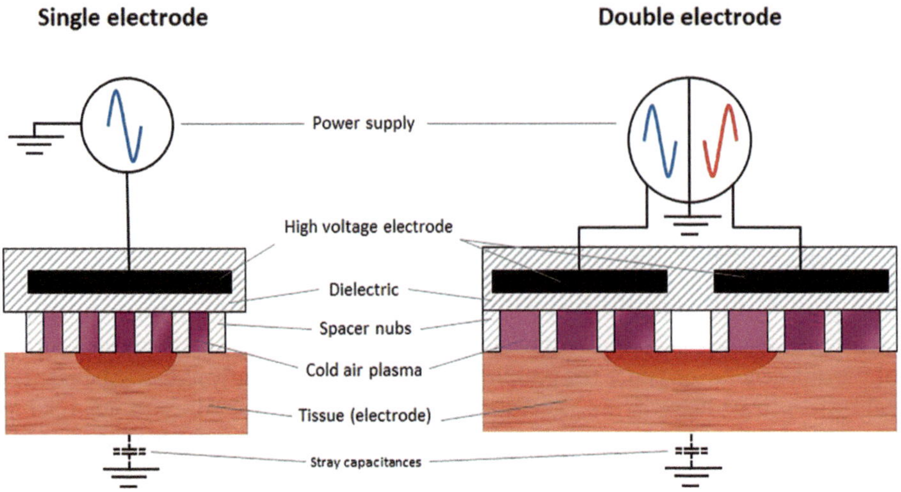

Single electrode   **Double electrode**

- Power supply -
- High voltage electrode
- Dielectric
- Spacer nubs
- Cold air plasma
- Tissue (electrode)
- Stray capacitances

Fig. 17.2 Configuration of electrodes (spacers) and concepts of power supplies of the Plasma-Derm® technology

This approach makes it possible to convert the existing layer of ambient air near the tissue surface into a cold air plasma, which means that no additional working gas is required. Furthermore, the full therapeutic potential of cold atmospheric pressure (CAP) can be harnessed due to the direct tissue contact with all plasma components (e.g., electric field, electric current, long-lived as well as short-lived gaseous species, UV photons). DBD-CAP provides the same physical principles as other CAP sources but, due to its unique electrode configuration, is also very effective in utilizing strong, pulsed electric fields in the treated tissue. It is assumed that this property can stimulate even deeper tissue layers (up to 2–4 mm), which in turn may explain the effectiveness of PlasmaDerm® technology in significantly increasing microcirculation.

Since its market launch in spring 2013, the device technology has been continuously improved with the participation of medical users under the aspects of therapeutic effectiveness and usability in therapeutic workflows. In addition to aspects of miniaturization, ease of use and applicability to the patient, the treatment area in particular, has been continuously enlarged. Beginning with an area of 1 cm², the electrodes of the PlasmaDerm® Dress can meanwhile cover 100 cm² treatment area.

All medical devices based on the PlasmaDerm® technology share the same usability concept – a disposable spacer pad (PlasmaDerm® Flex or Cutan) or dressing (PlasmaDerm® DRESS) needs to be connected to the correspondent base device (Fig. 17.3). Spacer pad or alternatively dressing are designed for flexible adaptation to the anatomical curved body surfaces and shall be aligned directly to the body area which shall be treated. Protrusions of the spacer or dressing ensure, that the correct distance and gap with ambient air is maintained between the device and the body surface. Once the device is activated the treatment can be started with

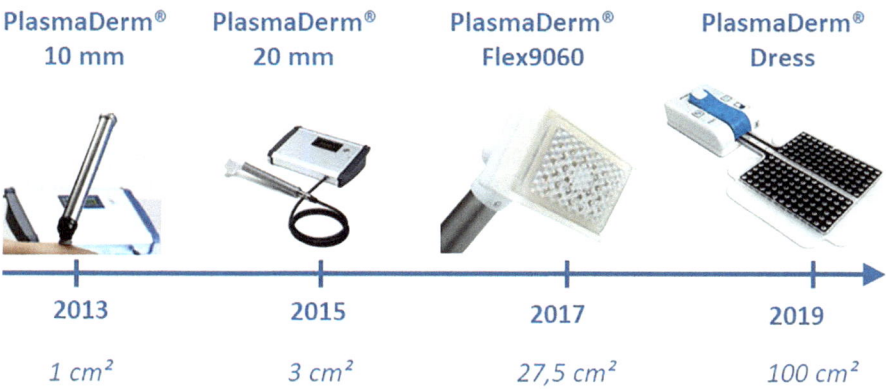

PlasmaDerm®   PlasmaDerm®   PlasmaDerm®   PlasmaDerm®
10 mm   20 mm   Flex9060   Dress

2013   2015   2017   2019

1 cm²   *3 cm²*   *27,5 cm²*   *100 cm²*

◻ **Fig. 17.3** History of PlasmaDerm® medical products

a single button technology with a fixed treatment duration (90 s). When the treatment area extends the area covered by the spacer, the position shall be changed and the procedure repeated until all intended areas received the DBD-CAP treatment. A small overlap of treatment areas can be performed without harm. Within a single treatment session, the same area can be treated repetitively up to three times. Spacer and dressing are delivered single packed and sterile to allow the treatment of open wounds and shall be disposed in a safe manner after the treatment is finished.

17.2.1.1 PlasmaDerm® Vario, Flex and Cutan

The system consists of three components:
- A mobile base unit (placed nearby the patient on a table) which needs to be connected to the power supply network (100–240 V)
- Handset variant Flex or Cutan which is connected to the base unit via a power cord and allows the placement of the applied part to the region of interest
- The disposable correspondent spacer type

The device can be operated by healthcare professionals or trained lay users for intermittent DBD-CAP treatments (e.g., in the course of a wound dressing change).

17.2.1.2 PlasmaDerm® DRESS

The system consists of two components:
- A small mobile base unit (placed nearby the patient) which needs to be connected to the power supply network (100–240 V)
- A disposable dressing made from silicone which is directly connected to the base unit and can be fixed on the body surface by use of a tape or bandage where it may remain for up to 7 days before it may be exchanged.

The device can be applied by healthcare professionals or trained lay users and operated by the patient or lay user without the need for a wound dressing change.

17.2.2 General Parameters

The PlasmaDerm® technology originates from research activities of the HAWK University of Applied Sciences and Arts in Germany, which successfully filed a basic patent on the arrangement and application of the DBD arrangement on living biological tissue (WO 2004/105810 A1). As soon as the technical implementation into the first, battery-powered generation of devices was completed, studies were carried out on their efficacy and safety. Since then, the device technology has been continuously developed further incorporating competent partners such as the Ruhr-University Bochum in Bochum, Germany, and the Fraunhofer-Institute for Surface Engineering and Thin Films in Braunschweig, Germany.

It is necessary to prevent excessive heating of gas and tissue while maintaining stable plasma formation. Power supplies which generate damped sinusoidal voltage pulses of about 10 us duration with amplitudes up to 17 kV at pulse repetition rates of about 100 Hz are effective for this purpose. At these operating parameters, electrical powers of up to some 100 mW are coupled into the electrode configurations. As a result, the air plasma can be maintained at mean gas temperature at the level of room temperature and locally heat the treated tissue to temperatures well below 40 °C and thus does not lead to thermal damaging [1–4].

Due to the choice of ambient air as the medium for plasma generation combined with the relatively low gas temperatures, the generation of ozone is prominent in every device generation of the PlasmaDerm® technology. When operating ceramic electrodes at input power densities of 150–400 mW/cm^2, the ozone concentration directly in the discharge volume is of the order of 200–1100 ppm [5]. For the product Flex9060 operating at significantly lower power densities of 12–20 mW/cm^2, ozone concentrations of up to 300 ppm in proximity to the treated surface were recorded. However, at a distance of 20 cm to the Flex9060 electrode, the ozone concentration is well below the guide value of 100 μg/m^3 as proposed by the WHO [6].

Furthermore, ambient air as the working gas also defines the characteristics of electromagnetic emission. Given the high amount of molecular nitrogen in air combined with mean electron energies of 6–12 eV in the plasma as well as low gas temperatures, the emission of all devices of the PlasmaDerm® technology is dominated by the second positive system of N$_2$ [5, 7–9]. Hence, spectral line emission appears in the range of 295–434 nm (UV-VIS) with a maximum between 312 nm and 358 nm (UV-B and UV-A, no UV-C). The intensities of this emission, however, are relatively sparse whereas the discharge can hardly be detected by the eye at daylight conditions. Parametric studies at input power densities of 150–400 mW/cm^2 have revealed, that even a continuous daily exposure of the human skin for up to 6 hours does not lead to UV-related, long-term risks [5].

17.2.3 Risk Assessment and Product Safety

Due to its classification as a medical device (class IIa/IIb), a wide range of requirements must be implemented from a regulatory perspective. The CE conformity process in the EU is governed by a comprehensive set of regulations with (EU) 2017/745 being in force during the production of this book.

According to its features, the PlasmaDerm® system is used to promote the healing of chronic wounds, in preventive surgical site care, for dermatological applications and in chronic inflammatory diseases (tendinosis). These benefits have to be weighed against the risks and mitigation measures as well as potential side effects:

- Electrical shock due to limited electrical safety
- Disturbance of other active devices due to limited electromagnetic compatibility
- Skin and tissue toxicity, sensitization or irritation due to limited biocompatibility
- Use errors due to inadequate usability
- Burns due to increased temperature

Electrical safety and EMC are achieved by compliance with, for example, IEC 60601-1, -1-2. Biocompatibility is achieved by compliance with, for example, ISO 10993-1, -5, -8 and -10 and USP class VI. The impact of UV-light emission, local temperature increase, reactive gas species and electrical fields and currents applied to the body were qualified in preclinical in vitro and animal studies and associated risks excluded by device design and limitation of the treatment duration (see ► Sect. 17.2.5). Up to now, the PlasmaDerm® System can be sold into the EU market without limitations. No known side effects compromise its distribution.

17.2.4 Indications

The PlasmaDerm® system is intended to be used in the treatment and management of chronic wounds:

- Chronic venous ulcers
- Arterial ulcers
- Mixed arterial-venous ulcers
- Ulcers as complication of diabetic foot syndrome
- Burn wounds
- Pressure ulcers
- Lymphatic ulcers
- Pyoderma gangraenosum
- Secondary wound healing situations

In addition, the device is used for improved wound healing or management after surgical interventions:

- Flap graft ingrowth promotion
- Healing of mesh graft donor sites
- Surgical incision wounds
- Transcutaneous conduits
- Surgical lesions after treatment of acne inversa

17.2.5 Use and Treatment Recommendations

The general workflow for a DBD-CAP treatment includes the preparation of the body site where the treatment shall be applied (e.g., undressing of a wound, cleaning of the wound), assembly of handset and spacer, activation of the base generator, placement of the spacer to the treatment site by gentle pressure and start of a 90-s DBD-CAP period (◘ Fig. 17.4). If the treatment area is larger than the spacer area, the application is repeated after the spacer has been moved to the next area. The positive effects on microcirculation, tissue oxygen saturation and hemoglobin content can be increased and prolonged when the 90-s treatment is repeated up to three times for the same area [10].

The frequency and overall duration of the DBD-CAP treatment depend on the underlying disease, condition and size of the wound, and condition, medication, and comorbidity of the patient, and last but not the least, wound healing phase. However, some general recommendations can be concluded from clinical experience and rationale:

Infected wounds should be treated with DBD-CAP 1–2× daily if possible and this scheme shall be continued until the infection disappeared.

Heavily secreting wounds should be treated every 2 days with a single DBD-CAP application until the exudation ceases and granulation is initiated.

During the granulation phase, the frequency can be reduced to a single DBD-CAP treatment every 3 days until epithelization is satisfactory.

In conditions with heavily impaired microcirculation (e.g., diabetic foot syndrome, peripheral arterial insufficiency), it is recommended to treat in addition to the wound area also the surrounding skin and to repeat the DBD-CAP application two to three times in order to strengthen and prolong the positive effect on microcirculation.

It is important to integrate the DBD-CAP treatment in the overall treatment regimen (e.g., to apply compression therapy, physiotherapy and lymph drainage in chronic venous insufficiency as soon as the infection is overcome and exudation ceased).

◘ **Fig. 17.4**   Use of Plasma-Derm®

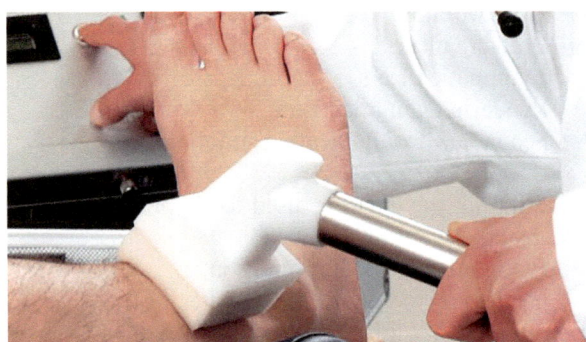

17

17.2.6 Successful Examples

A large number of treatments in the above-mentioned indications have been successfully carried out since market entry in Europe. The following treatment courses are examples of this (☐ Figs. 17.5, 17.6, 17.7, 17.8, and 17.9).

Indication	Peripheral vascular disease with exposed infected bone/tendon tissue
Comorbidities	Heart failure, COPD, psoriasis vulgaris
Treatment period	13 weeks
Number of treatments carried out	28

Indication	Diabetic foot syndrome, state after amputation
Comorbidities	Diabetes mellitus, PAD, polyneuropathy
Treatment period	6 weeks
Number of treatments carried out	6 (stationary) + 11 (ambulant)

Indication	Ulcus cruris venosum
Comorbidities	Chronic venous insufficiency
Treatment period	3 weeks
Number of treatments carried out	14

Indication	Ulcus cruris artriosum
Comorbidities	Diabetes mellitus, obesity
Treatment period	9 weeks
Number of treatments carried out	25

Indication	Postoperative wound healing disorder after surgery of a mandibular fracture
Comorbidities	Immunosuppression, renal anemia, hypertension, hyperthyroidism
Treatment period	4
Number of treatments carried out	4

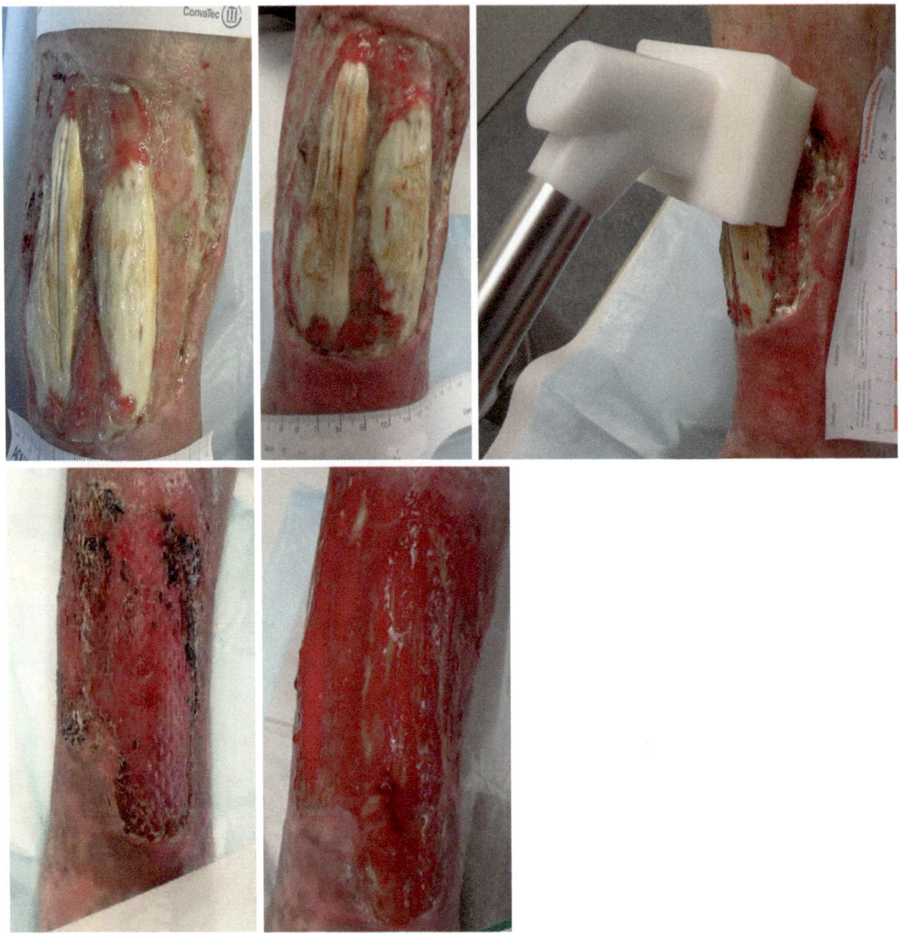

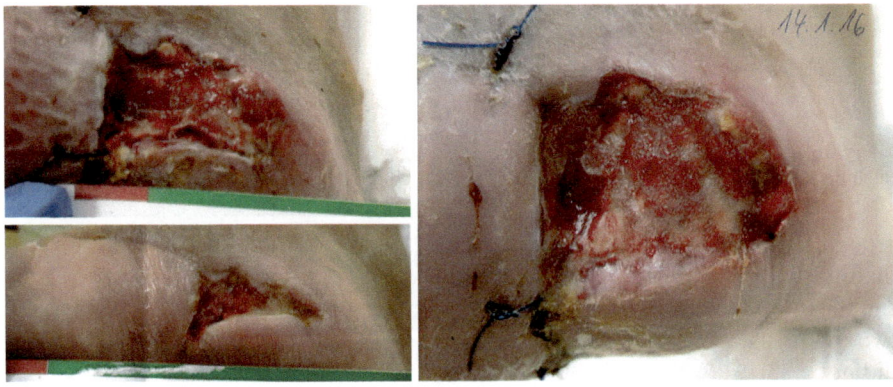

Fig. 17.5 Peripheral vascular disease with exposed infected bone/tendon tissue

17

Fig. 17.6 Diabetic foot syndrome, state after amputation

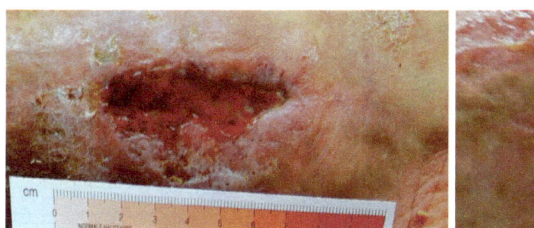 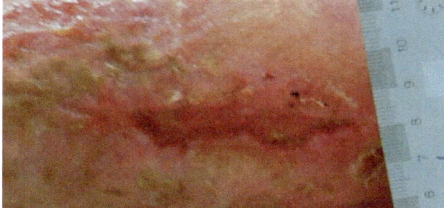

■ **Fig. 17.7** Ulcus cruris venosum

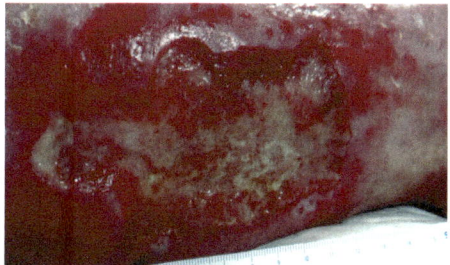 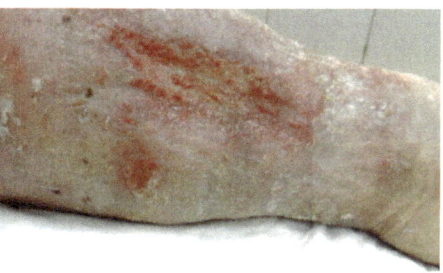

■ **Fig. 17.8** Ulcus cruris artriosum

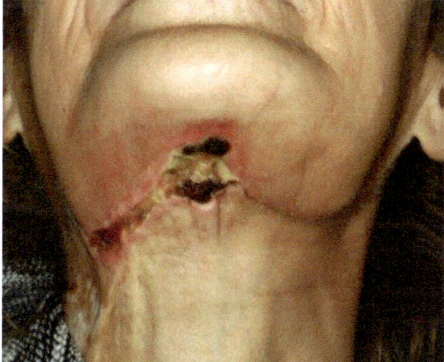 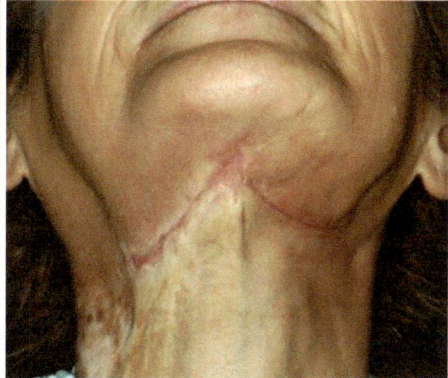

■ **Fig. 17.9** Postoperative wound healing disorder after surgery of a mandibular fracture

17.3 Clinical Trials

This chapter presents a small selection of clinical studies on the effectiveness of PlasmaDerm® Therapy and its properties of germ reduction, increase of microcirculation and wound healing.

Between 2011 and 2012, a first clinical investigation [11] was performed to investigate the safety and clinical performance in the application of the PlasmaDerm® VU2010 device for ulcers in chronic venous insufficiency.

The investigation was designed and executed as a single center, prospective randomized trial after approval by the responsible ethics committee and the Federal Institute for Drugs and Medical Devices (BfArM) in Germany. The investigation was performed to assess safety and, as secondary endpoints, efficacy and applicability of 45 s/cm^2 DBD-CAP as adjuvant therapy against chronic venous leg ulcers in addition to conventional wound treatment and compression therapy.

Subjects were randomized into two groups. The control group received standardized modern wound care ($n = 7$). The treatment group ($n = 7$) received in addition DBD-CAP 3× per week for 8 weeks.

The following parameters were analyzed:

The ulcer size was determined weekly (Visitrak®, photodocumentation). Bacterial load (bacterial swabs, contact agar plates) and pain during and between treatments (visual analogue scales) were assessed. Patients and doctors rated the applicability of plasma (questionnaires).

DBD-CAP was evaluated to display favorable antibacterial effects. The investigation demonstrated that plasma treatment with the PlasmaDerm® VU-2010 device is safe and effective in patients with chronic venous leg ulcers.

To achieve a larger treatment area and accommodate the need to provide disposable sterile devices, the development of the PlasmaDerm® Flex and Cutan devices were initiated.

The positive effect on elevation of microcirculation was confirmed in a study in 20 healthy volunteers [12] who received 90 s DBD-CAP (PlasmaDerm®) treatment. Oxygen saturation increased immediately after the treatment by about 24% and remained elevated for 8 minutes after application. Similar results were observed for cutaneous blood flow, which increased by 73% and remained elevated for 11 minutes.

The effect of repetitive DBD-CAP application on microcirculation and tissue oxygen saturation was investigated in another study in 20 healthy volunteers who received 3×90 s DBD-CAP (PlasmaDerm®) treatment with an intermediate gap of 10 minutes between the treatments respectively [10]. Tissue oxygen saturation and postcapillary venous filling pressure significantly increased after the first application and returned to baseline values within 10 minutes after treatment. After the second and third applications, both parameters increased significantly vs. baseline until the end of the 40-minute measuring period. Cutaneous blood flow was significantly enhanced for 1 minutes after the first application, with no significant differences found during the remainder of the observation period. The second application improved and prolonged the effect significantly until 7 minutes and the third application until 13 minutes.

With more sensitive optical investigation technologies, the microcirculatory effects of DBD-CAP were investigated in another study with 10 healthy volunteers [2]. The effect of DBD-CAP versus pressure application by placing the electrode alone was compared for application times of 90 s, 180 s and 270 s, respectively. Significant increases in microcirculation were only observed after plasma stimulation but not after pressure stimulus alone. For a period of 1 hours after stimulation, local relative hemoglobin was increased by 5.1% after 270 s DBD-CAP treatment. Tissue oxygen saturation increased by up to 9.4%, whereas blood flow was doubled (+106%). Skin pH decreased by 0.3 after 180 s and 270 s DBD-CAP treatment, whereas skin temperature and moisture were not affected.

The effect of DBD-CAP on physiological flora was studied in nine volunteers (four females and five males; mean age 29 years), and its effect on artificial contamination was studied in four volunteers (two females and two males; mean age 26.8 years). In this study [13] the effect of a jet plasma device was compared with the PlasmaDerm® VU2010 device. Both plasma devices led to a significant reduction physiological (PF) and artificially (AF) contaminated flora (Staphylococcus epidermidis and Micrococcus luteus). The maximum log reduction factors for PF were 1.3 for the DBD at 210 s and 0.8 for the APPJ at 60 s. For AF, the maximum log reduction factors were 1.7 for the DBD at 90 s and 1.4 for the APPJ at 120 s. Treatment with both devices was well tolerated.

The indications covered and successful treatments performed by DBD-CAP treatment in recent years included the healing intention of diabetic foot ulcers, treatment and recovery of infected and complicated amputation sites, treatment of ulcers due to peripheral arterial insufficiency (with or without revascularization), conversion of wounds due to lymphatic or venous congestion, pressure ulcers, burn wounds, secondary infected surgical wounds, pyoderma gangraenosum, necrobiosis lipoidica, epidermolysis bullosa, acne vulgaris, and others. Within the surgical disciplines, DBD-CAP is applied for ingrowth support of flap and mesh grafts, treatment of mesh graft and flap graft donor sites, treatments of suture defects and superficial surgical wound infections, treatment of larger dermatological biopsy areas, wound conditioning before mesh graft application, palliative treatment of exacerbated tumor wounds etc.

17.4 Outlook and Further Developments

Due to the large number of possible applications based on the DBD-CAP mechanism of PlasmaDerm® Therapy in various indications, further device and applicator modes will be developed and marketed in the future. That means, for example, a battery-powered device.

The requirements of the (EU) 2017/745 for the existing PlasmaDerm® Systems are already implemented since March 2020.

17.5 Conclusion

The medical products of the PlasmaDerm® technology are characterized by a high applicability in clinical workflows due to the particularly large treatment areas, the omission of a working gas to be supplied and the short treatment durations. In more than 30,000 treatments since 2013, no device-related complications have occurred, which proves the high level of application safety. The applications so far could be implemented in the hospital environment, general practitioner offices, outpatient wound centers as well as in home care environment.

Acknowledgments   The authors would like to thank all funding agencies and cooperation partners of the "BioLiP" research network, funded by the Federal Ministry of Education and Research (BMBF) under FKZ 13 N9089; the associated partners in the "PlaStraKomb" project, funded by the BMBF under FKZ PNT51501; the partners of the "Campus PlasmaMed II" research network, funded by the BMBF under FKZ 13 N11190; the partners of the research association "WuPlaKo", funded by the BMBF under FKZ 13GW0041D; the partners of the joint project "KonChaWu", funded by the State of Lower Saxony under FKZ ZW3-85006987 and the partners of the impulse projects "Therapy" & "MeWiFo" within the innovation partnership "Plasma for Life", funded by the BMBF under FKZ 13FH6I04IA & 13FH6I01IA.

Literature

1. Awakowicz P, Bibinov N, Born M, Busse B, Gesche R, Helmke A, Kaemling A, Kolb-Bachofen V, Kovacs R, Kuehn S, Liebmann J, Mertens N, Niemann U, Oplaender C, Porteanu HE, Scherer J, Suschek C, Vioel W, Wandke D. Biological stimulation of the human skin applying health promoting light and plasma sources. Contrib Plasma Physics. 2009;49:641–7.
2. Borchardt T, Ernst J, Helmke A, Tanyeli M, Schilling AF, Felmerer G, Viöl W. Effect of direct cold atmospheric plasma (diCAP) on microcirculation of intact skin in a controlled mechanical environment. Microcirculation. 2017;24:e12399.
3. Rajasekaran P, Opländer C, Hoffmeister D, Bibinov N, Suschek CV, Wandke D, Awakowicz P. Characterization of dielectric barrier discharge (DBD) on mouse and histological evaluation of the plasma-treated tissue. Plasma Process Polym. 2011;8:246–55.
4. Tuemmel S, Mertens N, Wang J, Viöl W. Low temperature plasma treatment of living human cells. Plasma Process Polym. 2007;4:465–9.
5. Helmke A, Mahmoodzada M, Wandke D, Weltmann KD, Viöl W. Impact of electrode design, supply voltage and interelectrode distance on safety aspects of a medical DBD plasma source. Contrib Plasma Physics. 2013;53:623–38.
6. Helmke A, Franck M, Wandke D, Viöl W. Tempo-spatially resolved ozone characteristics during single-electrode dielectric barrier discharge (SE-DBD) operation against metal and porcine skin surfaces. Plasma Med. 2014;4:67–77.
7. Kuchenbecker M, Bibinov N, Kaemling A, Wandke D, Awakowicz P, Viöl W. Characterization of DBD plasma source for biomedical applications. J Phys D Appl Phys. 2009;42:045212.
8. Rajasekaran P, Mertmann P, Bibinov N, Wandke D, Viöl W, Awakowicz P. DBD plasma source operated in single-filamentary mode for therapeutic use in dermatology. J Phys D Appl Phys. 2009;42:225201. (8pp).
9. Rajasekaran P, Mertmann P, Bibinov N, Wandke D, Viöl W, Awakowicz P. Filamentary and homogeneous modes of dielectric barrier discharge (DBD) in air: investigation through plasma characterization and simulation of surface irradiation. Plasma Process Polym. 2010;7:665–75.
10. Kisch T, Schleusser S, Helmke A, Mauss KL, Wenzel ET, Hasemann B, et al. The repetitive use of non-thermal dielectric barrier discharge plasma boosts cutaneous microcirculatory effects. Microvasc Res. 2016b;106:8–13.
11. Brehmer F, Haenssle HA, Daeschlein G, Ahmed R, Pfeiffer S, Görlitz A, et al. Alleviation of chronic venous leg ulcers with a hand-held dielectric barrier discharge plasma generator (PlasmaDerm® VU-2010): results of a monocentric, two-armed, open, prospective, randomized and controlled trial (NCT01415622). J Eur Acad Dermatol Venereol. 2015;29(1):148–55.

17

12. Kisch T, Helmke A, Schleusser S, Song J, Liodaki E, Stang FH, et al. Improvement of cutaneous microcirculation by cold atmospheric plasma (CAP): results of a controlled, prospective cohort study. Microvasc Res. 2016a;104:55–62.
13. Daeschlein G, Scholz S, Ahmed R, von Woedtke T, Haase H, Niggemeier M, et al. Skin decontamination by low-temperature atmospheric pressure plasma jet and dielectric barrier discharge plasma. J Hosp Infect. 2012;81(3):177–83.

SteriPlas® and PlasmaTact®

Jeiram Jeyaratnam and Mary McGovern

Contents

© Springer Nature Switzerland AG 2022
H.-R. Metelmann et al. (eds.), *Textbook of Good Clinical Practice in
Cold Plasma Therapy*, https://doi.org/10.1007/978-3-030-87857-3_18

⊜ Core Messages

- The Adtec SteriPlas is the only CE-certified, microwave-powered, cold atmospheric argon plasma medical device that offers the largest 12 cm² treatment area making it suitable for the treatment of large wounds.
- Smaller plasma pen devices such as the PlasmaTact offer a smaller 1 cm² treatment area, subsequently giving users a longer time to treat large wounds.
- Adtec Healthcare has been collecting clinical evidence for over a decade, documenting the proven antibacterial efficacy of the Adtec SteriPlas.
- Adtec has been developing plasma products for over 30 years.

18.1 Introduction

Adtec Healthcare began its journey into cold plasma medicine in 2002 when we designed our first cold plasma technology demonstrating its painless effect on contact with human skin. Studies and development continued into 2004 where we quickly learned that bacterial load reduction was possible through our technology. ◻ Figure 18.1 shows an Adtec plasma technician demonstrating the painless effect of Adtec cold plasma technology upon contact with skin.

In 2005, Adtec and the German scientific research organization, Max Planck Gesellschaft, formed a plasma medicine group to research the science of nonthermal argon plasma and investigate its potential medical applications. The research team led by Professor Gregor Morfill of the Max Planck Institute of Extra-

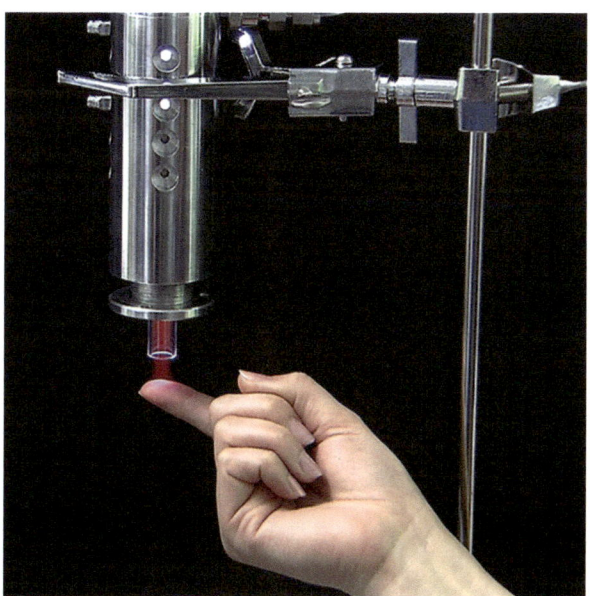

◻ **Fig. 18.1** Adtec's cold atmospheric plasma using helium gas

terrestrial physics included experts from various research organizations from Germany, Russia, the USA, and the United Kingdom.

The collaboration with the Max-Planck Gesellschaft led to the joint development of our shared patented 6-electrode plasma source (■ Fig. 18.2). The creation of this plasma source defined how our microwave argon plasma is generated. The remainder of the medical device including the aesthetics and critical components such as the generator, control box, and software were carefully designed by the dedicated development team at Adtec. This brought life to Adtec's first CE-certified medical device, the MicroPlaSter (■ Fig. 18.3).

The plasma medicine team carried out extensive research on the optimization of the MicroPlaSter, antibacterial efficacy in vitro, preclinical testing, safety of the plasma technology and they managed the first clinical trials. The scientific results and clinical evidence were used as the supporting Technical File information for the first Adtec medical device MicroPlaSter (Class IIa). Adtec's MicroPlaSter became the first cold plasma medical device in history to test the treatment of

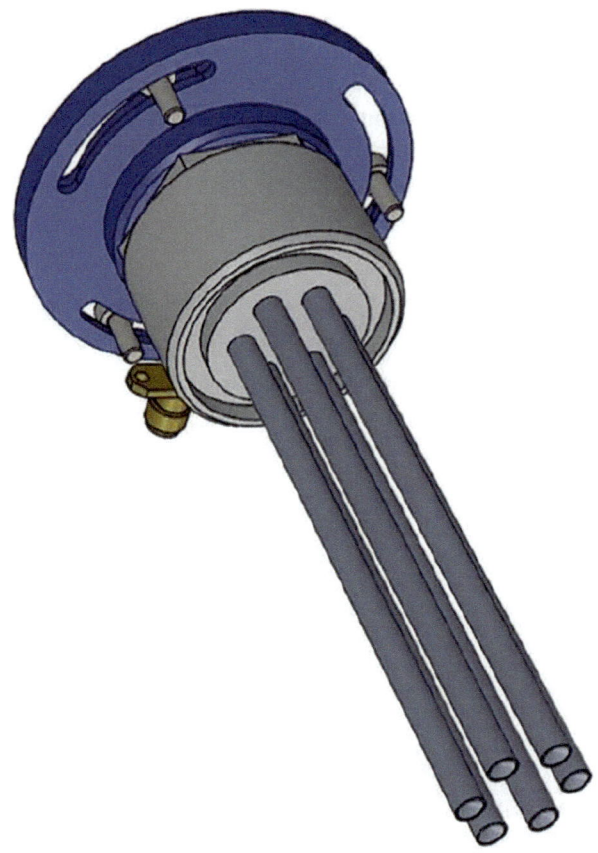

■ **Fig. 18.2** The patented six electrode plasma source which is currently used in the Adtec MicroPlaSter and Adtec SteriPlas

18

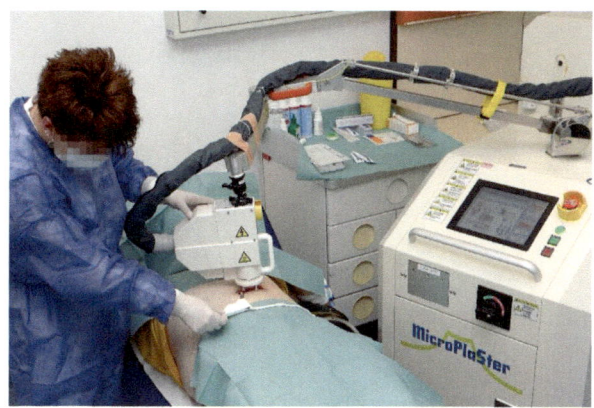

■ **Fig. 18.3** The Adtec MicroPlaSter: Adtec's first CE-certified cold plasma medical device in use at a German hospital

chronic wounds in clinical trials. The evidence generated from the studies had proven Adtec's patented plasma technology has antibacterial efficacy [1–8, 10–15]. This same plasma technology is incorporated in the second Adtec medical device – the Adtec SteriPlas.

18.2 About the Devices

18.2.1 Basic Principles

The Adtec SteriPlas has proven efficacy for the treatment of wounds, surgical site infections, and medical dermatology with a strong collection of clinical evidence [9, 16–22, 24–27]. The Adtec SteriPlas cold plasma has proven antibacterial efficacy including against antimicrobial-resistant bacteria both in vitro and in vivo. This includes wounds that are stalled by biofilm such as diabetic foot ulcers [20, 21] and deep sternum infections [16, 17, 22]. It has also shown strong efficacy for the treatment of dermatological conditions such as Hailey–Hailey Disease [13], Herpes Zoster [14], Actinic Keratoses [18, 19], and acne [27].

Like the Adtec SteriPlas (■ Fig. 18.4), the PlasmaTact (■ Fig. 18.5) is a reliable and robust plasma device that generates microwave cold atmospheric argon plasma. Its intended use is for sanitization, surface treatment for bonding or adhesion, and cleaning for plastic, metal, or ceramic surfaces. Although the PlasmaTact has been documented to show positive antimicrobial efficacy in vitro, it is not a registered medical device.

Cold plasma has been shown to demonstrate surface activation of materials such as plastic, metal, and textiles, which is a role that the PlasmaTact can achieve. ■ Figures 18.6 and 18.7 show the before and after results of using the PlasmaTact torch system on textile and metal, documenting a distinctive hydrophilic result after cold plasma application.

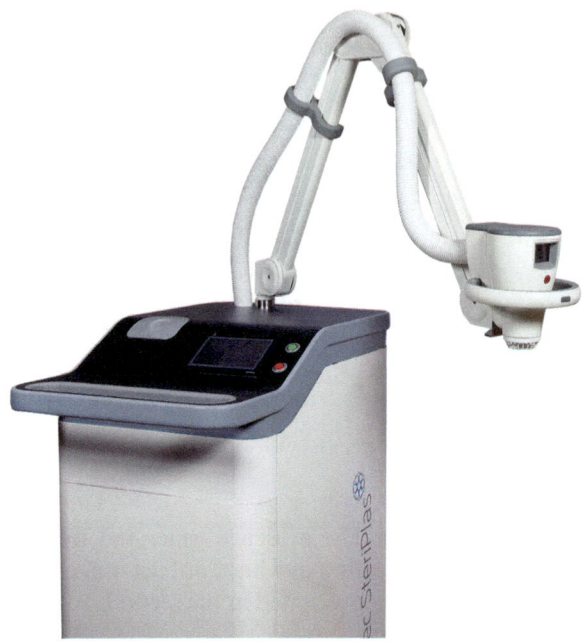

◘ Fig. 18.4 The Adtec SteriPlas cold plasma medical device with its flexible arm and plasma chamber

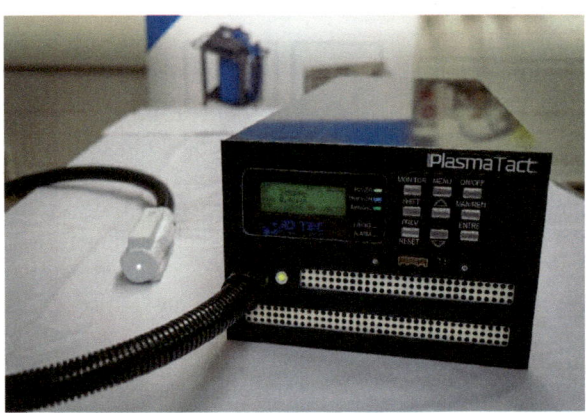

◘ Fig. 18.5 The portable PlasmaTact cold plasma device with its handheld plasma-pen style design

What separates the PlasmaTact from the Adtec SteriPlas is the advantage of being handheld and portable. It also offers users the ability to change power settings from 5 to 15 W, including the change of the gas flow rate. The PlasmaTact also operates using a single electrode allowing it to be contained within a handheld design, whereas the Adtec SteriPlas is composed of 6 electrodes carefully engineered into its plasma chamber. The PlasmaTact can also operate using Helium or Argon gas, whereas the Adtec SteriPlas remains fixed and is to only be used with Argon gas. But

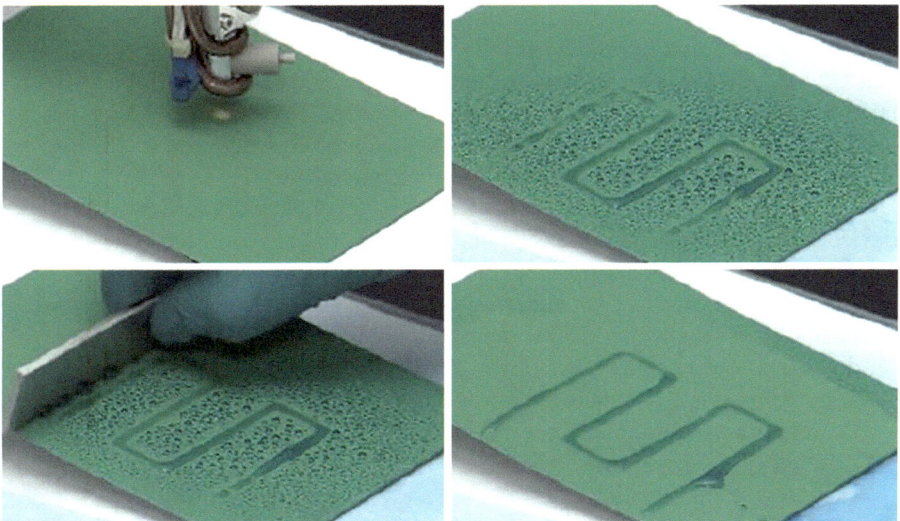

🔲 **Fig. 18.6** As the PlasmaTact follows a zigzag pattern, the scientist later applies water and removes the excess, leaving behind the distinctive hydrophilic result on the path that the PlasmaTact had followed on the treated textile

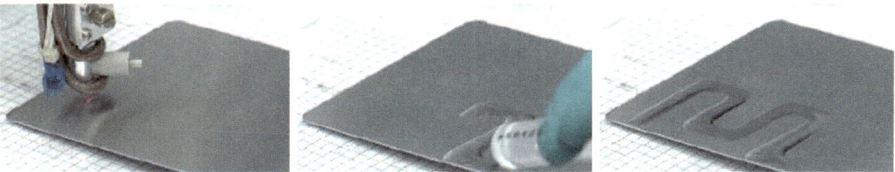

🔲 **Fig. 18.7** As the PlasmaTact follows a zigzag pattern, the scientist later applies water, which follows the path of the PlasmaTact showing the distinctive hydrophilic result on the treated metal sheet

delivering a 1 cm^2 treatment area of cold plasma with plasma pen devices like the PlasmaTact versus the larger 12 cm^2 treatment area of cold plasma with the Adtec SteriPlas suggests that the overall treatment time of the wound is extended.

Throughout the collection of our clinical evidence, Adtec has recommended a minimum treatment time of 2 minutes using our cold plasma technology. This means positioning the plasma chamber over the wound for 2 minutes to allow enough bombardment and rupture of the bacterial cells by the components of cold plasma to have them destroyed. A typical wound such as a diabetic foot ulcer may be larger than 1 cm^2 and therefore the user of the device would have to remain in position for 2 minutes for every 1 cm^2 of the wound covered with the PlasmaTact, meaning that the overall treatment time would be far more than 2 minutes in total. Using a plasma-pen-type design would mean the user would have to remain for longer to have achieved satisfactory coverage of the wound with cold plasma. However, the Adtec SteriPlas offers a much larger 12 cm^2 treatment area meaning every 2 minutes of cold plasma applied can cover 12 cm^2 of the wound each time. In a normal hospital setting, time is essential and clinicians may not be able to spend longer than necessary to cleanse the wound with cold plasma. Adtec Healthcare has opted to not register the PlasmaTact as a medical device as plasma pen devices with a small treatment area would take far longer to treat a typical large wound than the Adtec SteriPlas can. ◘ Figure 18.8 demonstrates the 12 cm² treatment area of the Adtec SteriPlas plasma chamber being used to treat a very large diabetic foot ulcer with multiresistant bacteria.

The Adtec SteriPlas boasts an array of advantages over plasma-pen-type devices such as the PlasmaTact. The main features of the Adtec SteriPlas include:

- 12 cm² treatment area (◘ Fig. 18.9).
- Flexible positioning of the arm allowing the plasma chamber to remain fixed in position over the wound whilst the treatment is conducted, giving the user freedom to complete other tasks.
- A short and simple 2-minute treatment time for every 12 cm² of the wound covered.
- Proven and patented plasma technology
- Contact-free and painless
- Harmless to mammalian cells [6]

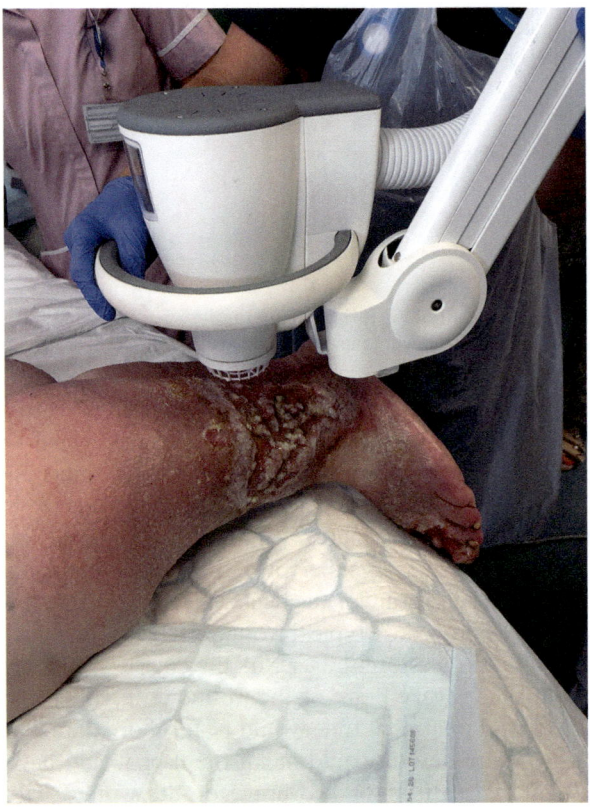

◘ **Fig. 18.8** The plasma chamber of the Adtec SteriPlas being used to treat a large diabetic foot ulcer at an NHS Hospital in the United Kingdom

18

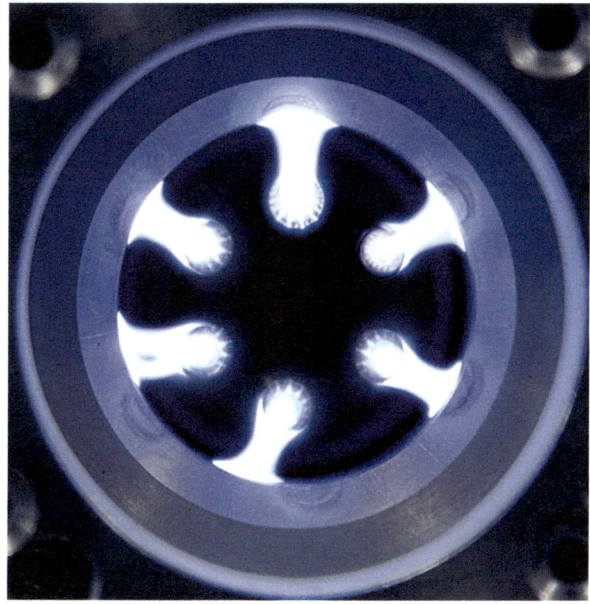

⬛ **Fig. 18.9** The Adtec SteriPlas boasts a large treatment area of 12 cm² comprising six electrodes

18.3 General Parameter: Physical Disruption of Bacterial Cells

Our research included a study of the mechanism of action of our argon microwave plasma device on bacteria and safety leading to the first clinical trials of gas plasma on wounds worldwide. The Adtec SteriPlas plasma chamber contains a patented ionization chamber that bombards argon gas with electrons emitted from multiple hot electric filaments. The resulting plasma includes ions and electrons, excited species, heat, electric fields, and UV radiation. Reactive oxygen and nitrogen agents may develop as the ions propelled by the argon gas exiting the treatment head bombard with the air between the plasma chamber and treatment area.

Adtec had carried out preclinical studies of the safety of the device for use on people. The plasma has proven antibacterial efficacy and does not harm mammalian cells [6]. The research findings were published, and the preclinical data was used to support our successful application to the ethics committee for the clinical trials in Germany.

It should also be noted that the concentration of each plasma component differs according to the plasma product design (how the plasma is generated). The plasma generated differs greatly if the carrier gas is air or argon gas and if it is a direct plasma source versus an indirect plasma source design.

To study the mode of action, we carried out a series of experiments to measure the antibacterial activity of the main components. As cold plasma has many components, it is difficult to isolate and measure the exact contribution of each component. The constituent agents cannot be reproduced on their own in the same form.

Professor Gregor Morfill, in his role as the Director and Professor of the Max Planck Institute for Extra-terrestrial Physics, has presented the plasma mode of action results of his research and other leading scientists [23]. The research was financed by the Max Planck Society. It can be shown that the main killing mechanism of the bacteria is physical in action [23].

Plasma Cell Interaction – How Does Plasma Work?

Active Agents for Cold Plasma:
Ions and electrons,
Reactive molecules,
Excited species,
Electric fields,
UV radiation.

Permeabilisation of cell membrane:
Electromechanical effects,
Local heating,
Chemical effects.

Penetration of reactive agents:
ROS and RNS.

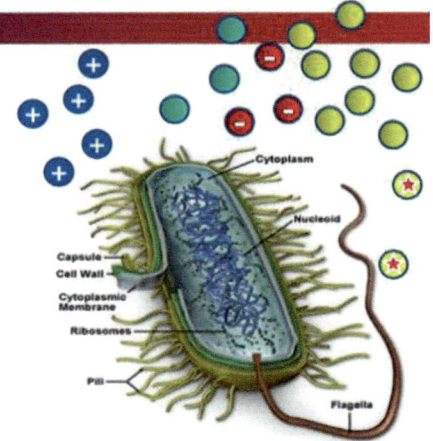

Yonson et al., J. Phys. D 2006, Halliwell and Gutteridge, Oxford Univ. Press 2007, Stoffels et al., IEEE Trans. Plasma Sci. 2008, Nosenko et al. NJP 2009, Leduc et al. NJP 2010, Liburdy and Vanek, Rad. Res. 1985, Kushner 2010, Puc et al., Radiol.Oncol. 2001, Kong et al. NJP 2010, Morfill et al. NJP 2010

Plasma Cell Interaction – How Does Plasma Work?

• **Electron-ion recombination** and **excited Atoms** can make the bacteria cell wall permeable (up to 5 nm) through local energy deposition and heating (+ 30°).

• **Cell charging** and disfigurement via Coulomb forces can induce shear stress and cell wall rupture (E ≥ 600 V/m).

• **Lipid peroxidation** can produce transient pores (through abstraction of H atoms from a methylene group through Hydroxyl radicals).

• **Electroporation** if the electric field exceeds ~ 50 kV/cm.

Kong et al. NJP 2009, Nosenko et al. NJP 2009, Leduc et al. NJP 2010, Graves et al. 2009, 2010, Kushner 2010

18

The "Electron-ion recombination and excited atoms" arises from local energy deposition and heating and is a physical effect that is achieved by physical bombardment (with ions and atoms) and rupturing of the cell wall. This physical action results in physical damage and rupture of the cell wall, compromising the cell structure and integrity of bacteria.

Likewise, the "Cell charging" effect of the plasma results in disfigurement due to physical forces (Coulomb forces are physical in nature) that cause shear stress. This physical action results in the disfigurement of the cell and in cell wall rupture, which is a physical outcome of a physical action.

The "Liquid Peroxidation" is a physicochemical action with a physical outcome in the creation of pores. This is not dissimilar to surfactant activity (primarily a physical, surface effect), which causes cell wall disfigurement and shear forces that can lead to cell wall damage and rupture.

Finally, "Electroporation" is a microbiology technique in which an electrical field is applied to cells in order to increase the permeability of the cell membrane. This is primarily a physical action (with the electrical field being a physical force) that has a physical effect on the integrity of the bacterial cell wall.

The components of cold atmospheric argon plasma are as equally important as each other for the destruction of bacterial cell walls.

18.4 Risk Assessment and Product Safety [28]

Adtec Healthcare had completed a full risk assessment under ISO 14971 to ensure that the medical device is safe for the user and the patient being treated. Data collected from the clinical trials, design process, and safety and EMC testing had been used to verify and check the data. All the data from clinical trial and research had been used as an input for the Adtec SteriPlas. Adtec Healthcare had conducted extensive tests regarding UV and Ozone gases in the clinical trials. This assessment had been reviewed constantly while the medical devices were in the field to ensure that they are always safe [25].

All medical devices should be designed by using the safety regulation in EN 60601. IEC 60601 is a series of technical standards for the safety and effectiveness of medical electrical equipment, published by the International Electrotechnical Commission. All devices must comply with EN 60601-1. Depending on the function of the device, it will apply to different families under the group. To ensure product safety, Adtec's nonthermal plasma devices have qualified under the following categories:

BS EN 60601-1 ed. 3.1 Medical electrical equipment—Part 1: General requirements for basic safety and essential performance.

A full safety test needs to be performed by a Test House.

IEC 60601-1-2:2014 Medical electrical equipment—Part 1–2: General requirements for basic safety and essential performance—Collateral standard: Electromagnetic compatibility—Requirements and tests.

A full EMC test needs to be performed by a Test House.

BS EN 62304:2006 + A1:2015—Medical device software. Software life-cycle processes.

A software assessment needs to be performed.

BS EN 62366-1:2015—Medical devices. Application of usability engineering to medical devices.

A usability file needs to be created using the above standard.

Pre-CE Mark: MicroPlaSter Alpha and Beta (Clinical Trials Version)

Name	MicroPlaSter -alpha	MicroPlaSter -Beta
Model	ARPP-MS-α Clinical trials version	ARPP-MS-β (Clinical trials version)
Plasma generation	Microwave argon plasma	Microwave argon plasma
Plasma recipe (Treatment)	Power – 80 ~ 110 W Gas flow-rate – 2 ~ 5 SLM Treatment time - 2-7 mins	Power – 80 ~ 85 W 2008 ~ 2009 Gas flow rate – 2-5 slm 2009 ~ 2013 Gas flow rate – 4 ~ 5 SLM Treatment time – 2–7 mins
Plasma source	6-electrode plasma torch 	6-electrode plasma torch
Plasma gas temperature	$\leq$48 °C at a distance of 20 mm from the plasma torch head	$\leq$48 °C at a distance of 20 mm from the plasma torch head
Safety tests		IEC60601-1 Test report 1601-1_C/97-04 EMC EN60601-1-2:2001 Test Report EMC08208

18 **CE Marked Medical Devices in Adtec NTGP Product Series**

Name	MicroPlaSter Class IIa	SteriPlas version 1 Class IIa Dec 2020 Class IIb	SteriPlas version 2 Class IIb
Model	ARPP-MS-02	ARPP-SP-01	ARPP-SP2-01
Plasma generation	Microwave argon plasma	Microwave argon plasma	Microwave argon plasma
Plasma recipe (Treatment)	Power – 80 W Gas flow rate – 4 SLM Treatment time- 2–5 mins	Power – 80 W Gas flow rate – 4 SLM Treatment time- 2–5 mins	Power – 80 W Gas flow rate – 4 SLM Treatment time- 2–5 mins
Plasma source	6-electrode plasma torch	6-electrode plasma torch	6-electrode plasma torch
Plasma gas temperature	≤48 °C (118 °F) at a distance of 20 mm from the plasma torch head	≤48 °C (118 °F) at a distance of 20 mm from the plasma torch grid	≤48 °C (118 °F) at a distance of 20 mm from the plasma torch grid
Safety tests	IEC60601-1 Test report E469793-D1 EMC EN60601-1-2:2001 Test Report EMC08208	IEC60601-1 Test report **TRA-027456-34-** EMC EN60601-1-2:2001 Test Report TRA027456-31-	≤48 °C (118 °F) at a distance of 20 mm from the plasma torch grid IEV60601-1 Test Report 01E46979D1000-1/AO/CO-informative EMC Test Report UL-EMC-RP13441367JD01A- and UL-EMC-RP11858484JD02A

18.5 Indications

18.5.1 Use and Treatment Recommendations

The Adtec SteriPlas cold plasma has proven antibacterial efficacy against antimicrobial-resistant bacteria both in vitro and in vivo. Its intended use is to manage the infections in wounds, surgical site infections, and dermatological conditions. Using clinical evidence collected with the Adtec MicroPlaSter and then the Adtec SteriPlas, scientists and clinicians were able to determine the recommended treatment time to achieve exceptional bacterial load reduction for every 12 cm² covered to be 2 minutes.

We have also determined that maintaining close proximity, within 2 cm, to the wound surface is recommended to achieve maximum efficiency during cold plasma treatment. Maintaining this distance throughout the treatment program has shown to achieve optimum results. Energy dissipation is a crucial factor to consider with distance. As expected with most medical devices using cold plasma, the further away the plasma source is from the wound surface, the less effective it can be. The plasma chamber of the Adtec SteriPlas is recommended to remain within 2 cm of the wound surface to allow interaction of the charged particles and UV light (all of which are important bactericidal components) for the maximum destruction of bacteria. The cold plasma generated in the Adtec SteriPlas is propelled with argon gas flow. ◘ Figure 18.10 shows the ideal distance from the plasma chamber to the surface of the wound.

Between each patient treatment, the Sensor Module is required to be replaced for hygiene purposes. The Sensor Module is the applied part (consumable) of the Adtec SteriPlas that features as a 2 cm depth spacer from the microwave double grid guard of the plasma chamber. The Sensor Module complies with the Essential Requirements and is CE marked in accordance with Annex II of the European Medical Devices Directive 93/42/EEC as modified by 2007/47/EC. The 2 cm distance separation from the plasma chamber and within 2 cm above the wound surface ensures the optimum distance from the wound surface to the plasma chamber (at 4 cm distance), allowing for reactive species to be created as a by-product of

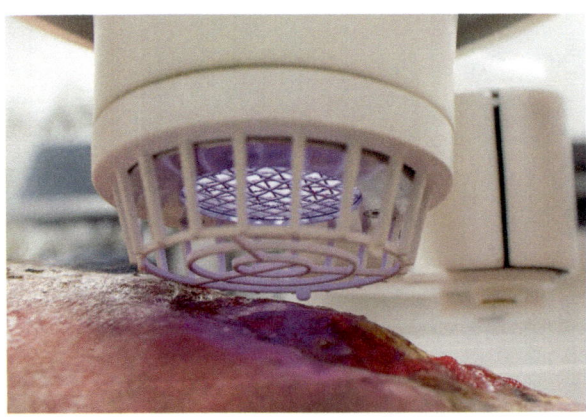

◘ **Fig. 18.10** The Adtec SteriPlas with its Sensor Module fixated above a chronic wound during a cold plasma treatment

18

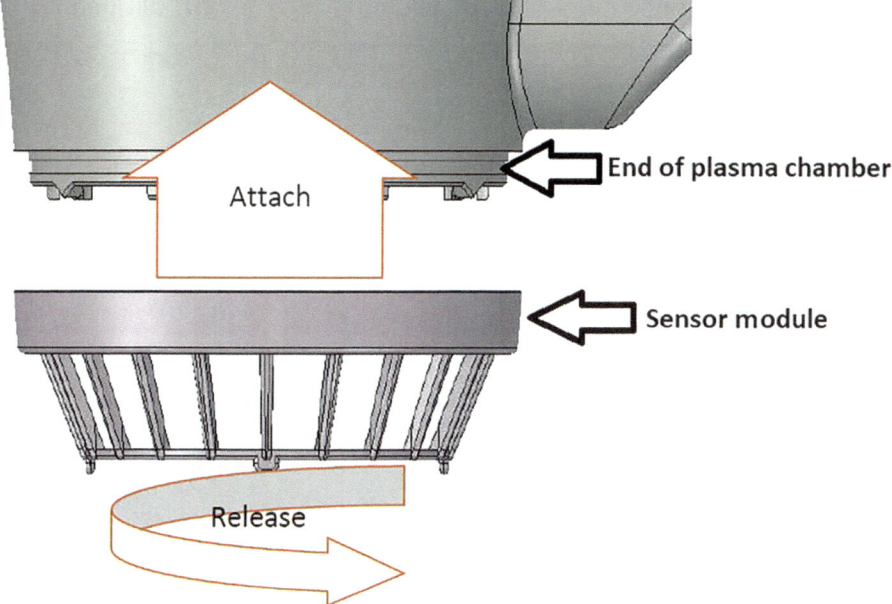

Attach

End of plasma chamber

Sensor module

Release

■ **Fig. 18.11** Illustration of the separation of the Sensor Module from the plasma chamber

cold plasma. Reactive oxygen and nitrogen species are also important bactericidal components for the destruction of bacteria. ■ Figure 18.11 demonstrates the separation of the Sensor Module from the Adtec SteriPlas plasma chamber.

Although not a registered medical device, the PlasmaTact has demonstrated antimicrobial efficacy in vitro for the treatment of multiresistant bacteria. Studies conducted involving inoculated agar plates of common multiresistant bacteria such as *Methicillin-resistant Staphylococcus aureus* (MRSA), *Escherichia Coli*, and *Vancomycin-resistant Enterococcus faecium* had shown significantly wide zones of inhibitions when treated with the PlasmaTact.

In ■ Fig. 18.12, the zones of inhibition can be observed on inoculated agar plates of *E. coli* following treatment with the PlasmaTact. The PlasmaTact remained at 15 W power and 3 cm distance from the surface of each agar plate. The variables included testing the difference using 1 standard liter per minute (slm) of cold plasma of 10^0 serial dilution of *E. coli*, 2 slm of cold plasma on 10^2 serial dilution of *E. coli* and 5 liters per minute of cold plasma at 10^4 serial dilution of *E. coli*. Like the Adtec SteriPlas, the optimum distance is within 2–4 cm of the subject to allow for optimum bacterial load reduction.

18.6 Successful Examples

Over the last decade, clinical evidence for the Adtec SteriPlas has shown its proven and patented plasma technology has the advantage to treat wounds, surgical site infections, and dermatological conditions.

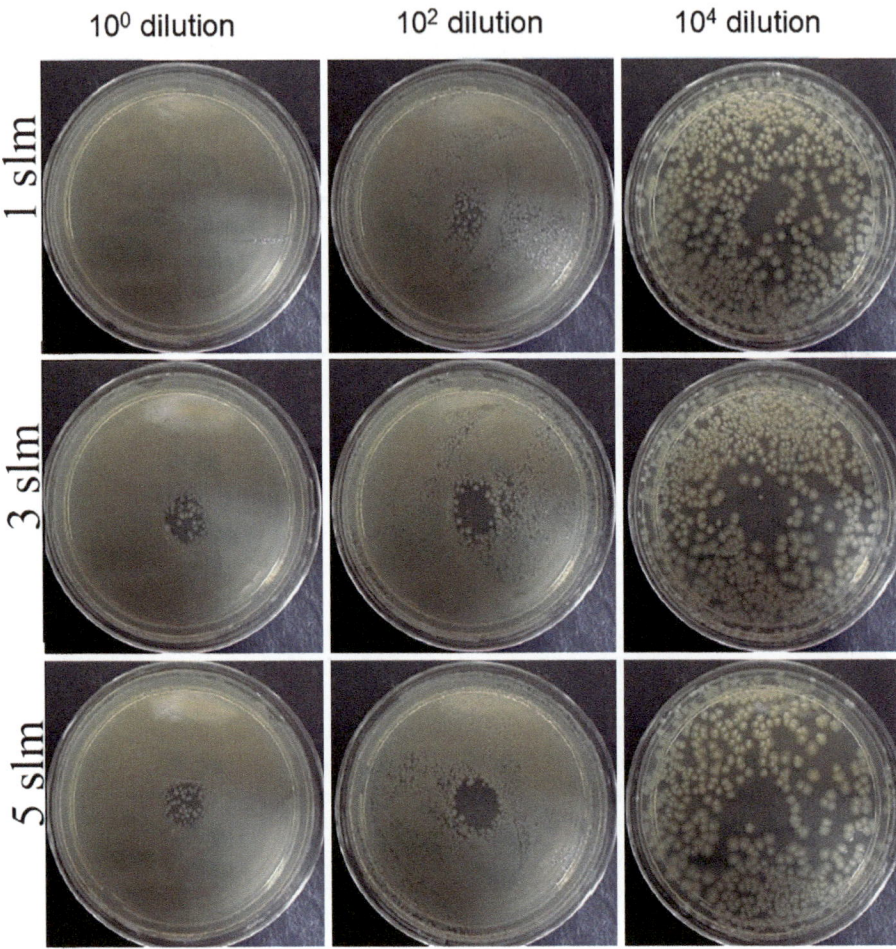

■ **Fig. 18.12** The antibacterial efficacy of the PlasmaTact in vitro

Recent clinical evidence includes efficacy for the treatment of infected diabetic foot ulcers, cardiac left ventricular assist devices (LVAD), cardiac surgical site infections, and actinic keratoses and acne.

18.6.1 Diabetic Foot Ulcers [20]

Diabetic foot ulcers are the most costly and devastating complication of diabetes, which affects 15% of diabetics during their lifetime. The annual incidence of foot ulceration in the UK varies from 1% to 3.6% with a prevalence of 5%. It is also a major source of morbidity and the leading cause of frequent hospitalization. Bacterial colonization of chronic diabetic wounds is a well-recognized contributor to impaired wound healing.

A retrospective case report review on the impact of the Adtec SteriPlas treatment on three diabetic foot ulcer patients all of whom have had Type 2 diabetes for over 10 years. All patients suffered from chronic, nonhealing foot and leg ulcers with multiresistant infection. All three patients had at least three courses of intravenous antibiotics for more than 6 weeks prior to treatment with the Adtec SteriPlas. Two out of the three patients had adequate vascular supply, based on vascular clinical assessment, arterial duplex +/− CT angiogram. Two out of the three patients had a HbA1c <55 mmol/mol with a combination of insulin, SGLT2 inhibitors, and GLP1 receptor agonist.

During treatment with the Adtec SteriPlas, all patients were treated for 5 minutes per head size area of the machine, twice a week (total of 8–11 sessions each) in addition to standard wound care. This was delivered by specialist diabetes podiatrists. The patients' wounds were regularly assessed by the podiatrist and the consultant based on clinical assessment, inflammatory markers, and microbial swab growth.

18.6.1.1   Patient 1

This patient had chronic left foot and leg ulcers for 2 years with severe pain which required multiple courses of antibiotics alongside a whole spectrum of analgesic modalities. The pain was so severe that her mobility was significantly reduced. The severity was such that she had been considered for a major amputation. Once treatment with the Adtec SteriPlas had started, there was significant improvement in foot and leg ulcers in terms of clinical appearance as well as with pain control. Her leg ulcers remain stable up to 8 months after treatment finished. ◘ Figure 18.13 illustrates the visual condition of the left foot ulcers before the treatment with the Adtec SteriPlas, and ◘ Fig. 18.14 illustrates the visual condition of the left foot ulcers after the final treatment with the Adtec SteriPlas.

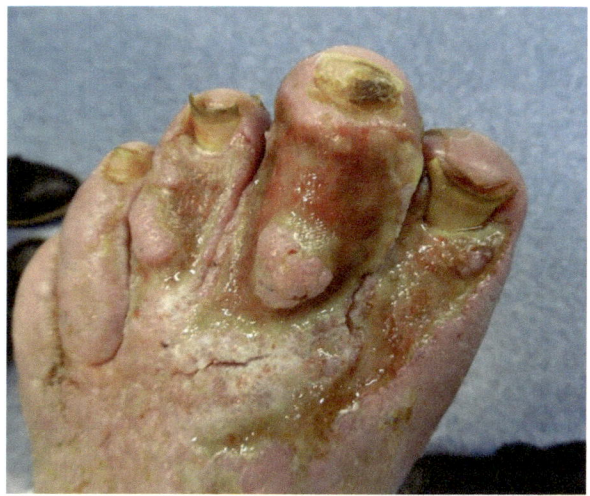

◘ **Fig. 18.13**   Before CAP

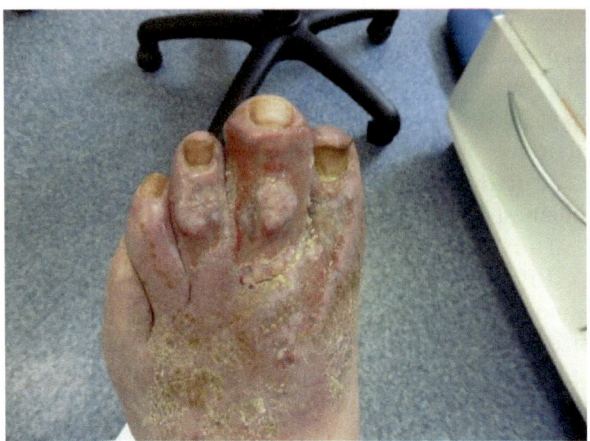

◘ Fig. 18.14   After CAP

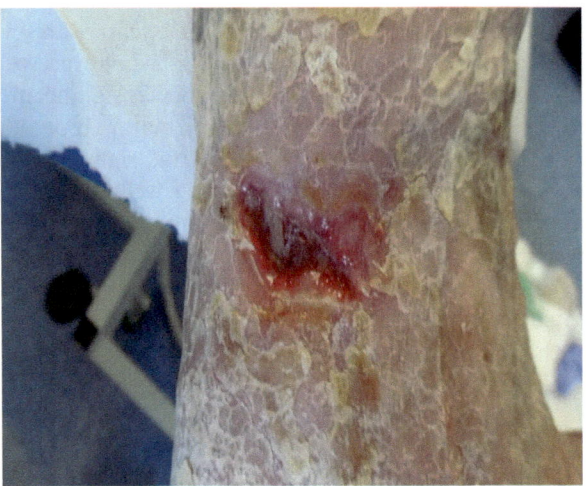

◘ Fig. 18.15   Before CAP

18.6.1.2   **Patient 2**

This patient had a right leg ulcer for 5 years which did not improve with regular dressings and/or multiple prolonged courses of antibiotics. When treatment with the Adtec SteriPlas began, there was a significant reduction in the size and severity of the wound and signs of healthy granulating tissues developing. The ulcer had completely healed during therapy and in the 12 months following the final treatment with the Adtec SteriPlas, his skin has remained intact with no further ipsilateral ulcerations. ◘ Figure 18.15 illustrates the visual condition of the leg ulcer prior to the start of treatment with the Adtec SteriPlas and ◘ Fig. 18.16 illustrates the visual condition of the leg ulcer at the end of the treatment.

18

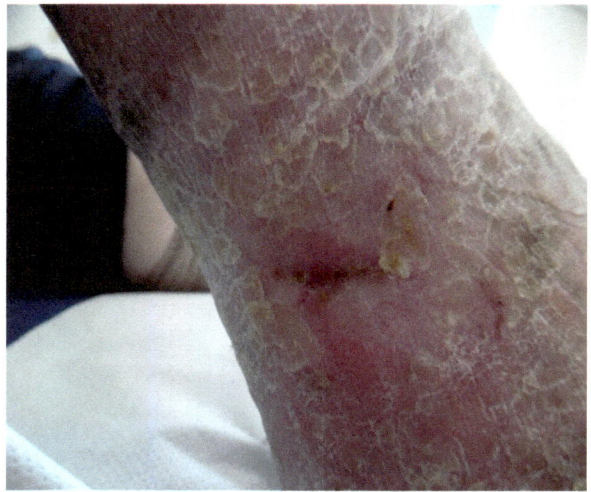

■ **Fig. 18.16**   After CAP

18.6.1.3   **Patient 3**

This patient had a background of stage 3 chronic kidney disease and congestive cardiac failure with chronic bilateral foot and leg ulcers for 9 years. He had regular dressings, multiple prolonged courses of antibiotics, optimization of his heart failure with a pacemaker, rate control, and anticoagulation. Despite all these interventions, his ulcers still persisted. He went onto have angioplasty of both lower limbs with temporary success.

During and after cold plasma treatment with the Adtec SteriPlas, there was a 20% reduction in wound size and severity. ■ Figure 18.17 illustrates the visual appearance of the ulcer before treatment with the Adtec SteriPlas, and ■ Fig. 18.18 illustrates the visual appearance of the ulcer after treatment with the Adtec SteriPlas.

Despite the limited number of patients in this short study, there is a potential benefit. A key limitation is vascular insufficiency and its severity. The improvement of diabetic foot and leg ulcers are postulated to be due to a reduction in the microorganism and infection load of the wound. This is achieved in a different mode of action to that of antibiotics (physical mode of action vs chemical mode of action). This suggests that resistance is unlikely to be generated.

18.6.2   **Surgical Site Infections [24]**

Adtec's medical device was used at the University Hospital Heidelberg in Germany to test the efficacy of gas plasma on 20 patients with infected drivelines. Amongst the 20 patients were 18 men and 2 women. Two hundred and five treatments were administered using the Adtec medical device amongst the 20 patients. The treatment count administered varied for each patient between 3 and 15 applications of

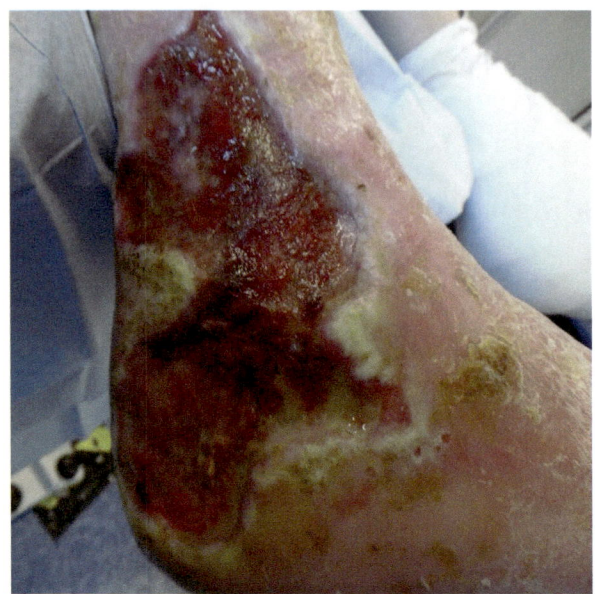

■ Fig. 18.17   Before CAP

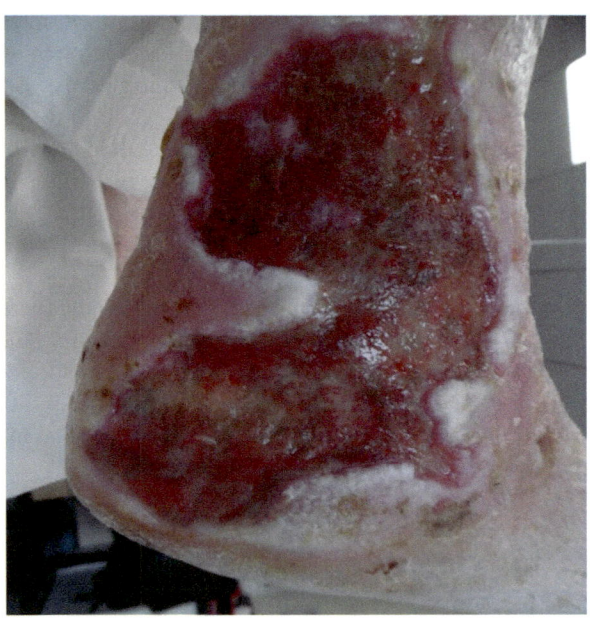

■ Fig. 18.18   After CAP

18

Adtec's cold atmospheric plasma. The treatment time also varied per patient and was between 4 and 8 minutes per application. Treatment with the Adtec medical device was given alongside standard treatment.

Wound protocol consisted of standardized routine treatment, inclusive of:

- The use of facemask, sterile gloves
- Disinfectant with Octenidin (Octenisept®)
- Treatment with the Adtec medical device (minimum 240 seconds per application)
- Bacteriostatic dressings with silver (Aquacel AG Extra®)
- Cover dressing with polyurethane foam (Mepilex Border®)
- Fixation with Foley Anchor®

18.7 Results

18.7.1 Patient 1

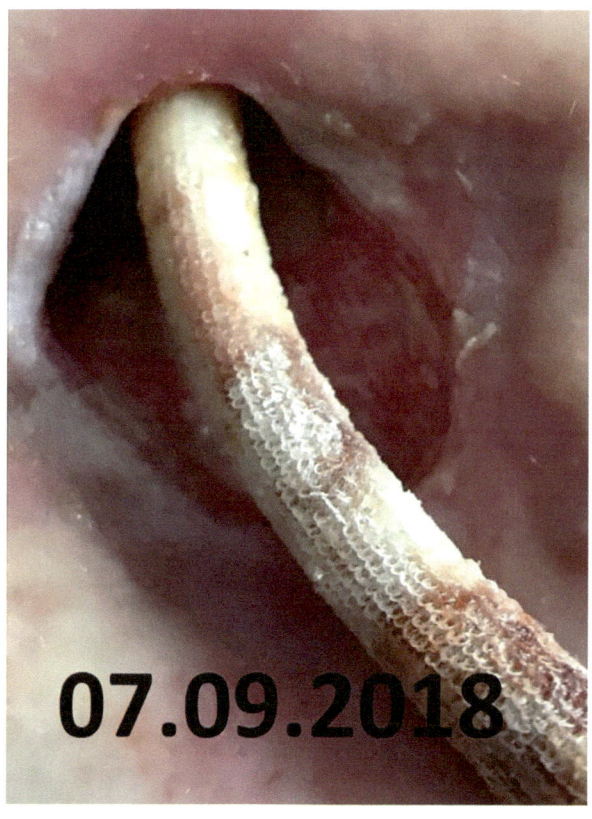

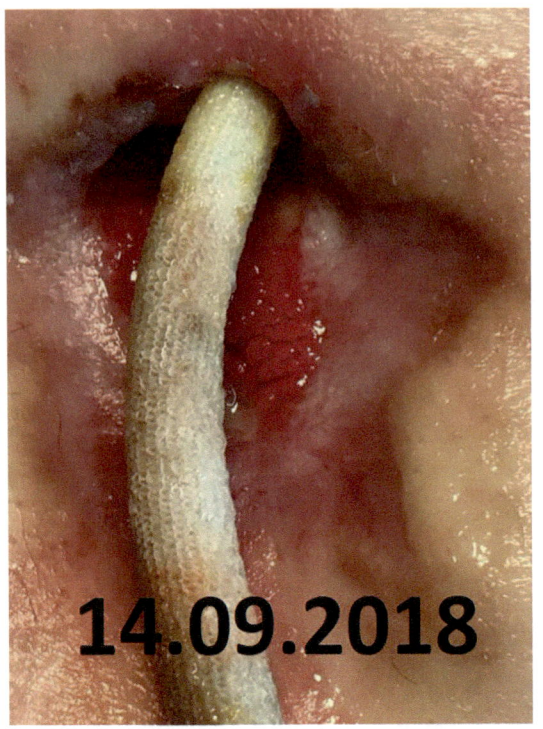

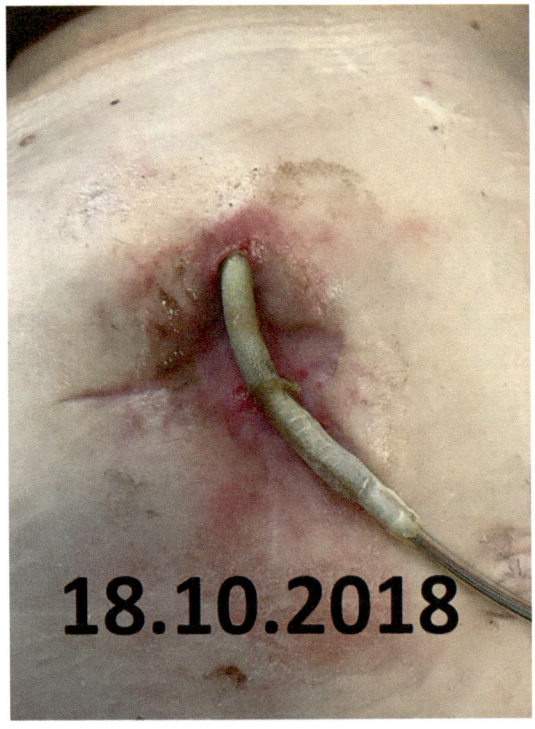

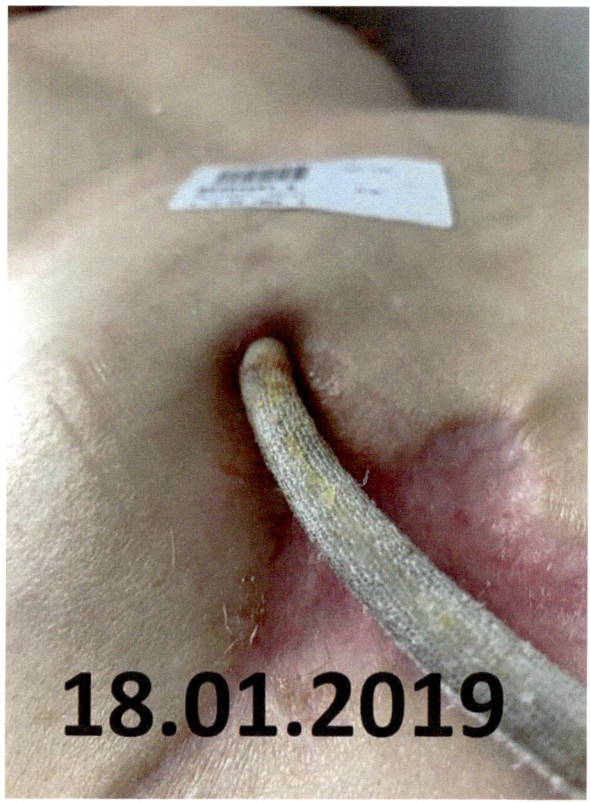

The first swab taken for this patient was on August 5, 2018 and contained traces of *Pseudomonas aeruginosa*. The initial therapy for this patient consisted of intravenous meropenem antibiotics, surgical debridement with VAC-therapy and 20 VAC-exchanges.

When the Adtec medical device was introduced, the treatment program consisted of no antibiotic use, cold atmospheric plasma and standard care twice a week out of hospital, and discharge and ambulatory conduction once a week.

There was a total of 12 applications of cold atmospheric plasma administered to this patient. The last swab recorded was on February 24, 2019, which consisted of *Staph. epidermidis* and still without the use of antibiotics.

18.7.2   Patient 2

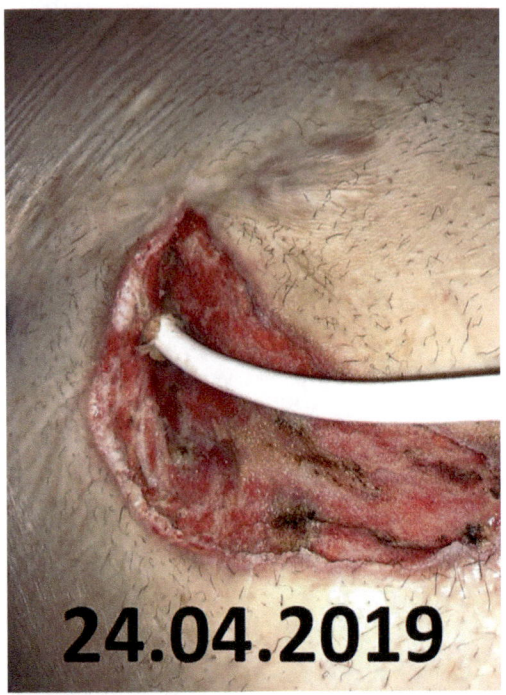

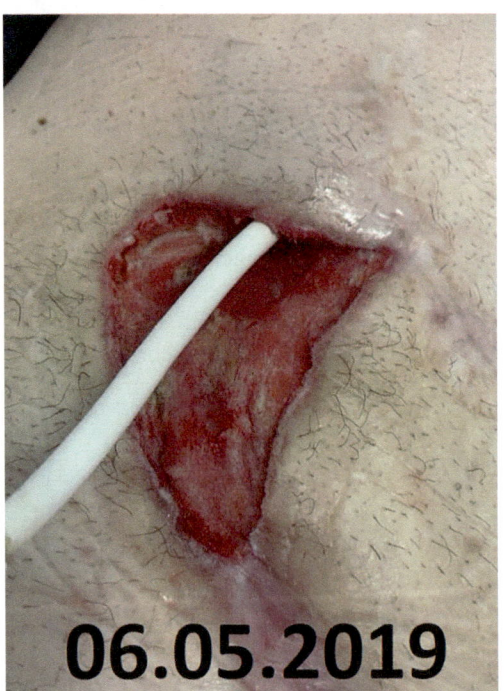

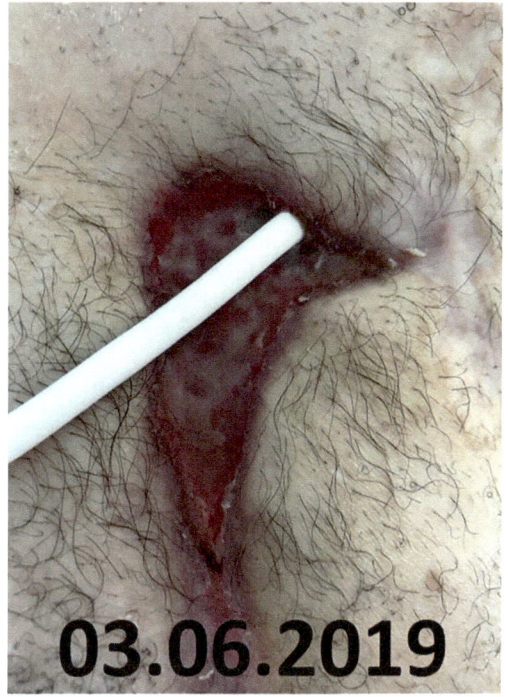

03.06.2019

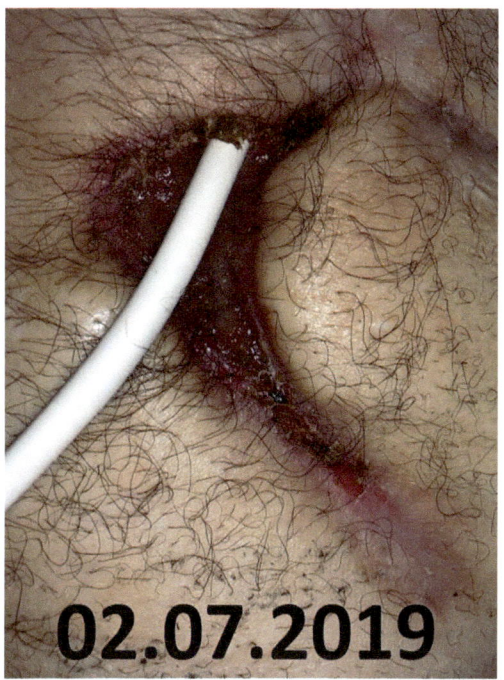

02.07.2019

The first swab taken for this patient was on March 2, 2019 and contained traces of *Staph. aureus.* The initial therapy for this patient consisted of intravenous flucloxacillin and rifampicin antibiotics, surgical debridement with VAC-therapy and 7 VAC-exchanges.

When the Adtec medical device was introduced, the treatment program consisted of doxycycline antibiotics for 4 weeks alongside cold atmospheric plasma and standard care. There were a total of nine applications of cold atmospheric plasma administered to this patient. The therapy had ended due to a heart transplant. The last swab recorded was on July 5, 2019, which contained no viable microorganisms whilst on no antibiotic use.

18.7.3   Patient 3

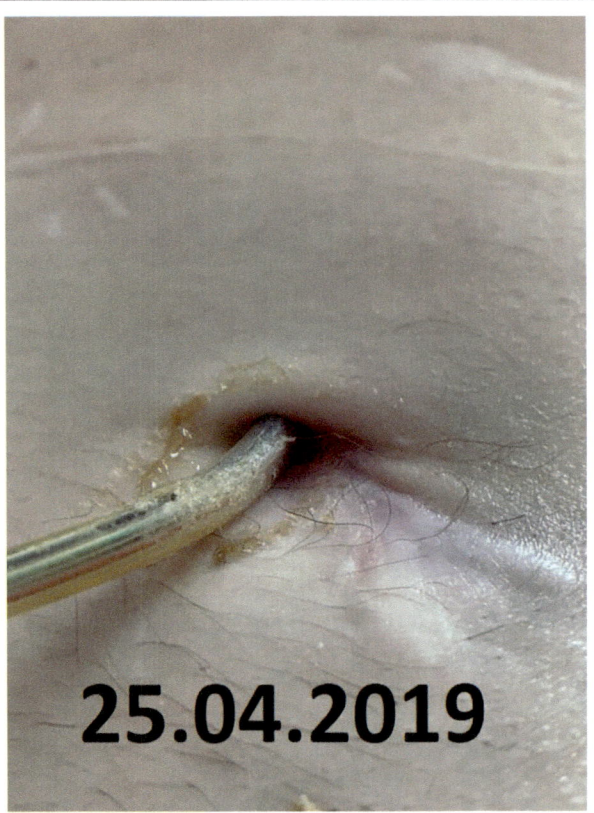

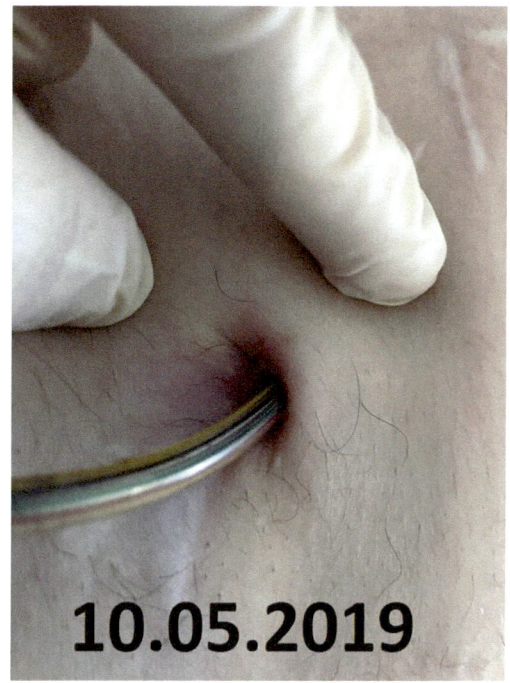

10.05.2019

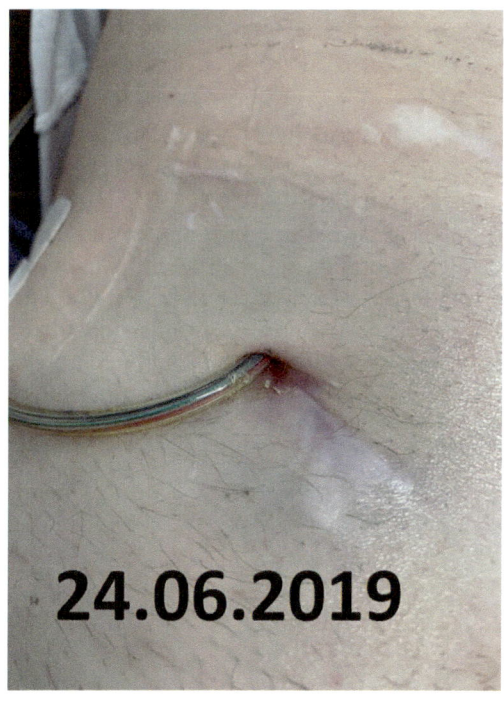

24.06.2019

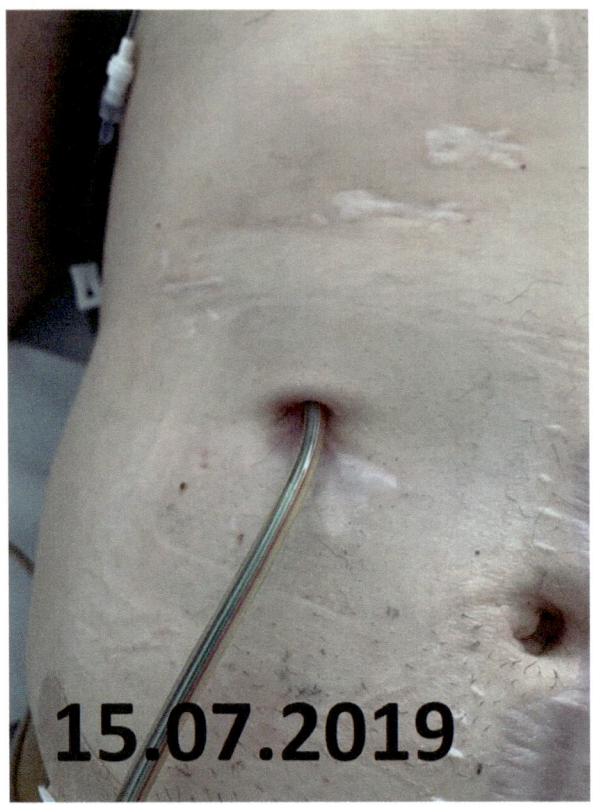

The first swab taken for this patient was on April 20, 2019 and contained traces of *Staph. aureus*. The initial therapy for this patient consisted of intravenous flucloxacillin and rifampicin antibiotics.

When the Adtec medical device was introduced, the treatment program consisted of cotrimoxazole antibiotics and the patient was discharged. Cold atmospheric plasma and standard care were given twice a week. There was a total of 15 applications of cold atmospheric plasma administered to this patient. The last swab recorded was on August 20, 2019, which contained no viable microorganisms whilst on no antibiotic use.

18.7.4 Patient 4

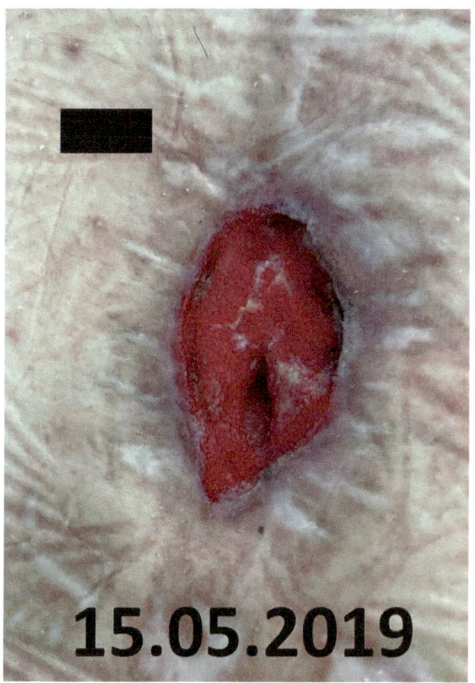

15.05.2019

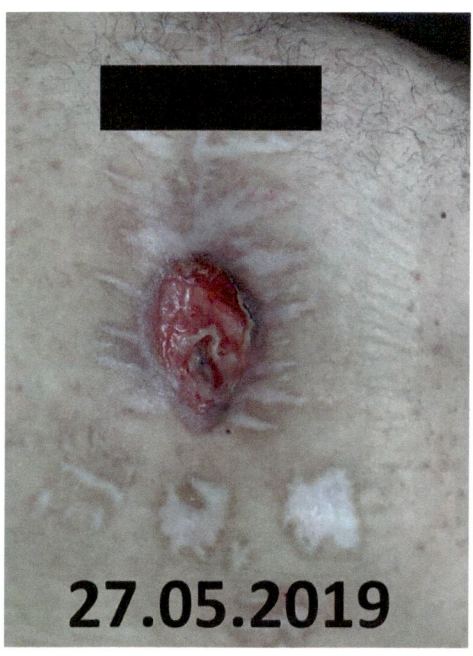

27.05.2019

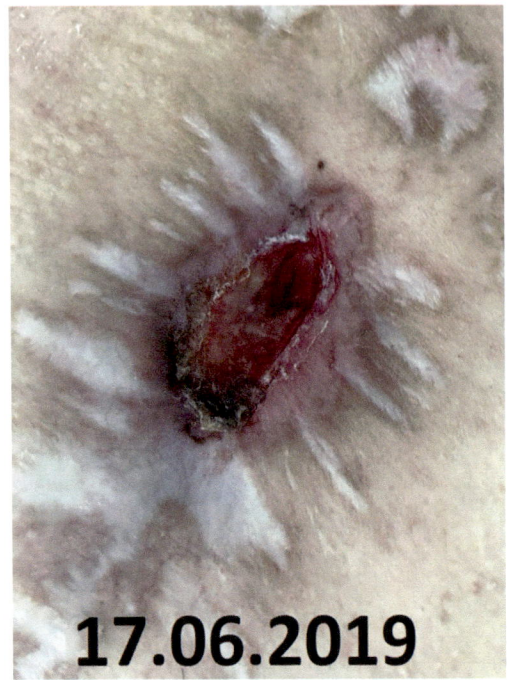

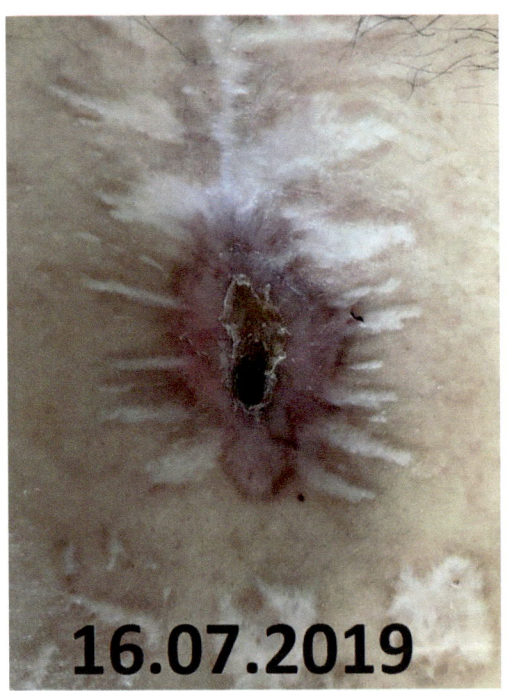

18

The first swab taken for this patient was on May 15, 2019 and contained traces of *Staph. aureus*. The initial therapy for this patient consisted of intravenous flucloxacillin and rifampicin antibiotics, surgical debridement with VAC-therapy and 6 VAC-exchanges.

When the Adtec medical device was introduced, the treatment program consisted of amoxicillin/ clavulanic acid alongside cold atmospheric plasma and standard care. There was a total of 10 applications of cold atmospheric plasma administered to this patient. The last swab recorded was on August 14, 2019, which contained no viable microorganisms whilst on no antibiotic use.

18.7.5 Patient 5

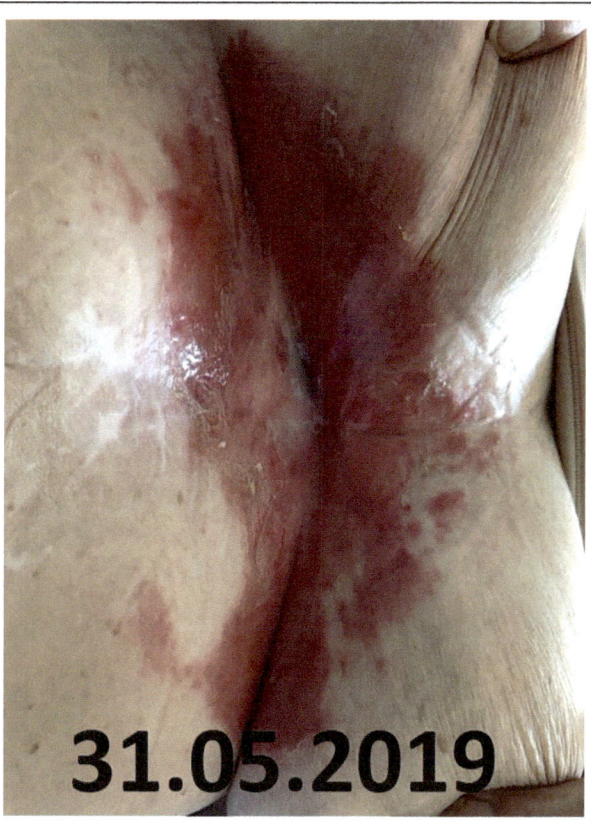

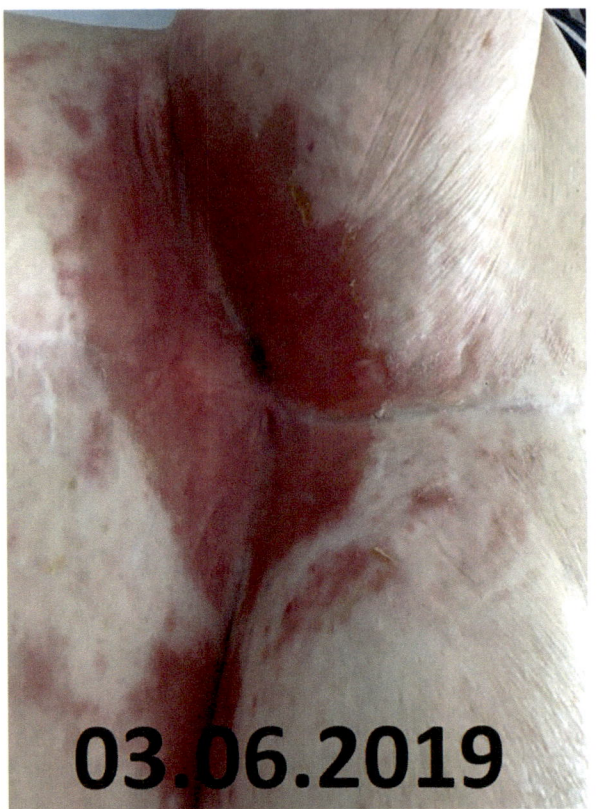

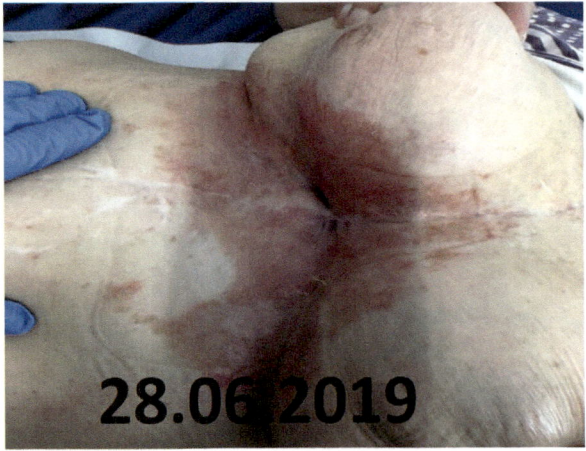

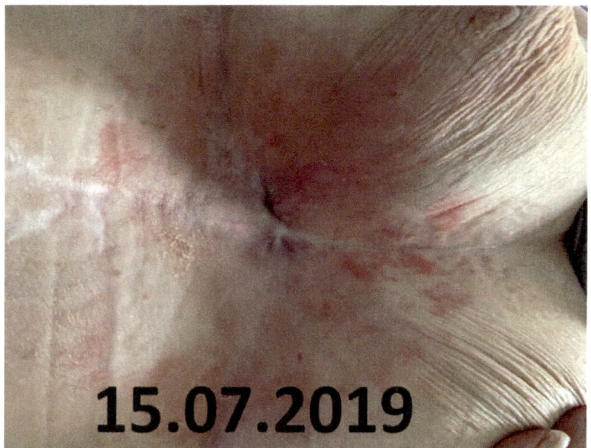

The first swab taken for this patient was on May 25, 2019 and contained traces of *Pseudomonas aeruginosa*. The initial therapy for this patient consisted of intravenous meropenem antibiotics, surgical debridement with VAC-therapy and 20 VAC-Weschel.

When the Adtec medical device was introduced, the treatment program consisted of no antibiotics alongside cold atmospheric plasma and standard care 1–2 times per week. There was a total of 16 applications of cold atmospheric plasma administered to this patient. The last swab recorded was on September 16, 2019, which contained no viable microorganisms whilst on no antibiotic use.

Conclusion

Cold atmospheric plasma is an already tested procedure in other applications of wound care and dermatology. It is a simple and effective method of therapy for managing infected drivelines with accelerated healing and significant microbial load reduction. It is a painless procedure and can save costs and time. A further study by the Department of Cardiac Surgery at the University Hospital Heidelberg [25] demonstrates the data as being the first study to analyze the safety and efficiency of the Adtec SteriPlas in the treatment of driveline infections.

18.7.6 Dermatology [29]

18.7.6.1 Introduction

Actinic keratoses (AK) represent the most common skin malignancy worldwide and are considered the earliest stage of squamous cell carcinoma (SCC). Importantly, up to 20% of AK transform into invasive SCC within 10–25 years.

Conventional treatment therapies for AK and field cancerization bear significant side effects and/or are restricted to small skin areas. Thus, there is a continuing need for effective as well as nontoxic lesion and field-directed therapies for AK.

In addition to the well-documented antimicrobial properties of CAP, growing evidence points to antitumoral effects in vitro and in vivo as well as in clinical settings. Moreover, anecdotal observations suggested promising clinical response in several subjects with AK treated with various CAP devices.

18.7.6.2 Objective

Comparison of clinical efficacy and safety of cold atmospheric argon plasma versus diclofenac 3% gel in patients with AK/field cancerization.

18.7.6.3 Materials and Methods

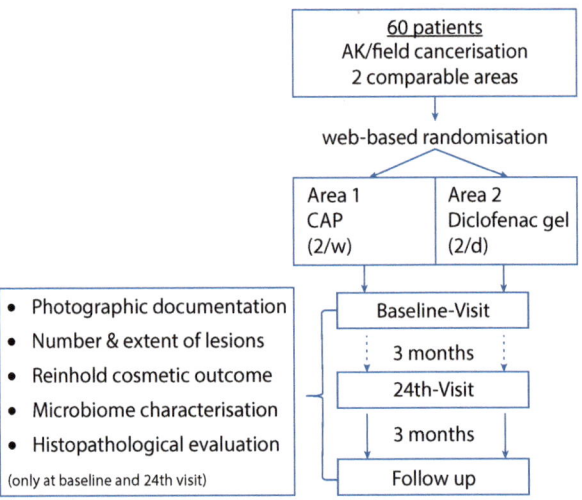

Patients with field AK/field cancerization are randomly assigned into two groups for the study: to be treated with CAP twice a week or diclofenac 3% gel twice daily. Photographic documentation, the number and extent of lesions, Reinhold cosmetic outcome, microbiome characterization, and the histopathological evaluation will be documented.

18.7.6.4 Results

CAP treatment showed significantly better effectiveness over diclofenac in reducing the lesion count (33%, 95% CI 20–45%, vs. 21%, 95% CI 9–33%; $P = 0.048$, Wilcoxon signed-rank test) and the AK-affected area (41%, 95% CI 28–54%, vs. 27%, 13–42%; $P = 0.033$, Wilcoxon signed-rank test) by the end of treatment (visit 24). A complete field clearance was observed in one CAP-treated patient at visit 24 and at 3-month follow-up in four CAP-treated patients (◘ Fig. 18.19).

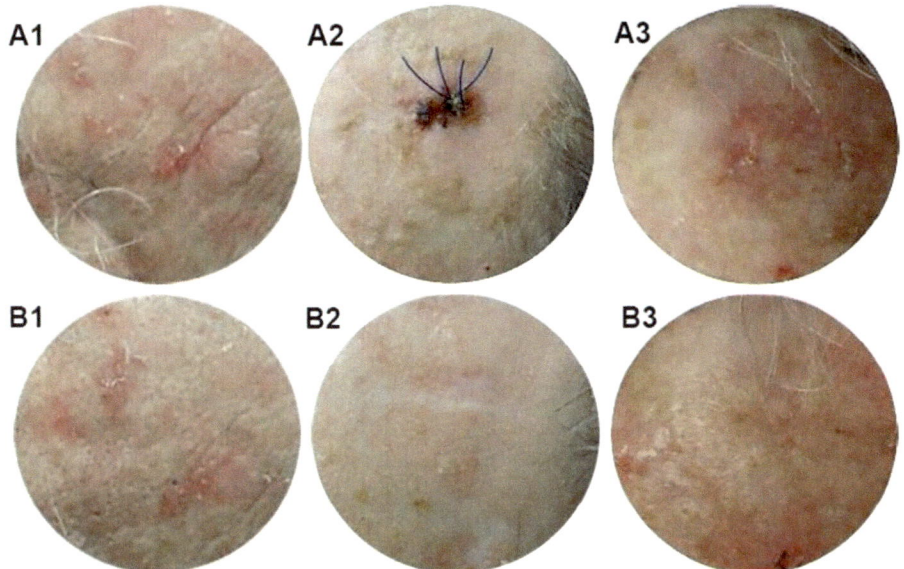

◘ Fig. 18.19   Images A1–3: before CAP; B1–3: after CAP (24th visit)

Conclusions

The data demonstrates that the Adtec SteriPlas represents an effective tool for the management of AK/field cancerization. The clinical efficacy of this modality is comparable to that of diclofenac gel. However, unlike diclofenac, CAP showed no side effects. Thus, this modality might be especially well suited for patients who require nontoxic treatment options, particularly immunocompromised patients and those with extensive field cancerization.

18.8   Clinical Trials

Adtec's patented cold plasma technology has been featured in a variety of clinical trials including:

- Isbary G, Morfill GE, Schmidt H-U, Georgi M, Ramrath K, Heinlin J, Karrer S, Landthaler M, Shimizu T, Steffes B, Bunk W, Monetti R, Zimmermann JL, Pompl R, Stolz W. A first prospective randomized controlled trial to decrease bacterial load using cold atmospheric argon plasma on chronic wounds in patients. Br J Dermatol. 2010;163(1):78–82.

- Study objective – The first ever clinical trial recorded to test the efficacy of cold plasma on bacterial load reduction in wounds.
- Number of patients treated – 36
- Any side effects observed – None

- Isbary G, Heinlin J, Shimizu T, Zimmermann JL, Morfill G, Schmidt H-U, Monetti R, Steffes B, Bunk W, Li Y, Klaempfl T, Karrer S, Landthaler M, Stolz W. Successful and safe use of 2 min cold atmospheric argon plasma in chronic wounds: results of a randomized controlled trial. Br J Dermatol. 2012;167(2):404–10.

- Study objective – Having already demonstrated efficacy with 5 minutes of cold plasma treatment, this study objective is to test any efficacy at 2 minutes of treatment with the same Adtec medical device.
- Number of patients treated – 24
- Any side effects observed – None

- Heinlin J, Zimmermann JL, Zeman F, Bunk W, Isbary G, Landthaler M, Maisch T, Monetti R, Morfill GE, Shimizu T, Steinbauer J, Stolz W, Karrer S. Randomized placebo-controlled human pilot study of cold atmospheric argon plasma on skin graft donor sites. Wound Repair Reg. 2013;21(6):800–7.

- Study objective – Having already shown cold plasma's positive response to bacterial load reduction in wounds, this study objective was to show if cold plasma can improve wound healing.
- Number of patients treated – 40
- Any side effects observed – None

- Isbary G, Stolz W, Shimizu T, Monetti R, Bunk W, Schmidt H-U, Morfill GE, Klaempfl TG, Steffes B, Thomas HM, Heinlin J, Karrer S, Landthaler M, Zimmermann JL. Cold atmospheric argon plasma treatment may accelerate wound healing in chronic wounds: results of a retrospective in vivo randomized controlled study. Clin Plasma Med. 2013;1(2):25–30.

- Study objective – The study objective was to measure the differences in wound healing (in wound width and length) before and after each cold plasma treatment, which varied from 3–7 minutes per treatment.
- Number of patients treated – 70
- Any side effects observed – None

- Isbary G, Shimizu T, Zimmermann JL, Heinlin J, Al-Zaabi S, Rechfeld M, Morfill GE, Karrer S, Stolz W. Randomized placebo-controlled clinical trial showed cold atmospheric argon plasma relieved acute pain and accelerated healing in herpes zoster. Clin Plasma Med. 2014;2(2):50–5.

- Study objective – The study objective was to assess the safety, pain reduction, and healing rates of patients with Herpes Zoster with weekday 5 minutes Adtec cold plasma treatment.

18

- Number of patients treated – 37
- Any side effects observed – None

- Moelleken M, Jockenhöfer F, Wiegand C, Buer J, Benson S, Dissemond J. Pilot study on the influence of cold atmospheric plasma on bacterial contamination and healing tendency of chronic wounds. JDDG. 2020. ► https://doi.org/10.1111/ddg.14294

- Study objective – In this randomized clinical pilot study (RCT) patients with therapy-refractory chronic wounds were examined over a maximum of twelve weeks. Groups 1 and 2 were treated with the Adtec SteriPlas once and twice a week, respectively. Patients in Group 3 received placebo therapy once a week.
- Number of patients treated – 37
- Any side effects observed – None

- Koch F, Salva KA, Wirtz M, Hadaschik E, Varaljai R, Schadendorf D, Roesch A. Efficacy of cold atmospheric plasma vs. Diclofenac 3% gel in patients with actinic keratoses: a prospective, randomized and rater-blinded study (ACTI-CAP). JEADV. 2020. ► https://doi.org/10.1111/jdv.16735

- Study objective – To assess the clinical response of the Adtec SteriPlas vs. Diclofenac 3% gel in patients with Actinic Keratoses (aged 56–91 years).
- Number of patients treated – 60
- Any side effects observed – None

18.9 Outlook and Further Developments

Adtec Healthcare has invested significantly in scientific studies to support the safety, efficacy, and application of cold plasma in medicine. The body of evidence is constantly growing for the effectiveness and application of Adtec plasma in a wide range of therapies, particularly in wound care, surgical site infection, and dermatological applications.

> **Conclusion**
> Microwave-generated Argon Gas Plasma has proven anti-bacterial clinical efficacy in the treatment of wounds, surgical site infections, and dermatological conditions. There are many more potential clinical indications that need to be properly investigated with clinical trials to prove efficacy. The safety of cold plasma and new regulatory standards for the plasma generated by the medical devices is required to establish plasma medicine as a routine medical treatment.

References

1. Shimizu T, Steffes B, Pompl R, Jamitzky F, Bunk W, Morfill GE, Ramrath K, Georgi M, Stolz W, Schmidt H-U, Urayama T, Fujii S. Characterization of microwave plasma torch for decontamination. Plasma Process Polym. 2008;5:577–82. https://doi.org/10.1002/ppap.200800021.
2. Sato T, Miyahara T, Doi A, Ochiai S, Urayama T, Nakatani T. Sterilization mechanism for Escherichia Coli by plasma flow at atmospheric pressure. Appl Phys Lett. 2006;89:73902.
3. Sato T, Fujioka K, Ramasamy R, Urayama T, Fujii S. Sterilization efficacy of a coaxial microwave plasma flow at atmospheric pressure. IEEE Trans Ind Appl. 2006;42:399–404.
4. Sato T, Doi A, Urayama T, Nakatani T, Miyahara T. Inactivation of Escherichia Coli by a coaxial microwave plasma flow. IEEE Trans Ind Appl. 2007;43:1159–63.
5. Maisch T, Bosserhoff AK, Unger P, Heider J, Shimizu T, Zimmermann JL, Morfill GE, Landthaler M, Karrer S. Investigation of toxicity and mutagenicity of cold atmospheric argon plasma. Environ Mol Mutagen. 2017;58(3):172–7.
6. Heinlin J, Isbary G, Stolz W, Morfill G, Landthaler M, Shimizu T, Steffes B, Nosenko T, Zimmermann J, Karrer S. Plasma applications in medicine with a special focus on dermatology. J Eur Acad Dermatol Venereol. 2010. https://doi.org/10.1111/j.1468-3083.2010.03702.x.
7. Isbary G, Heinlin J, Shimizu T, Zimmermann JL, Morfill G, Schmidt H-U, Monetti R, Steffes B, Bunk W, Li Y, Klaempfl T, Karrer S, Landthaler M, Stolz W. Successful and safe use of 2 min cold atmospheric argon plasma in chronic wounds: results of a randomized controlled trial. Br J Dermatol. 2012;167(2):404–10.
8. Ermolaeva SA, Varfolomeev AF, Yu M, Chernukha DS, Yurov MM, Vasiliev AA, Kaminskaya MMM, Romanova JM, Murashev AN, Selezneva II, Shimizu T, Sysolyatina EV, Shaginyan IA, Petrov OF, Mayevsky EI, Fortov VE, Morfill GE, Naroditsky BS, Gintsburg AL. Bactericidal effects of non-thermal argon plasma in vitro, in biofilms and in the animal model of infected wounds. J Med Microbiol. 2011;60:75–83.
9. Booth R, Wounds UK. Antibiofilm activity demonstrated following treatment with a novel plasma device (Poster presentation). 2015.
10. Isbary G, Morfill GE, Schmidt H-U, Georgi M, Ramrath K, Heinlin J, Karrer S, Landthaler M, Shimizu T, Steffes B, Bunk W, Monetti R, Zimmermann JL, Pompl R, Stolz W. A first prospective randomized controlled trial to decrease bacterial load using cold atmospheric argon plasma on chronic wounds in patients. Br J Dermatol. 2010;163(1):78–82.
11. Heinlin J, Zimmermann JL, Zeman F, Bunk W, Isbary G, Landthaler M, Maisch T, Monetti R, Morfill GE, Shimizu T, Steinbauer J, Stolz W, Karrer S. Randomized placebo-controlled human pilot study of cold atmospheric argon plasma on skin graft donor sites. Wound Repair Regen. 2013;21(6):800–7.
12. Isbary G, Stolz W, Shimizu T, Monetti R, Bunk W, Schmidt H-U, Morfill GE, Klaempfl TG, Steffes B, Thomas HM, Heinlin J, Karrer S, Landthaler M, Zimmermann JL. Cold atmospheric argon plasma treatment may accelerate wound healing in chronic wounds: results of a retrospective in vivo randomized controlled study. Clin Plasma Med. 2013;1(2):25–30.
13. Isbary G, Morfill G, Zimmermann J, Shimizu T, Stolz W. Cold atmospheric plasma: a successful treatment of lesions in Hailey-Hailey disease. Arch Dermatol. 2011;147(4):388–90.
14. Isbary G, Shimizu T, Zimmermann JL, Heinlin J, Al-Zaabi S, Rechfeld M, Morfill GE, Karrer S, Stolz W. Randomized placebo-controlled clinical trial showed cold atmospheric argon plasma relieved acute pain and accelerated healing in herpes zoster. Clin Plasma Med. 2014;2(2):50–5.
15. Isbary G, Shimizu T, Zimmermann J, Hubertus T, Morfill G, Stolz W. Cold atmospheric plasma for local infection control and subsequent pain reduction in a patient with chronic post operative ear infection. New Microbes New Infect. 2013;1(3):41–3.
16. Rotering H. EWMA 2016. Cold Atmospheric Plasma - New options for infection control in wound management (Oral presentation).
17. Rotering H. EACTS 2017. Cold atmospheric plasma and Advanced NPWT - New option for complex wounds in cardiac surgery (Oral presentation).

18

18. Wirtz M, Stoffels I, Dissemond J, Schadendorf D, Roesch A. Actinic keratoses treated with cold atmospheric plasma. J Eur Acad Dermatol Venereol. 2018;32(1):37–9. https://doi.org/10.1111/jdv.14465.

19. Salva K, Wirtz M, Koch F, McGovern M, Schadendorf D, Roesch A. EADV 2018. Efficacy of cold atmospheric plasma versus diclofenac 3% gel in patients with actinic keratoses/field cancerization: preliminary results of a prospective, randomized, rater-blinded study (ACTICAP) [Poster presentation].

20. Thant A. ISDF 2019. Adtec Cold Plasma treatment to assist in treating diabetic foot with multiresistant infection (Poster presentation).

21. Pierides M. EWMA 2019. The Gas Plasma device a novel therapy in treating non resolving infected diabetic foot and leg ulcers (Poster presentation).

22. Rotering H, Hansen U, Welp H, et al. Cold atmospheric plasma and advanced negative pressure wound therapy – treatment concept for complicated wounds in cardiac surgery. Z Herz- Thorax-Gefäßchir. 2020;34:52.

23. Morfill G. Plasma medicine with particular emphasis on hygiene and medicine. Max Planck Institute (extract of Plasma Medicine Team report).

24. Mueller F. EACTS 2019. Cold atmospheric plasma for driveline infections (Oral presentation).

25. Kremer J, et al. Wound management of driveline infections with cold atmospheric argon plasma - proof of concept. J Heart Lung Transplant. 2020;39(4S). Section S488, Chapter (1249).

26. Moelleken M, Jockenhöfer F, Wiegand C, Buer J, Benson S, Dissemond J. Pilot study on the influence of cold atmospheric plasma on bacterial contamination and healing tendency of chronic wounds. J Dtsch Dermatol Ges. 2020. https://doi.org/10.1111/ddg.14294.

27. Arisi M, et al. Cold atmospheric plasma (CAP) as a promising therapeutic option for mild to moderate acne vulgaris: clinical and non-invasive evaluation of two cases. Clin Plasma Med. 2020. ISSN: 2212-8166.

28. Herbst F, Van Schalkwyk J, McGovern M. MicroPlaSter and SteriPlas. Comprehensive clinical plasma medicine. Springer International Publishing AG, part of Springer Nature; 2018. https://doi.org/10.1007/978-3-319-67627-2_34.

29. Koch F, Salva KA, Wirtz M, Hadaschik E, Varaljai R, Schadendorf D, Roesch A. Efficacy of cold atmospheric plasma vs. Diclofenac 3% gel in patients with actinic keratoses: a prospective, randomized and rater-blinded study (ACTICAP). J Eur Acad Dermatol Venereol. 2020. https://doi.org/10.1111/jdv.16735.

Plasma Care®

Julia L. Zimmermann,
Claudia C. Roskopf, Sylvia Cantzler,
Jens Kirsch, Rico Unger,
Hannes Weilemann, Maximilian Cantzler,
Michael Linner, Martin Wunderl,
and Tim Maisch

Contents

© Springer Nature Switzerland AG 2022
H.-R. Metelmann et al. (eds.), *Textbook of Good Clinical Practice in Cold Plasma Therapy*, https://doi.org/10.1007/978-3-030-87857-3_19

📧 **Core Messages**
- The plasma care® is the first CE-mark approved portable, battery-operated CAP medical device that is based on the SMD technology.
- Within the enclosed volume of a sterile, disposable spacer the plasma care® generates plasma-activated air with long-lived RONS that inactivate bacteria and can stimulate wound healing.
- Extensive preclinical tests have shown the plasma care® to be effective and safe, a clinical trial has commenced and initial results from case studies (human and veterinary practice) are encouraging.

19.1 Introduction

Cold plasma therapy for the treatment of infected chronic wounds has been shown to be effective and safe in the clinic setting [1–4]. However, many patients with nonhealing wounds receive outpatient care [5]. Due to their limited mobility, the repetitive clinic visits, which are necessary in the course of cold plasma therapy, pose a problem for them. To therefore make cold plasma therapy also available for chronic wound patients, who are treated at home, a miniaturized cold atmospheric plasma (CAP) device – the plasma care® – was developed.

19.2 About the Device

The plasma care® is portable, battery-operated, and easy to use, which also makes it suitable for outpatient care [6]. It received CE-mark approval on June 13th, 2019 as a class IIa medical device. The device has approximately the size and weight of an old telephone handset and is constructed from four components (◘ Fig. 19.1): (1) the body contains the high voltage power supply and the hardware which is necessary to control and monitor the plasma production. (2) The control panel, which covers the body of the plasma care®, serves as a user interface and possesses a single touch button to power the device on and off and to start the plasma treatment. Moreover, the charging state can be monitored via the battery symbol on the display. The charging process is wireless, which enables a device design without any openings for plugs or wired contacts so that a quick and thorough cleaning process by means of wipe disinfection is possible. This is particularly important, as the plasma care® can potentially encounter pathogenic microorganisms during wound treatment. (3) In order to charge or store the device, it is placed into its docking station. (4) Finally, the core of the plasma care® is its plasma source unit (PSU) which incorporates the Surface Micro-Discharge (SMD) technology [7, 8]. The PSU is responsible for generating CAP straight from the ambient air and can be exchanged, if necessary (i.e., in case of heavy contamination or mechanical damage).

19

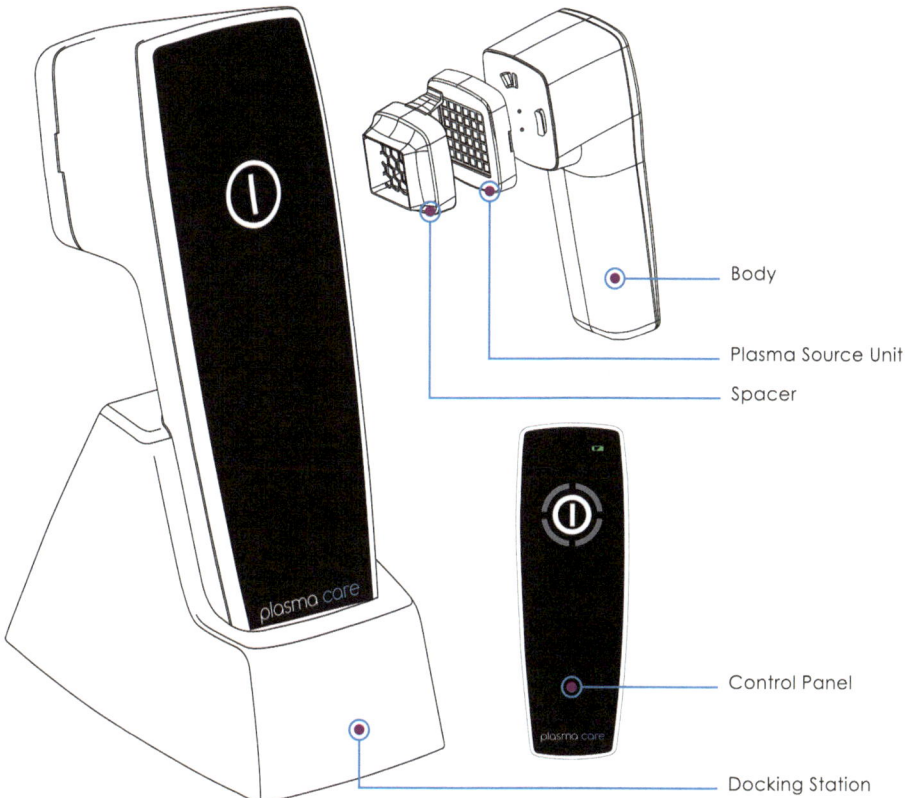

Fig. 19.1 The plasma care® and its components

The plasma care® itself does not come in contact with the skin or wound surface of the patient. The only part, which touches the patient's skin or wound is a sterile, disposable spacer, which is attached to the device to make it operable. The plasma care® spacer has multiple functions with respect to hygiene, safety and plasma chemistry. Firstly, hygienic treatment of the patient is guaranteed, because the sterile spacer can only be used for the treatment of one single patient (i.e., six 1-minute treatments within a total time of 10 minutes). Due to the integrated RFID-tag the spacer cannot accidentally be used for a second time and thus cross-contamination between patients is almost excluded. Secondly, the outer walls as well as the mesh grid of the spacer – integrated for safety reasons – (■ Fig. 19.1) prevent any direct contact between the patient's skin and the plasma source. And thirdly, the spacer provides a defined air volume for the generation of a specific mix of plasma species and for the diffusion of these species to the wound surface.

The plasma care® is approved for the therapeutic treatment of chronic and acute, open wounds with critical colonization or infection with bacteria as well as for the prophylactic treatment of wounds to prevent infection. It can be used by healthcare professionals in clinics, by physicians, in homes for the elderly, and by homecare medical services.

19.2.1   Basic Principles/Technology

As mentioned before, the plasma care® uses the so-called SMD technology for the production of CAP [8]. The plasma source itself is composed of a high voltage sheet electrode – made out of copper, an insulator – composed of ceramic, and a grounded structured stainless-steel electrode (mesh grid) [9]. The plasma source is incorporated into the PSU (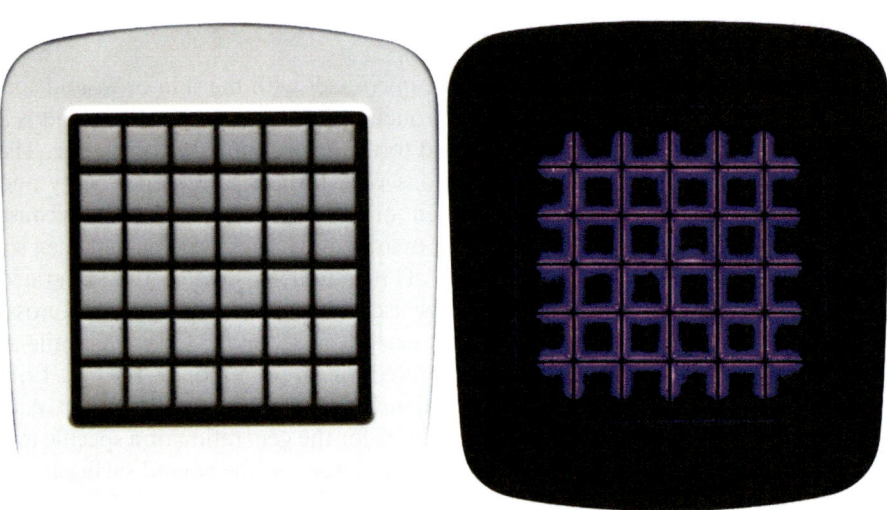 Fig. 19.2), which can be removed from the body of the plasma care® as necessary (e.g., for cleaning purposes).

The following parameters are used for plasma production (■ Table 19.1):

By applying a voltage of only $3.5 \, kV_{pp}$ at a frequency of 4 kHz so-called micro-discharges are produced on the mesh grid of the structured electrode of the plasma source. These micro-discharges interact with the ambient air in the plasma care® spacer thereby producing more than 600 chemical reactions leading to a mix of electrons and ions, excited atoms and molecules, and reactive oxygen and nitrogen species (RONS) [10]. This reactive mix of species within the volume enclosed by the spacer is transported to the wound surface of the patient by diffusion (■ Fig. 19.3).

19.2.2   General Parameter

The plasma care® was carefully developed according to the regulatory require-ments of the Medical Device Directive 93/42/EEC and complies with the essential requirements by following the applicable guidelines, specifications, and standards like the IEC 60601-1 for electrical medical devices [11] and others such as the DIN SPEC 91315 on "general requirements for plasma sources in medicine" [12], the

plasma source unit, off: left – on: right

19

■ **Fig. 19.2** The Surface Micro-Discharge (SMD) plasma source unit (PSU) of the plasma care®. Left: mesh grid electrode and insulator of the PSU. Right: powered PSU in the dark. The character-istic purple glow of the CAP is visible

◻ **Table 19.1** Technical data of the SMD PSU of the plasma care®

Technical data, PSU of plasma care®

Voltage	$3.5\,kV_{pp}$
Frequency	4 kHz
Plasma power consumption	0.4–1.5 W
Gas	Ambient air
Gas flow	None

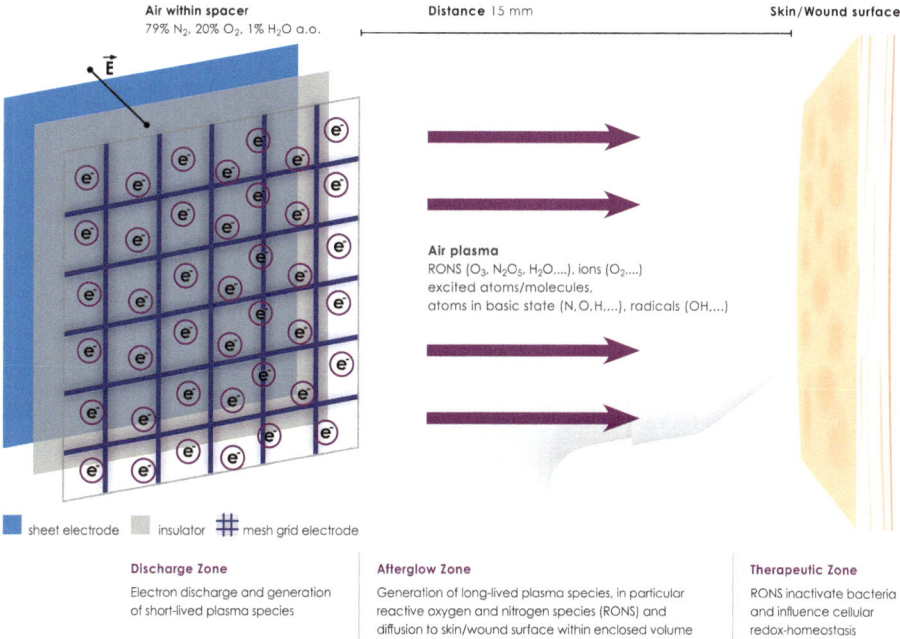

◻ **Fig. 19.3** The SMD PSU of the plasma care® turns the enclosed air within the spacer into plasma-activated air. Within the spacer, this plasma-activated air including the reactive oxygen and nitrogen species (RONS) diffuses from the SMD PSU to the skin/wound surface

IEC 62304 on medical device software [13], the EN ISO 10993 on the biological evaluation of medical devices [14], and MEDDEV 2.7/1 Revision 4 on the clinical evaluation.

19.2.2.1 Mechanical Parameter

The plasma care® is designed for use as a portable medical device, which can be taken to the patient by any physician, nurse, or other healthcare professional rather than requiring the patient to be moved to the device. The mechanical parameter of the plasma care® and the plasma care® spacer are given in ◘ Tables 19.2 and 19.3.

The plasma care® was designed without any openings for plugs, so that it can be cleaned and disinfected easily and thoroughly on the go. Its casings as well as those of the plasma care® spacer are made of plastics that meet the biocompatibility requirements for the intended use.

As already described, the plasma is produced by an SMD plasma source incorporated in an exchangeable PSU. To prevent contamination of the PSU and direct contact between patient and micro-discharges the plasma care® is used in combination with the sterile, disposable spacer. The plasma care® spacer provides an air volume of approx. 18.4 cm³, which ensures the specific production of a certain plasma species mix as well as defined diffusion of these species to the wound surface. The area of the SMD plasma source and the size and volume of the plasma

◘ **Table 19.2** Mechanical parameter of the plasma care®

Name	plasma care®
Plasma production	SMD
Time of operation	Up to 3 min/13 cm²
Operational control	LED-touch panel
Control	Semi-automatic
Power supply voltage	100–240 V
Power supply frequency	50 Hz/60 Hz
Outer dimensions [$L \times W \times H$]	16 cm × 5.5 cm × 6 cm
Weight	320 g
Surface material	ABS PC 3010

◘ **Table 19.3** Mechanical parameter of the plasma care® spacer

Name	plasma care® spacer
Identification	RFID
Time of operation	Up to 3 min/13 cm²
Outer dimensions [$L \times W \times H$]	6.7 cm × 5.5 cm × 4.1 cm
Treatment area	16 cm²
Weight	14 g
Material	ABS 8391 MED

19

care® spacer were chosen in order to maximize the size of the wound treatment area, while maintaining a comfortable device size for outpatient care. Within a single patient treatment session, the plasma care® spacer can be used for up to six 1-minute plasma treatments, so that it can be applied in a pattern across the entire wound. This is necessary if the wound is larger than 16 cm². An RFID-tag, which is marked as invalid once the spacer has been used, is integrated into the flap of the plasma care® spacer. Thus, accidental cross-contamination between patients by using the same spacer is prevented. Since the spacer has direct contact with the (potentially infected) wound surface and/or skin of the patient, it must be disposed of after use.

To charge the plasma care® wirelessly, it is placed into its docking station. The double-cell battery is fully recharged within 5 hours and lasts for up to 200 1-minute treatments at full capacity. The charging status of the device is indicated by the color of the battery symbol in the top right corner of the touch display: green – fully charged, yellow – halfway charged, red – recharging necessary.

19.2.2.2 Physicochemical Parameters

Plasma is a mixture of different components including free electrons, ions, and reactive species, irradiation in the form of heat and light in the UV, and visible spectrum as well as an electromagnetic field. In CAP that is generated from ambient air – as is the case for the plasma care® – more than 600 chemical reactions occur that give rise to an entire cocktail of RONS [10]. When a CAP is used for therapeutic purposes, the amount of potentially harmful components of the plasma, such as UV irradiation, heat, and ozone emission, need to be within nonhazardous ranges. Such nonhazardous ranges are defined by different guidelines, standards, and committees, some of which are referred to in the DIN SPEC 91315 [12].

The results from the physicochemical characterization of cold plasma that is generated by the plasma care® and the respective publicly available limits are given in ◘ Table 19.4. The measurements were performed as recommended in the DIN SPEC 91315 with adaptations, if necessary. (The DIN SPEC 91315 suggests adaptations for different medical plasma sources.) Regarding physical parameters, such as temperature, artificial optical irradiation (including UV light) and electrical currents, the plasma from the plasma care® is well within the safe range. The same is true for the emission of ozone and nitrogen dioxide during plasma production.

19.2.2.3 Biological Characteristics

In addition to their safety, electrical medical devices also need to display a high level of performance. The purpose of the plasma care® is the painless reduction of bacteria in infected wounds and the prevention of infection in wounds that may get infected. Thus, the plasma that is produced by the plasma care® was preclinically evaluated regarding its anti-microbial efficacy and its safety upon application to the exposed human tissues (wound surface and surrounding skin).

In extensive preclinical tests that followed DIN SPEC 91315, the plasma care® was proved effective against ten bacterial strains from risk groups I and II including *S. aureus*, *E. faecalis*, *P. aeruginosa*, *E. coli*, *C. propinquum* and MRSA. For this purpose, a bacterial suspension with a concentration of 10^8/ml was prepared. A

■ **Table 19.4** Methods, results, and limits from the physicochemical characterization of the cold plasma that is generated by the plasma care®

Parameter	Method	Result (mean values)	Limit(s) by the authorities	Conclusion
Temperature	Measurement of the air temperature within the closed volume of the plasma care® spacer as only the plasma-activated air comes into direct contact with the skin/wound surface	**Max. 1 °C/min; 40 °C is not reached at operating temperatures of up to 35 °C**	40 °C	The temperature increase produced by the plasma care® is well below the limits set by the authorities
Thermal performance	Not applicable, as there is no contact between the SMD plasma and human skin/wound surfaces	n/a	n/a	
Artificial optical irradiation	Measurement of emitted UV-irradiation (UV-A, UV-B and UV-C) at wavelengths of 180–400 nm for maximum treatment interval of 3 minutes. Measurements weighted according to ICNIRP-weighting function and compared with known limits	**Light output (E_{eff}) = 0.0011 µW/cm^2 Effective irradiation = 0.198 µJ/cm^2 in 3 min = 0.00198 J/m^2 in 3 min**	TROS IOS [15]: Exposure limit = 30 J/m^2·day (180–400 nm) ICNIRP [16]: Light output limit (E_{eff}) = 50 µW/cm^2 in 1 min Exposure limit = 30 J/m^2 (180–400 nm) Exposure limit = 104 J/m^2, nonweighted (315–400 nm)	The UV emission produced by the plasma care® is well below the limits set by the authorities

19

| Acoustic energy | Measurement of acoustic energy emitted by the device during plasma generation for a cumulative exposure of 24 hours over a 24 hours period (dBA). This continuous exposure is a worst-case scenario, which is not expected in practice | **Emitted acoustic energy of the plasma care® is 67.2 dBA for a cumulative exposure of 24 hours over a 24 hours period (dBA)** | DIN EN ISO 60601-1 [11]: 80 dBA for a cumulative exposure of 24 hours over a 24 hours period (dBA) | The acoustic energy emitted by the plasma care® is below the limits set by the authorities even with regards to the continuous worst-case scenario |
| Electrical current | Measurement following DIN SPEC 91315 using an electrically conductive surface. Earth leakage current, touch current, and patient leakage current need to be below the limits according to DIN EN 60601-1 and DIN EN 60601-2-57 | **Earth leakage current is not applicable due to the medical device design Touch current and patient leakage current are 2.2 µA max (measured by TÜV Rheinland)** | DIN EN ISO 60601-1 [11]: 100 µA | The electrical currents produced by the plasma care® are well below the limits set by the authorities |

(continued)

Table 19.4 (continued)

Parameter		Method	Result (mean values)	Limit(s) by the authorities	Conclusion
O₃ concentration	Closed spacer volume (approx. 18.4 cm³)	(1) Plasma care® with attached spacer is placed on a flat surface and plasma treatment is started. (Accumulation of ozone within closed spacer volume for 1–3 minutes) (2) Lifting of the spacer and immediate ozone concentration measurement with 20 cm distance at 0°, 45° and 90° (distance and angles chosen as suggested in DIN SPEC 91315, represent "worst case" as the distance between plasma care® and operator is more likely to be 80 cm)	**0° angle:** **Immediate [O₃] = 0.11 ppm/1 min treatment** **[O₃] after 15 min = 0.0014–0.089 ppm (depending on no. of applications, that is, 1 to 6 1-minute treatments)** **45° angle:** **Immediate [O₃] = 0.012 ppm/1 min treatment** **[O₃] after 15 min = 0.0000–0.0047 ppm (depending on no. of applications)** **90° angle:** **Immediate [O₃] = 0.0007 ppm/1 min treatment** **[O₃] after 15 min = 0.0000–0.0003 ppm (depending on no. of applications)**	NIOSH [17]: 0.3 ppm short-term-dose (respiratory intake within 15 minutes)	The ozone emission produced by the plasma care® is below the limits set by the authorities
	20 m³ standard room	Measurement of ozone emission in an environmental chamber (0.5 m³) according to UBA-FB-001159 (guideline from environmental agency) and upscaling to a standard room with a volume of 20 m³	0.5 m³, 90° angle, 6× 1 min treatments: 0.548 ppm **Upscaling to 20 m³ = 0.0137 ppm**	NIOSH [17]: 0.05 ppm long-term-dose (respiratory intake within 8 hours)	The ozone emission produced by the plasma care® is below the limits set by the authorities

19

Plasma Care®

50 m³ standard room (typical treatment room)	Measurement of ozone emission in an environmental chamber according to UBA-FB-001159 (guideline from environmental agency) and upscaling to a standard room with a volume of 50 m³	0.5 m³, 90° angle, 6× 1 min treatments: 0.548 ppm **Upscaling to 50 m³ = 0.0055 ppm**	NIOSH [17]: 0.05 ppm long-term-dose (respiratory intake within 8 hours)	The ozone emission produced by the plasma care® is below the limits set by the authorities
NO_2 concentration	Closed spacer volume (approx. 18.4 cm³)	Measurement of NO_2 concentration within the closed spacer volume via absorption spectroscopy	**Below measurement limit of 5 ppb**	NIOSH [18]: 1 ppm long-term-dose (respiratory intake within 8 hours)	The nitrogen dioxide emission produced by the plasma care® is below the limits set by the authorities

defined volume thereof was applied to CASO agar plates, allowed to dry, and then treated with plasma for 1–5 minutes. After a 24-hour incubation period at 37 °C surviving CFUs (colony-forming units) within the zone of inhibition were counted. All tested bacterial strains were reduced by 5.4–6 logs within 1 minute of CAP treatment (◘ Table 19.5). There was no significant difference in their sensitivity toward CAP. Similarly, a 4.6 log-reduction of planktonic cells from the yeast *C. albicans* that were cultivated on Sabouraud-Bouillon-agar plates was obtained after a 1-minute plasma treatment (◘ Table 19.5).

The plasma care® was, moreover, effective upon application to biofilms of *E. faecalis*. To test this, experiments were carried out as described by Theinkom et al. 2019 [19]. Briefly, a defined quantity of bacteria was suspended in modified com-

◘ **Table 19.5** Selected methods and results from the performance tests (anti-microbial efficacy) of the plasma care® PSU

Efficacy testing on prokaryotic cells	Method	Results
Bactericidal efficacy	Treatment of risk group I and II bacterial strains on agar	*Log-reduction after 1 min* E. coli → 5.8 S. aureus → 5.6 P. aeruginosa → 5.9 MRSA → 6.0 E. faecalis → 5.4 C. propinquum → 5.8 and others
	Treatment of *E. faecalis* biofilm	*24-hour biofilm: Log-reduction/ treatment* 3.28 log/1 min 4.73 log/3 min 3.52 log/5 mJ/cm³ UV-C 5.63 log/CHX 0.2% 6-hour biofilm: 8.3 log/5 min 24-hour biofilm: 5 log/5 min 48-hour biofilm: 2.3 log/5 min
Fungicidal efficacy	Treatment of planktonic *Candida albicans* on agar	*Log reduction/treatment time* 4.6 log/1 min 5.3 log/3 min 5.4 log/5 min 5.8 log/10 min
Bactericidal efficacy on ex vivo skin	Artificial contamination and treatment of porcine or human skin	*% reduction/treatment time* (1) S. aureus: 69%/1 min and 95%/5 min (2) E. coli: 83%/1 min and 99%/5 min (3) E. faecalis: 69%/1 min and 91%/5 min

The plasma care® displayed a high-performance level of antimicrobial activity.

plete saliva broth with fetal calf serum (FCS) to generate a 24 hours, 48 hours or 72 hours biofilm [20, 21]. In a 24-hour biofilm of *E. faecalis*, which contained 8.6×10^{13} bacteria, a 3.28 log reduction was achieved after 1 minute of plasma treatment compared to the untreated control. A reduction of 4.73 logs was achieved after a 3-minute plasma treatment. (Please note that the quality of biofilms varies between experiments and thus strongly affects the achieved log-reduction. In the tests with the plasma care®, very high log-reductions were achieved.)

To investigate the efficacy of the plasma from the plasma care® under more life-like conditions, bacterial inactivation experiments on porcine (female or castrated male, 6-months-old pigs) and human skin biopsies were carried out. The samples were washed, shaved and the subcutaneous tissue was removed. Subsequently, the biopsies were embedded in HEPES-agar and contaminated with bacteria (*S. aureus*, *E. faecalis* and *E. coli*). Plasma was applied and surviving bacteria were collected and incubated overnight at 37 °C. The CFU count yielded a reduction of 69% (*S. aureus* and *E. faecalis*) and 83% (*E. coli*) on artificially contaminated skin biopsies within 1 minute of plasma treatment (◘ Table 19.5).

The plasma treatment in principle is not a targeted therapy which attacks pathogens exclusively. Healthy human tissue also comes into contact with the plasma. Therefore, it was carefully examined whether the plasma treatment from the plasma care® causes any changes in vitro in both, single-layer primary human fibroblasts and keratinocytes, or in ex vivo human skin. Plasma treatments of up to 3 minutes had no impact on metabolic activity, vitality, or migration behavior of primary human fibroblasts and keratinocytes in vitro (◘ Table 19.6). Furthermore, no histological or pro-apoptotic changes were observed in "normal" or "sensitive" skin from healthy donor biopsies (◘ Table 19.6). Because these results indicate a safe therapeutic window, the longest permissible treatment period for a single wound area with the plasma care® within 24 hours was fixed at 3 minutes.

Mutagenicity studies (*hypoxanthine-guanine phosphoribosyltransferase* [HGPRT] assay using V79 cells) with the plasma source from the plasma care® were carried out as described by Maisch et al. 2017 [22]. The cells were treated with plasma for 30 seconds, 1 minute, 3 minutes, or 5 minutes (longer treatment periods are not possible due to the limitations in cell tests; positive control = UV-C irradiation at 1 mJ/cm^2). Surviving cells (= mutants) were enumerated multiple times.

The results showed that the number of surviving clones in previous toxicity tests was sufficient for evaluation (i.e., cell survival was not inhibited by the plasma treatment). Thus, the analysis of the HPRT test was valid. According to Bradley et al. 1981 [23], a substance or combinations of substances are mutagenic, when the spontaneous mutation rate (mutation frequency of untreated control) is exceeded threefold. For the plasma treatment with the plasma care® this was not the case (◘ Table 19.6). Thus, no elevated mutation rate following plasma treatment with the plasma care® plasma source is observed. The HGPRT test provided no evidence of any genotoxic potential of the plasma from the plasma care®.

In summary, the results from extensive preclinical studies of the plasma care® show that this medical device is effective and safe within a therapeutic window of 1–3 minutes.

□ **Table 19.6** Selected methods and results from preclinical safety tests (eukaryotic cell culture and histology) of the plasma care® PSU

Safety testing on eukaryotic cells	Method	Results	
Metabolic activity	MTT assay (% reduction in mitochondrial activity in monolayer cultures)	*Primary human fibroblasts* Untreated = 0% reduction 1 min = 20% reduction 2 min = 21.4% reduction 3 min = 61.4% reduction 5 min = 88.6% reduction UV-C (10 mJ/cm^3) = 100% reduction	*Primary human keratino-cytes* Untreated = 0% reduction 1 min = 0% reduction (2.2% increase) 2 min = 5.4% reduction 3 min = 20.7% reduction 5 min = 55.4% reduction UV-C (10 mJ/cm^3) = 96,7% reduction
Vitality	LUNA assay (live/dead staining, provided as % alive)	*Primary human fibroblasts* Untreated: 91% 1 min: 83% 2 min: 77% 3 min: 79% 5 min: 82% UV-C (10 mJ/cm^3): 8%	*Primary human keratino-cytes* Untreated: 92% 1 min: 82% 2 min: 82% 3 min: 76% 5 min: 40% UV-C (10 mJ/cm^3): 25%
Cell migration	Scratch assay	Cell migration of primary human keratinocytes, that is, closure of scratch in cell monolayer, is not affected by 1–3 min plasma treatment - time to closure: 24–28 hours Scratch closure is slightly delayed after 5 min plasma treatment	
Mutagenic-ity	HGPRT test using V79 hamster cells	Neg. control = 2.05 mutants/10^6 cells 30 sec = 0.62 mutants/10^6 cells 1 min = 0.86 mutants/10^6 cells 3 min = 0.64 mutants/10^6 cells 5 min = 0.27 mutants/10^6 cells Pos. control (UV-C) = 15.74 mutants/10^6 cells	
Ex vivo skin	Histology		
	HE staining (macroscopic damage)	No macroscopic damage detectable immediately after or 4 hours after plasma treatment of 1–5 minutes	
	TUNEL assay (apoptosis)	No induction of apoptosis immediately after or 4 hours after plasma treatment of 1–5 minutes in "normal" or "stripped" skin biopsies	

The preclinical evaluation of the safety of plasma from the plasma care® revealed a therapeutic window of 1–3 minutes

19

19.2.3 Risk Assessment and Product Safety

Risks associated with the use of and treatment with the plasma care® were minimized and product safety was maximized during its development. The following clinical risk factors were identified and addressed.

1. Cross-contamination between two patients via the plasma care®: this potential risk has been almost excluded, because the sterile, disposable plasma care® spacer cannot be reused once a treatment was performed (integrated RFID-security). The plasma care® itself does not come into direct contact with the patient's skin or wound surface due to the spacer. Moreover, the protection grid within the spacer prevents any direct contact between PSU and contaminated skin. Cleaning and disinfection of the plasma care® by wipe disinfection is easy and thorough due to the smooth surfaces of the housing without any openings.

2. Mechanical damage to the PSU leads to a change in the chemical plasma composition: the protection grid within the plasma care® spacer prevents mechanical damage to the plasma care® during its operation. Furthermore, the correct plasma composition is ensured via a monitoring system that is integrated into the hard- and firmware of the plasma care®. If the plasma production parameters deviate from the preset values, then the treatment cannot commence – the PSU has to be exchanged [24].

3. Mis-application of the plasma care® that leads to treatment times of more than 3 minutes (maximum permissible treatment time): a single treatment period with the plasma care® is set to 1 minute and a spacer can only be used for six consecutive 1-minute treatments, so that no unintentional excessive application can occur.

4. Skin irritation of operator or patient by contact with the plasma care® or the plasma care® spacer: biocompatible plastics are used for the casing of the plasma care® and the spacer. Skin irritations resulting from the plasma treatment are currently investigated in a post-market clinical follow-up (PMCF) trial, and a post-market surveillance (PMS) system is in place.

5. Use of the plasma care® on wounds with thick biofilms, fibrin layers, and/or necrotic tissue: the manual of the plasma care® states explicitly that the current standard-of-care according to the German S3 guideline on wound treatment needs to be adhered to, which includes careful wound debridement.

The following physical and technological risk factors were identified and addressed:

1. A short circuit of the PSU leads to an electrical shock to the user or patient: If a short circuit of the PSU occurs, the high voltage power supply has a safety switch that blocks the flow of electricity. Moreover, electricity is only applied to the PSU, if a valid spacer is attached, so that no physical contact between the operator/patient and the PSU can happen during its operation.

2. Electrical stray radiation from the plasma care® disrupts other medical devices: The electrical stray radiation that is emitted from the plasma care® – as from any other electrical device – is within official limits. Furthermore, there is a warning in the manual that covers the topic of potential electrical stray radiation from the plasma care®.

3. Electrical stray radiation from other devices disrupts the plasma care® and prevents its operation: The plasma care® adheres to official limits for robustness toward electrical stray radiation. If a treatment is interrupted, it can be continued upon restart of the plasma care®. Furthermore, there is a warning in the manual that covers the topic of potential disruptions of medical devices due to electrical stray radiation from other high-frequency devices.

19.3 Indications

Like other forms of physical wound therapy, such as low-level laser and hyperbaric oxygen/carbon dioxide therapy, CAP therapy is used to impact the microenvironment of hard-to-heal wounds so that microbial contamination is controlled, and wound healing is stimulated. The mechanism of action in plasma therapy, however, is based on the interaction of a complex mixture of RONS species amongst other cold plasma components with both prokaryotic and eukaryotic cells. The plasma care® in combination with the plasma care® spacer, its sterile disposable attachment, is approved for the painless cold plasma treatment of chronic and acute, open wounds with the potential indication of a bacterial load (prophylactic) as well as for wounds that are already colonized and infected with bacteria. It can be used for infection prophylaxis and as an add-on treatment in addition to the standard-of-care, in wounds that are already critically colonized or infected. There are only a few contraindications: wounds with heavy and acute bleeding are excluded because the plasma species are carried away by the blood flow. Wounds at exposed inner organs (in surgery), wounds in the head and neck area, and pediatric wound patients under the age of 12 are excluded for lack of data. And finally, wounds involving mucous membranes – especially in the nose and mouth – are excluded, because the produced ozone could lead to respiratory irritation. The area of indication is shown in ◘ Table 19.7.

Many patients with infected chronic wounds involve the elderly population. These patients often possess co-morbidities or disabilities such as limited mobility, sensory disorders, metabolic disorders, circulatory disorders, venous insufficiency or veins damaged by thrombosis, peripheral artery disease (PAD), diabetes mellitus, and neoplastic diseases. Wound treatment is symptomatic, and it is essential to treat the underlying disease as well to prevent future relapses as much as possible.

19.3.1 Use and Treatment Recommendations

The plasma care® was designed to be user-friendly. Thus, it only has a single touch button, which is used to power the medical device on or off and to start the plasma treatment. No pressure is necessary to operate the device. It is enough to gently place a thumb on the touch button and wait for the device to power on, which is indicated by the lighting up of the touch button.

Once the plasma care® is activated the sterile package of a plasma care® spacer is opened and the spacer is attached to the medical device. Subsequently, an initialization process is started automatically, which lasts for 15–45 seconds. Throughout

19

■ **Table 19.7** Area of indication and contraindications for the therapeutic application of the plasma care® on chronic and acute, open wounds

Indication			Contraindication
Etiology/cause	*Disease/condition*	*Symptoms and aspects*	
Chronic wounds			**Wounds with heavy and acute bleeding**
Arterial, venous, infectious, diabetic, neuropathic, traumatic, vasculitic	Ulcers, decubitus or pyoderma gangrenosum	Potential indication of bacterial load (prophylactic), colonization, and infection with bacteria	**Wounds at exposed inner organs (surgical area)**
Acute, open wounds			**Wounds involving mucous membranes**
Mechanical cause	Abrasions, cuts, stab wounds, lacerations, contused wounds, avulsions, fissures, bites, gunshot wounds, impalement injuries, amputation of extremities	Potential indication of bacterial load (prophylactic), colonization, and infection with bacteria	**Wounds in the head and neck area** **Children under the age of 12 years**
Thermal cause	Burns, frostbite		
Surgical	Surgery wounds, secondary healing surgery wounds, split-thickness skin graft sites		

initialization, the "plasma ring" that surrounds the touch button flashes blue. During this process, the so-called "burn-in," the PSU, and the generated mix of plasma species are monitored: the composition of the plasma mix affects its efficacy and is dependent on many operating and environmental parameters. Since the plasma mix is a result of more than 600 reactions in the air, it is not possible to check every single component. Instead, certain electrical values are measured, and a monitoring value is computed which correlates with the specified plasma composition and thus with the anti-bacterial efficacy of the plasma source. As soon as this quality test during the burn-in process is completed, the plasma ring stops flashing and radiates a constant blue light. The plasma care® is now ready for use. The spacer is placed gently onto the wound surface so that a certain volume of air is enclosed in the process. Plasma production is started by touching the on/off button briefly (for about 1 second). The long-lived plasma species that are generated at the PSU then travel from the plasma source to the wound surface through the volume of air that is enclosed by the spacer. Once these plasma species come into contact with the microorganisms that colonize the wound, the microbes are inactivated (■ Fig. 19.4). This process is highly effective when bacteria are freely accessible.

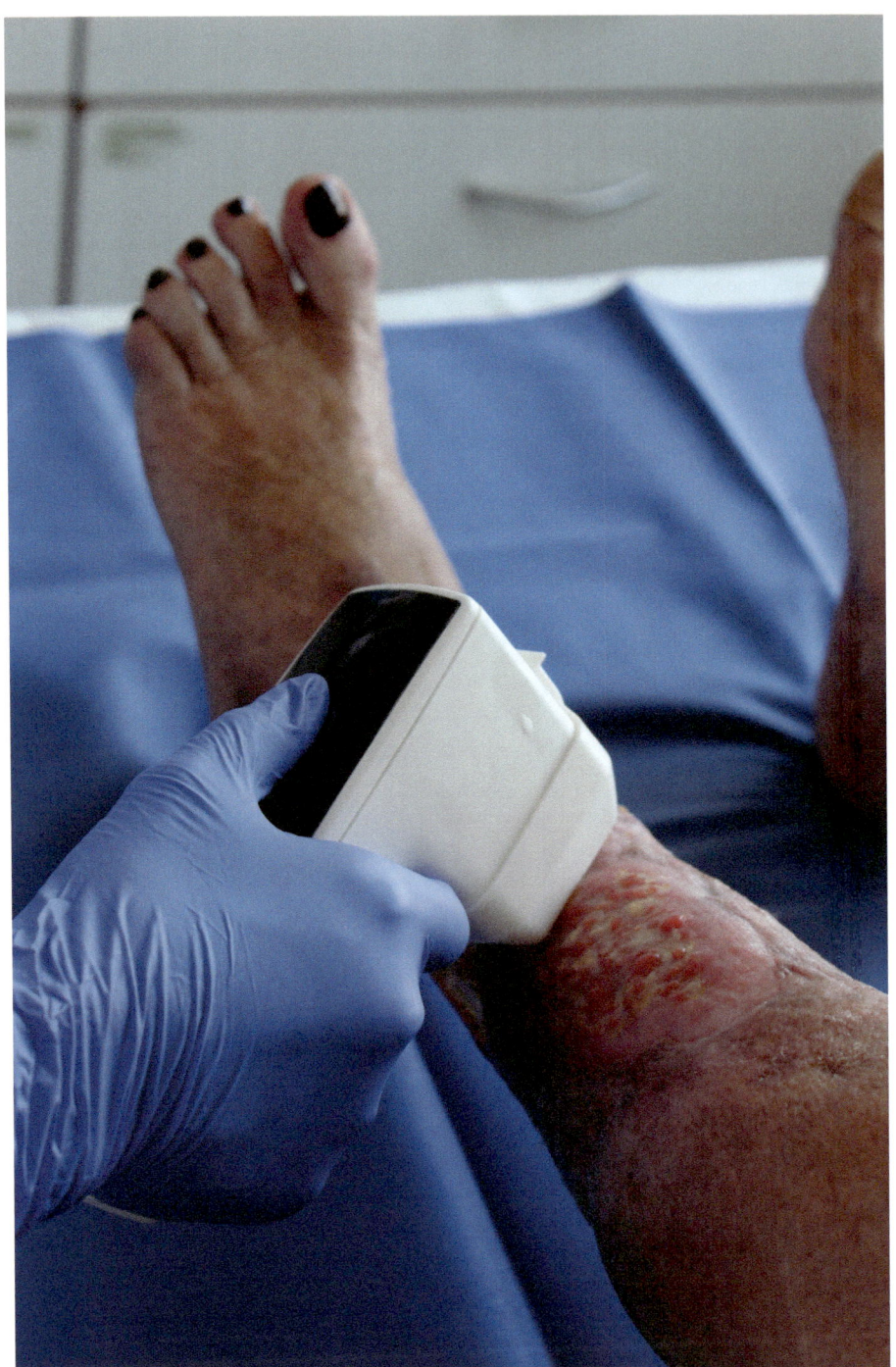

19

■ **Fig. 19.4**   Wound treatment with the plasma care®

Several requirements must be met to achieve efficient bacterial reductions: (1) the wound surface needs to be freely accessible (i.e., ointment residues, wound exudate, fibrin layers, necrotic tissue, etc.). need to be removed thoroughly. (2) The wound surface needs to be cleaned with a reagent-free wound irrigation solution such as Ringer's solution or physiological sodium chloride solution. This is advisable, because a thin film of humidity increases the efficacy of the plasma species mix as efficient reactive species such as hydrogen peroxide are generated from interactions between plasma and water molecules. (3) The temperature and humidity must not fall below 10 °C and 25% RH, or rise above 35 °C and 70% RH, respectively.

Preclinically, the plasma mix from the plasma care® already showed a very high level of bactericidal activity after only 1 minute of application (5–6 log reduction on agar irrespective of the bacterial strain). In an actual wound setting, however, the plasma treatment will be less efficient due to the uneven surface, which makes some bacteria less accessible than others, and due to shielding effects when bacteria grow in layers on top of one another. As a result, the plasma treatment needs to be performed several times to fully control an infection.

Based on experience with other cold plasma medical devices, one to two CAP treatments per week in the course of regular wound dressing changes are recommended at present. The total number of treatments that are required can vary and must be decided by the physician, veterinarian, or wound expert. The treatment duration for a single wound area of 16 cm^2 in 12 hours can be up to 3 minutes (= three 1-minute treatments with the plasma care®). More specific treatment recommendations for the plasma care® will be provided when more clinical evidence has been collected.

19.3.2 Successful Examples

The plasma care® has been CE-mark approved in June 2019 and clinical evidence is accumulating. While writing the summary of this article, the plasma care® was already employed successfully by several physicians, nurses, veterinarians, and other healthcare professionals. Four successful examples of wound treatment with the plasma care® in veterinary as well as in human medicine are presented here:

Case report, veterinary practice An 8-year old paint horse mare, which had median nerve neurectomy in the left foreleg performed in March 2019, developed traumatic neuromas on both ends of the injured nerve tissue. In a second operation, eleven and a half weeks later, the neuromas were removed. Intraoperatively, the lateral tissue appeared to be strongly edematous and partially necrotic. It was resected as extensively as possible. Following the operation, however, suture dehiscence occurred laterally due to the tissue inflammation and an open, purulent wound developed (☐ Fig. 19.5, Day 0), in which a high burden of *E. coli* was detected that was partially resistant to common antibiotics including cephalosporins, lincosamides, fluorochinolones, and intermediary tetracyclines. After the operation, the wound was treated with a ketanserine ointment and dressed daily. Additionally, the mare was first started

VETERINARY MEDICINE

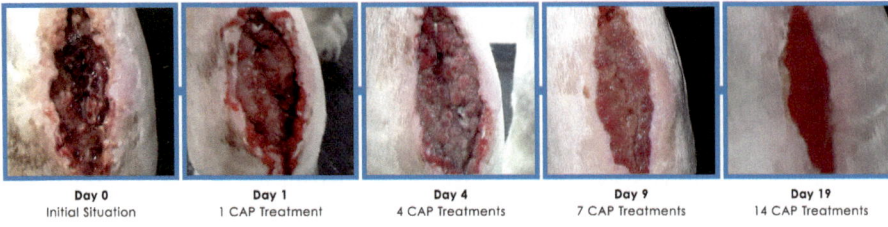

| Day 0 | Day 1 | Day 4 | Day 9 | Day 19 |
| Initial Situation | 1 CAP Treatment | 4 CAP Treatments | 7 CAP Treatments | 14 CAP Treatments |

▣ Fig. 19.5 Wound progression in an 8-year-old paint horse mare with postoperative wound infection. The mare was treated with cold plasma 14 times in the course of 3 weeks. (Images courtesy of Pferdeklinik am Kirchberg GmbH)

on an antibiosis with penicillin and gentamicin for 5 days and then switched to sulfonamide-trimetoprim as wound healing did not improve. On day nine, cold plasma therapy was initiated in parallel to the antibiosis. Shortly before the plasma treatment, the wound was cleaned with physiological sodium chloride solution, and after plasma treatment, ketanserine ointment and new wound dressing were applied as before. The mare was treated with plasma for 2 minutes on each wound area for seven consecutive days and received another course of plasma treatment for 7 days after a two-day break.

Upon initiation of cold plasma therapy, the infection was controlled and wound healing reinitiated. A clear improvement was already visible after the first day of CAP therapy (▣ Fig. 19.5, Day 1). Surprisingly, the wound started granulating from the inside without displaying signs of hypergranulation (▣ Fig. 19.5, Day 4) and the tissue tightened visibly. On the third day of the second course of plasma treatment, the antibiosis was discontinued. The mare was released 4 weeks after the operation with full wound closure (▣ Fig. 19.5, Day 19).

Case report, outpatient care   A 61-year-old female patient had suffered a traumatic trans-tibial amputation and developed a nonhealing postoperative wound in January 2018 after a skin flap had been transposed over the stump. In the course of the following one and a half years, the patient was cared for by a professional homecare service. The wound situation and the pain intensity described by the patient kept alternating between improvement and worsening. Wound exudate was mostly moderate and reddish. The skin environment of the wound remained intact.

At the age of 63, the patient was started on plasma therapy as an add-on in August 2019. At initiation of the plasma therapy, the wound area (▣ Fig. 19.6, Day 0) had a length of 2.04 cm and a width of 1.87 cm, displayed several small skin lesions, and wound exudate was moderate. The patient was treated with plasma for 1 minute per treatment area nine times over the course of three and a half weeks (twice a week). A detailed description of the changes in the wound situation is given in ▣ Table 19.8. On the last day of CAP treatment, the length and width of the wound had decreased to 0.48 cm and 0.51 cm, respectively (▣ Fig. 19.6, Day 25). The surrounding skin was intact, and the patient had not experienced pain during any of the plasma treatments.

HUMAN MEDICINE

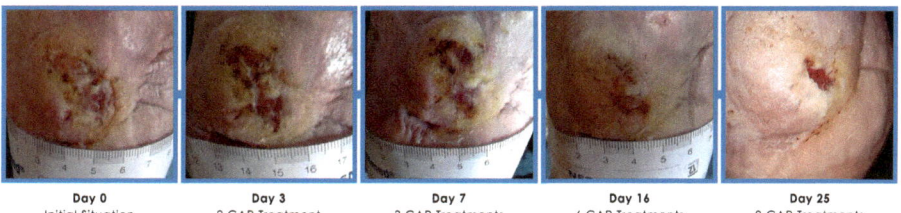

Day 0	Day 3	Day 7	Day 16	Day 25
Initial Situation	2 CAP Treatment	3 CAP Treatments	6 CAP Treatments	9 CAP Treatments

◘ **Fig. 19.6**   Wound progression in a left lower limb amputee with a nonhealing wound. The patient achieved almost full wound closure after nine treatments. (Images courtesy of Ellipsa Medical Services GmbH)

◘ **Table 19.8**   Detailed description of plasma treatment and wound progression in a left lower limb amputee and changes in length and width of the wound over the course of plasma therapy

CAP treat-ment #	Wound size		Exudate		Surrounding skin	Comment
	Length	*Width*	*Amount*	*Color*		
1	2.04	1.87	Moder-ate	Mixed	n/a	Small skin lesions in wound area, no pain during treatment
2	2.48	2.27	n/a	n/a	n/a	Wound area displays redness, fewer skin lesions, no odor, no layers, no pain
3	2.16	1.78	n/a	n/a	n/a	Redness declines, lower tissue appears smooth and homogeneous, no odor, no layers
4	2.09	2.28	Reduced	n/a	Wound edges display yellow discoloration and are slightly tougher	Open wound areas appear to shrink, no odor, no layers
5	2.57	2.71	n/a	n/a	Maceration, because patient did not apply biatain Adh correctly	Wound area appears to be reduced, no odor, no pain
6	0.69	1.4	n/a	n/a	No more maceration	Wound area shrinks
7	0.35	0.58	n/a	n/a	Keratinous and slightly macerated pain outside of the wound area	Wound base inconspicuous and clean, appointment with podologist to remove keratoses
8	0.86	0.79	n/a	Trans-parent	Painful pinhead lesion	Wound area shrinks
9	0.48	0.51	n/a	n/a	n/a	n/a

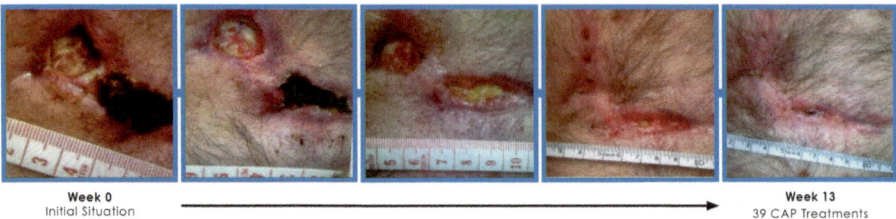

Week 0
Initial Situation

Week 13
39 CAP Treatments

◘ **Fig. 19.7** Wound progression in a cancer survivor with an infected nonhealing wound at the sternum. The patient achieved full wound closure after 13 weeks. (Images courtesy of Dr. med. Clemens Witzenhausen)

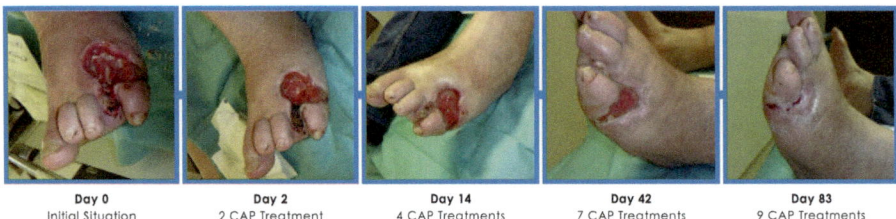

Day 0
Initial Situation

Day 2
2 CAP Treatment

Day 14
4 CAP Treatments

Day 42
7 CAP Treatments

Day 83
9 CAP Treatments

◘ **Fig. 19.8** Wound progression in a patient with diabetic foot syndrome after amputation of the left digitus pedis IV. The patient achieved full wound closure after 12 weeks. (Images courtesy of Klinikum am Steinenberg, Reutlingen)

Case report, physician's practice   Two months after the removal of a liposarcoma at the sternum and partial rib resection of C2-C5 on the right and C2-C4 on the left, a 40-year-old male patient presented with a putrid wound abscess cavity at the surgical site in August 2019. The wound was revised and a vacuum seal applied; however, the wound remained infected and did not heal (◘ Fig. 19.7, Week 0). In October 2019, cold plasma therapy was initiated. The patient was treated for 1–2 minutes per wound area three times per week. Necrotic tissue and blood crusts were removed regularly. Over the course of 13 weeks, the necrotic tissue areas reduced visibly in size, the wound became smoother and started to heal from the edges (◘ Fig. 19.7). In January 2020, the wound had healed completely.

Case report, hospital   In June 2019, a 50-year-old male patient who suffered from diabetes mellitus type II, presented with a diabetic ulcer on metatarsal IV and V and with a necrotic fourth toe at the left foot (digitus pedis IV sinistra). The wound was initially infected with *Klebsiella pneumoniae spp. pneumoniae*, which was superseded by an infection with partially resistant *Corynebacterium striatum* and *Enterococcus spp.* Accordingly, the initial intravenous antibiosis with piperacillin/tazobactam was switched to ciprofloxacin and then to vancomycin as the inflammation parameters elevated and the results from the bacterial swab became available. Moreover, the patient had to observe strict bed rest during his hospitalization period of 44 days and received biosurgical debridement. However, the wound situation did not improve, salvation of the toe was unsuccessful, and the digit had to be amputated after one month (◘ Fig. 19.8, Day 0). Subsequently, cold plasma therapy was initiated and

19

performed as adjunct after mechanical debridement for 2 minutes per wound area at each change of dressing and ambulatory follow-up visit of the patient. During the first 5 weeks, plasma treatments were carried out once or twice a week and afterward once every 2–4 weeks. The bacterial burden in the wound that was detected via a bacterial swab, semi-quantitatively was significantly reduced in Week eight. In total, nine plasma treatments were carried out over the course of 12 weeks. Within this period, the ulcer healed (◻ Fig. 19.8), and the patient did not experience pain during any of the plasma treatments.

19.4 Clinical Trials

The results regarding safety and efficacy of the plasma care® from preclinical tests, clearly showed that SMD cold plasma technology was successfully integrated into a battery-operated portable medical device. To further investigate the performance and safety of the medical device in a clinical setting, a PMCF trial was started in the summer of 2019, which is registered at the ISRCTN database with the ID ISRCTN98384076.

The primary outcome parameter in the plasma care®-study is the reduction of the bacterial load in treated wounds. Secondary outcome parameters are the intensity of pain during treatment with the plasma care® and the safety of the treatment based on serious adverse events (SAEs) and adverse events of special interest (AEosi, i.e., local skin reactions). Furthermore, 3D photographic records of the treated wounds including their respective dimensions and the development thereof are obtained to document the wound healing process. The plasma care®-study is a prospective, parallel-group, randomized, placebo-controlled, single-blinded, multi-center superiority medical device trial with an adaptive multi-arm multistage design. It is an exceptional and challenging trial considering that all patients serve as their own controls: each patient included in the trial must have two comparable treatment sites that are colonized with bacteria. One treatment site is treated with the plasma care®, the other with a placebo device that looks and sounds the same as the plasma care®, but that does not produce any plasma. The first patient in the trial was recruited in July 2019. Results from the plasma care®-study are expected to be published in 2021.

In parallel to the above-mentioned clinical trial three observational studies including 30 hard-to-heal wounds (in 28 patients), prevailing for several months to several years, with various genesis such as venous and arterial leg ulcers, diabetic foot ulcers, postoperative wound healing disorders, and surgical site infections were conducted. The patients were treated over a period of 4–10 weeks with 1–2 plasma treatments per week, each treatment lasting for 1–2 minutes. The results revealed that the plasma treatment was well tolerated by all patients. No pain or side effects were reported. The majority of the wounds significantly improved in response to the plasma treatment: For 20 patients, the wounds changed their "status" from nonhealing to healing thereby reaching the epithelialization phase after only a few weeks of treatment. Furthermore, a significant reduction in wound fibrine and wound secretion was observed. All in all, the plasma treatment for these

20 patients led to a wound size reduction of approximately 50% in 4 weeks and up to 100% at the end of the treatment period ranging from 4 to 10 weeks. For eight patients, wound size reduction stagnated even under the plasma treatment.

19.5 Outlook and Further Developments

Currently, terraplasma medical focuses on the collection of clinical data with the plasma care® to further show the efficacy and safety of the plasma treatment. More detailed use and treatment recommendations can thus be provided to health-care professionals in the future, and the benefits for the patients can be described more closely. Furthermore, adaptations of the plasma care® spacer are planned, so that larger wound areas, entry sites of catheters and drivelines, and wounds at poorly accessible locations may be treated even better. Since the air volume enclosed by the spacer and the design, size, and operating parameters of the PSU affect the plasma composition, an adaptation of the spacer, and/or the PSU require careful development. Finally, additional areas of indication, such as dermatological skin disorders, will be explored in the future.

References/Further Reading/Additional Resources

1. Brehmer F, Haenssle HA, Daeschlein G, Ahmed R, Pfeiffer S, Görlitz A, Simon D, Schön MP, Wandke D, Emmert S. Alleviation of chronic venous leg ulcers with a hand-held dielectric barrier discharge plasma generator (PlasmaDerm ® VU-2010): results of a monocentric, two-armed, open, prospective, randomized and controlled trial (NCT01415622). J Eur Acad Dermatol Venereol. 2015;29:148–55.
2. Daeschlein G, Scholz S, Ahmed R, et al. Cold plasma is well-tolerated and does not disturb skin barrier or reduce skin moisture. J Dtsch Dermatol Ges. 2012;10:509–15.
3. Heinlin J, Zimmermann JL, Zeman F, et al. Randomized placebo-controlled human pilot study of cold atmospheric argon plasma on skin graft donor sites. Wound Repair Regen. 2013;21:800–7.
4. Isbary G, Heinlin J, Shimizu T, et al. Successful and safe use of 2 min cold atmospheric argon plasma in chronic wounds: results of a randomized controlled trial. Br J Dermatol. 2012;167:404–10.
5. Heyer K, Herberger K, Protz K, Glaeske G, Augustin M. Epidemiology of chronic wounds in Germany: analysis of statutory health insurance data: epidemiology of chronic wounds in Germany. Wound Repair Regen. 2016;24:434–42.
6. Wunderl M, Unger, R, Kirsch J, Zimmermann JL. Plasmaeinrichtung zur Behandlung von Körperoberflächen. (DE 10 2018 209 735 A1) Deutsches Patent- und Markenamt. 2019. https://depatisnet.dpma.de/DepatisNet/depatisnet?action=bibdat&docid=DE102018209735A1
7. Shimizu T, Lachner V, Zimmermann JL. Surface microdischarge plasma for disinfection. Plasma Med. 2017;7:175–85.
8. Morfill GE, Shimizu T, Steffes B, Schmidt H-U. Nosocomial infections—a new approach towards preventive medicine using plasmas. New J Phys. 2009;11:115019.
9. Morfill G, Schimizu T, Li Y. Elektrodenanordnung und Plasmaquelle zur Erzeugung eines nicht-thermischen Plasmas sowie ein Verfahren zum Betreiben einer Plasmaquelle. (DE 10 2015 213 975 A1) Deutsches Patent- und Markenamt. 2018. https://depatisnet.dpma.de/DepatisNet/depatisnet?action=bibdat&docid=DE102015213975A1.
10. Sakiyama Y, Graves DB, Chang H-W, Shimizu T, Morfill GE. Plasma chemistry model of sur-

face microdischarge in humid air and dynamics of reactive neutral species. J Phys D Appl Phys. 2012;45:425201.

11. International Organization for Standardization. IEC 60601-1-11:2015: medical electrical equipment - part 1–11: general requirements for basic safety and essential performance - collateral standard: requirements for medical electrical equipment and medical electrical systems used in the home healthcare environment, 2nd ed. 2015.

12. von Woedtke T, Mann MS, Ahmed R, Dürr U, Gavenis K, Wurster S, Daeschlein G, Emmert S, Tiede R. DIN SPEC 91315: Allgemeine Anforderungen an medizinische Plasmaquellen. DIN Deutsches Institut für Normung e.V. 2014.

13. International Organization for Standardization. IEC 62304:2006: medical device software - software life cycle processes. International Organization for Standardization. Geneva. 1st ed; 2006.

14. International Organization for Standardization. ISO 10993-1:2018: biological evaluation of medical deices - part 1: evaluation and testing within a risk management process. International Organization for Standardization. Geneva. 5th ed; 2018.

15. Bundesanstalt für Arbeitsschutz und Arbeitsmedizin. TROS Inkohärente Optische Strahlung - Teil 2: Messungen und Berechnungen von Expositionen gegenüber inkohärenter optischer Strahlung. 2013.

16. International Commission on Non-Ionizing Radiation Protection. Guidelines on limits of exposure to ultraviolet radiation of wavelengths between 180 nm and 400 nm (incoherent optical radiation). Health Phys. 2004;87:171–86.

17. OSHA. The National Institute for Occupational Safety and Health (NIOSH) (1989) Ozone.

18. OSHA. The National Institute for Occupational Safety and Health (NIOSH). Nitric Oxide and Nitrogen Dioxide - Method 6014. NIOSH Man Anal Methods (NMAM) 1–4. 1994.

19. Theinkom F, Singer L, Cieplik F, Cantzler S, Weilemann H, Cantzler M, Hiller K-A, Maisch T, Zimmermann JL. Antibacterial efficacy of cold atmospheric plasma against Enterococcus faecalis planktonic cultures and biofilms in vitro. PLoS One. 2019;14:e0223925.

20. Cieplik F, Späth A, Regensburger J, Gollmer A, Tabenski L, Hiller K-A, Bäumler W, Maisch T, Schmalz G. Photodynamic biofilm inactivation by SAPYR—an exclusive singlet oxygen photosensitizer. Free Radic Biol Med. 2013;65:477–87.

21. Cieplik F, Pummer A, Regensburger J, Hiller K-A, Späth A, Tabenski L, Buchalla W, Maisch T. The impact of absorbed photons on antimicrobial photodynamic efficacy. Front Microbiol. 2015. https://doi.org/10.3389/fmicb.2015.00706.

22. Maisch T, Bosserhoff AK, Unger P, Heider J, Shimizu T, Zimmermann JL, Morfill GE, Landthaler M, Karrer S. Investigation of toxicity and mutagenicity of cold atmospheric argon plasma. Environ Mol Mutagen. 2017;58:172–7.

23. Bradley MO, Bhuyan B, Francis MC, Langenbach R, Peterson A, Huberman E. Mutagenesis by chemical agents in V79 Chinese hamster cells: a review and analysis of the literature. Mutat Res/Rev Genet Toxicol. 1981;87:81–142.

24. Zimmermann J, Linner M, Cantzler S, Morfill G, Weilemann H, Cantzler M. Verfahren zum Prüfen und/oder Überwachen einer Elektrodenanordnung zur Erzeugung eines nicht-thermischen Plasmas. (DE 10 2018 209 729 A1) Deutsches Patent- und Markenamt. 2019. https://depatisnet.dpma.de/DepatisNet/depatisnet?action=bibdat&docid=DE102018209729A1.

Organization

Contents

Who Belongs to a Good Cold Plasma Practice Team?

*Steffen Emmert, Lars Boeckmann,
Tobias Fischer, Thomas von Woedtke,
Klaus-Dieter Weltmann,
Stefanie Kirschner, Anne Kirschner,
and Hans-Robert Metelmann*

Contents

© Springer Nature Switzerland AG 2022
H.-R. Metelmann et al. (eds.), *Textbook of Good Clinical Practice in
Cold Plasma Therapy*, https://doi.org/10.1007/978-3-030-87857-3_20

☺ Core Messages

- A "basic" plasma clinic should provide all patient care settings: inpatient, day-care, outpatient, as well as homecare settings within a collaborative network that fits the patients' needs according to their individual disease situation.
- For this setting, a "basic" plasma team consisting of trained doctors and nurses or medical physician assistants may be mandatory.
- For a CPC, further requirements in research, teaching, and development may be necessary.
- For this setting, a comprehensive plasma team consisting of a wide spectrum of specialists may be needed: medical doctors, dental doctors, plasma nurses, plasma health physicists, plasma engineers, plasma biologists, and not least plasma marketers.

20.1 Introduction

This comprehensive book is all about the new field of plasma medicine. This field was established 5–10 years ago with the first devices that have been licensed as medical devices for the therapy of wounds in 2013. Both devices were established in Germany which currently can still claim the lead in plasma medicine development. The development of plasma medicine in recent years may bring to mind the development of the laser technology some decades ago and, thus, envisage the potential future success of this field.

As depicted in this book in Part I, cold atmospheric plasma (CAP) can be viewed as a leap innovation in basic research for patient benefit. It has been well established that cold physical plasma contains a cocktail of diverse physico-electro-chemical substances and parameters that in concert exert medical effects. What cold plasma is, how it works in medicine, how safe it is in medical use, and which plasma technologies are approved to date are discussed in Part II of this book. Part III focuses on basic aspects of good clinical practice in plasma medicine: choice of device, selection of patients suitable for plasma therapy, general aspects of treatment, as well as handling complications during cold plasma treatment. Most importantly also with respect to the needs of a plasma team, Part IV discerns the different indications for which a plasma treatment has been established so far. The indications range from treating chronic and acute wounds, infected skin and/or mucosa, cancer ulcers, surgical sites that are already infected, or pose a risk for such complications including artificial fistulas to aesthetic medicine applications and dental aesthetics. This already gives a hint of the diverse needs of a plasma team needed for handling the respective indications. Surely, for further developments of plasma medicine in the respective indications, a broader team of plasma specialists is needed. Part of such a comprehensive plasma team are developers of new indication-specific devices who see the foundation of start-up companies to market such new devices on the horizon. To this end, Part V summarizes the devices and companies that market medically licensed plasma devices but are also keen on developing the field of plasma medicine further with respect to devices, indications, standardization and norms, and treatment reimbursement.

This all said it is evident that plasma medicine covers a wide variety of technical, physical, biological, chemical, and medical aspects that raise the question: What is needed to properly perform plasma treatments. This is covered in this last book Part VI and clearly, the team that assures good clinical practice in cold plasma therapy is very closely connected to the requirements of a cold plasma medicine clinic. We propose, as done with other medical fields, for example oncology, the distinction into "basic" team and clinic that would correspond to a certified skin or head and neck cancer center in oncology and "comprehensive" plasma team and clinic that would correspond to a comprehensive cancer center (CCC) including research, teaching, and entrepreneurship.

20.2   Requirements for a Basic Plasma Team

As outlined above and in the succeeding chapters, plasma medicine may be currently divided into three main action fields: Clinical Dermatology including tissue regeneration and wound healing [1, 2]; Microbiology and Hygiene and Dental Medicine including disinfection/antimicrobial treatments and implantology [3]; Oncology which might impose the most promising potential in the future [4–7]. At least one certified doctor and a trained nurse in the action field who are also experienced in plasma medicine should compose the minimum core group of a basic plasma team.

Depending on these indications specially trained and experienced doctors with board exams in the respective specialty are certainly mandatory (◘ Fig. 20.1). However, is a board certification sufficient or should a doctor also have a certain amount of experience in plasma medicine? In other words, is special training and certification in plasma medicine needed?

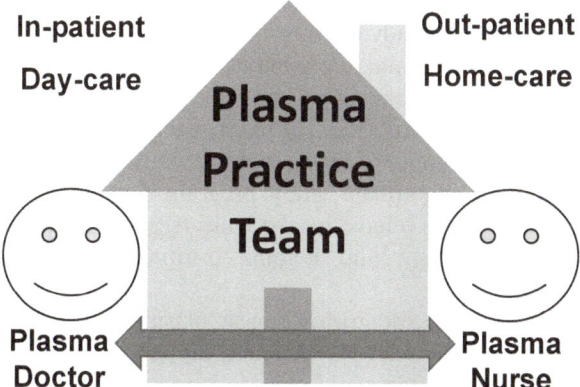

◘ **Fig. 20.1**   Requirements for a plasma practice team: medical doctor and nurse to serve the patient needs in all patient care settings (inpatient, day-care, outpatient, home care)

To this end, there is a current initiative in Germany to establish guidelines for the application of cold physical plasma in medicine. The landscape of guidelines in Germany is orchestrated by the AWMF: A working association of all medical specialties including the German Dermatological Society or the German Society for Oral and Maxillofacial Surgery. The AWMF combines a total of 179 Medical Specialty Societies plus three associated societies from all areas of medicine. In addition, the AWMF represents Germany in the Council for International Organizations of Medical Sciences (CIOMS). The responsibility of the AWMF is to establish medical guidelines in an interdisciplinary setting with the participation of all medical societies involved in the respective topic.

Already in 2018, an initiative to establish rationales for the therapeutic use of cold physical plasma was made under the guidance of Prof. Hans-Robert Metelmann and the German Society of Oral and Maxillofacial Surgery. As this is and must be an interdisciplinary effort further Medical Societies are involved: German Dermatological Society, German Society for ENT including Neck Surgery, German Society for Plastic, Reconstructive, and Aesthetic Surgery, German Society for Trauma Surgery, German Society for Burns, German Society for Family Practitioners, German AIDS-Society, German Diabetic Society, German Society for Dental and Oral Medicine, German Society for Geriatrics, German Society for Surgery, German Society for Wound Healing and Wound Treatment, German Society for Palliative Treatment, German Society for Adiposity, German Society for Vascular surgery, German Cancer Society, German Society for Laser Medicine, German Society for Nursing, German Society for Parodontology, German Society for Plastic Surgery, German Ophthalmological Society, and German Society for Orthodontics. Another scientific partner of this guideline project is the Leibniz-Institute for Plasma Science and Technology (INP Greifswald) as well as the National Center for Plasma Medicine (NZPM). This German guideline practically mirrors the content of this internationally oriented book.

To extrapolate this into the future, it appears obvious that if a distinct guideline for plasma medicine exists, a distinct certification for doctors to apply cold physical plasma in medicine also has to be established to demonstrate to patients the experience not only in the respective medical specialty but also in the plasma medicine specialty. In line with this, an already existing study program was recently extended to allow for the earning of a diploma in plasma medicine (DPM) by attending lectures (dies academicus), practical training in plasma clinics, and literature studies (▶ https://laserstudium.com/index.php?title=DALM_Struktur#Mit_Schwerpunkt_PlasmaMedizin). This possibility to earn a diploma in plasma medicine is embedded into the international postgraduate study program for aesthetic laser medicine (▶ https://laserstudium.com/) offered by the University of Greifswald, the German Dermatological Laser Society, and Leibniz Institute for Plasma Science and Technology e.V.

Given all these efforts, the doctor of a basic plasma team will have to earn his board exam in his medical specialty as well as a diploma in plasma medicine.

However, also nurses applying cold physical plasma should not only be trained in nursing but also applying plasma treatment appropriately within the given indication. It can be envisaged that in parallel with a doctoral diploma in plasma medicine also a nursing diploma in plasma medicine will have to be established. This seems appropriate as the work setting of a plasma nurse in a basic plasma team and clinical setting may be diverse: Nurses use cold plasma in the clinic and day-care clinic. This will require a full degree in nursing plus experience in the correct plasma treatment. In this setting, a close collaboration with the plasma doctor who is also present in the clinic will be possible (■ Fig. 20.1). However, in a home-care setting, the nurse or even a medical physician assistant by degree will have to perform a plasma treatment at the patient at home without the help of a doctor. To this end, a certificate in plasma medicine is certainly helpful.

> **Tip**
>
> Wound management is a multi-modal therapy including CAP. Nurses and medical assistance personnel involved should have an education which entitles them to work according to the recommendations of the European Wound Management Association or comparable organizations.

Another development to foster the collaboration between plasma doctors and plasma nurses especially in a home-care setting will be the implementation of digital technologies. This will include telemedicine, but also the development of digital devices that automatically scan the performance of plasma application as well as the medical results thereof (e.g., the progress in wound healing). Such automated "plasma pocket" devices as additional tools on the plasma device used will, in addition, ascertain the correct application of cold plasma. And to also include patient apprehension, the development of a specific plasma app or ePRO (electronic patient-reported outcome) may help not only to assure good quality in plasma medicine but also to establish new procedures or procedural changes more quickly as comparisons are easier with big data sets.

> **❶ Caution**
>
> Nurses and medical assistance personnel involved in wound treatment should report any adverse effect in association with CAP therapy to the supervising doctor. Adverse effects in association with plasma therapy are extremely rare, always raising suspicion that they are not caused by plasma therapy.

20.3 Requirements for a Comprehensive Plasma Team

In parallel with the establishment of CCC, we propose comprehensive plasma teams in comprehensive plasma clinics (CPC). Basic teams may consist of a plasma-certified consultant, a plasma-certified nurse or medical physician assistant, and certain telemedical devices that are being currently developed.

As outlined in ▶ Chap. 22, a CPC should include an interdisciplinary research unit. Ideally, such a plasma research unit may contain a center to perform clinical phase I–II trials as well as investigator-initiated trials (IITs). A CPC should also offer enough lab space to perform biomedical, chemical, and engineering research as well as offices as think-tanks for research beyond the wet-lab including nursing, administration, and health in a broader sense. The possibilities to perform a minimum of animal experiments needed to bring a new plasma treatment into human use may also be advisable. Of course, teaching is another prerequisite of an interdisciplinary research unit. Therefore, a comprehensive plasma team may perform an internationally visible plasma medical translational teaching in all plasma application fields including dermatology, oral and maxillofacial surgery, oncology, microbiology, hygiene, biology, chemistry, physics, engineering, and nursing. To round up the circle and to bring plasma medical knowledge to routine clinical use people with the spirit for entrepreneurship should not be missing. New plasma technological devices need to be patented and spin-off companies established.

To combine all these aspects comprehensively, in addition to a plasma doctor and a plasma nurse (◘ Fig. 20.1), plasma health physicists, plasma engineers, plasma biologists, and last not least plasma marketers should be part of a comprehensive plasma practice team (◘ Fig. 20.2). The beauty (and innovativeness) of this concept is that not only different disciplines are combined under one roof. Each specialty trains and teaches its own specialists. Plasma medicine is the retaining clip that fosters interdisciplinary work and inspires each discipline involved. This bears the excitement that disciplines that usually do not work together are brought onto one table. The collaboration between doctors, nurses, and biologists with engineers and marketers who all speak different languages (i.e., have different perspectives and importance in their field) is the real excitement. And especially such collaborations are the backgrounds that pave the way for real new developments: leap innovations like plasma medicine.

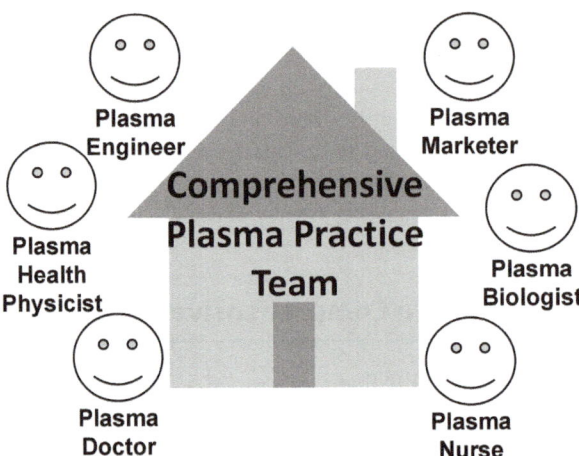

◘ **Fig. 20.2** Requirements of a comprehensive plasma practice team: medical doctor and nurse supported by plasma biologists, plasma health physicists, plasma engineers, and plasma marketer

Conclusion

It is obvious that within the developing and broad field of plasma medicine the team who performs the plasma treatment is closely connected with the requirements of a plasma clinic. A "basic" plasma clinic depending on the respective spectrum of indications treated with plasma should provide all patient care settings: inpatient, day-care, outpatient, as well as home-care settings within a collaborative network that fits the patients' needs according to their individual disease situation. For this setting, a "basic" plasma team consisting of trained doctors in the respective specialized field and nurses or medical physician assistants may be mandatory. For a CPC, further requirements in research, teaching, and development may be necessary as depicted in ▶ Chap. 22. For this setting, a comprehensive plasma team consisting of a wide spectrum of specialists may be needed: medical doctors, dental doctors, plasma nurses, plasma health physicists, plasma engineers, plasma biologists, and not least plasma marketers.

Acknowledgments This work is partly supported by the European Social Fund (ESF), reference: ESF/14-BM-A55-0001/18, ESF/14-BM-A55-0005/18, ESF/14-BM-A55-0006/18, and the Ministry of Education, Science and Culture of Mecklenburg-West Pomerania, Germany. S.E. is supported by the Deutsche Forschungsgemeinschaft (DFG EM 63/13-1) and the Damp Foundation. L.B. is supported by the Dermatological Society of Mecklenburg-West Pomerania.

References

1. Bernhardt T, Semmler ML, Schäfer M, Bekeschus S, Emmert S, Boeckmann L. Plasma medicine: applications of cold atmospheric pressure plasma in dermatology. Oxidative Med Cell Longev. 2019;3873928:1–10.
2. Boeckmann L, Bernhardt T, Schäfer M, Semmler ML, Kordt M, Waldner AC, Wendt F, Sagwal S, Bekeschus S, Berner J, Kwiatek, Frey A, Fischer T, Emmert S. Current indications for plasma therapy in dermatology. Hautarzt. 2020;71:109–13.
3. Metelmann R, von Woedtke T, Weltmann KD, editors. Comprehensive clinical plasma medicine. Heidelberg: Springer; 2018.
4. Metelmann H-R, Seebauer C, Miller V, Fridman A, Bauer G, Graves DB, et al. Clinical experience with cold plasma in the treatment of locally advanced head and neck cancer. Clin Plasma Med. 2018;9:6–13.
5. Witzke K, Seebauer C, Jesse K, Kwiatek E, Berner J, Semmler M, Böckmann L, Emmert S, Weltmann KD, Metelmann H, Bekeschus S. Plasma medical oncology: immunological interpretation of head and neck squamous cell carcinoma. Plasma Process Polym. 2020;17:e1900258. (1–9).
6. Berner J, Seebauer C, Sagwal S, Boeckmann L, Emmert S, Metelmann H, Bekeschus S. Medical gas plasma treatment in head and neck cancer – challenges and opportunities. Appl Sci. 2020;10:1944. (1-14).
7. Semmler MS, Bekeschus S, Schäfer M, Bernhardt T, Fischer T, Witzke K, Seebauer C, Rebl H, Grambow E, Vollmar B, Nebe B, Metelmann HR, von Woedtke T, Emmert S, Boeckmann L. Molecular mechanisms for the efficacy of cold atmospheric pressure plasma (CAP) in cancer treatment. Cancers. 2020;12:e269. (1–19).

How to Assure Good Clinical Practice in Plasma Therapy?

*Hans-Robert Metelmann, Stefan Hammes,
Kristina Hartwig, Christian Seebauer,
Ajay Rana, Eun Ha Choi, Masaru Hori,
Hiromasa Tanaka, Oksana Wladimirova,
Vu Thi Thom, Vandana Miller,
Anne Kirschner, Stefanie Kirschner,
and Thomas von Woedtke*

Contents

© Springer Nature Switzerland AG 2022
H.-R. Metelmann et al. (eds.), *Textbook of Good Clinical Practice in
Cold Plasma Therapy*, https://doi.org/10.1007/978-3-030-87857-3_21

📘 Core Messages
- Clinical plasma medicine at bedside and at bench is a teamwork including plasma doctors responsible for the patients' benefit, plasma nurses carrying out the treatment, plasma natural scientists supervising patient-related studies, and plasma engineers developing the devices.
- Patients' safety matters and quality assurance of research require adequate education and training of all team members.
- The modules of the international postgraduate Master of Science Study Program "Plasma and Aesthetic Laser Medicine - PALM" (Greifswald University Medicine) provide adequate education and training by tailored courses for the different needs of the different members of the clinical plasma medicine team.

21.1 Introduction

Good Clinical Practice (GCP) in plasma therapy is a matter of education. Recent genuine and significant progress in cold physical plasma research has intensified the scientific development of plasma medicine worldwide and subsequently promising treatment concepts with medical plasma devices have been approved by legal authorities' permission. To use plasma technology to treat patients in an effective and nonhazardous manner requires the adequate training of doctors and nurses. However, clinical plasma medicine is a teamwork not only including plasma doctors responsible for the patients' benefit and plasma nurses carrying out the treatment, but plasma natural scientists supervising related studies and plasma engineers developing the appropriate device as well. The considerable demand for qualified staff both at bedside and at bench in an extremely innovative field calls for continuing and postgraduate education programs as a matter of quality assurance.

⚠ Caution
Especially in new, very innovative and fast-developing fields of medicine like clinical plasma medicine, scientifically based university-level education is important to assure good clinical practice!

Greifswald University was the first in Europe to establish in 2001 a university-based postgraduate medical education program focused upon clinical application of photonic energy devices [1, 2]. Recently, this program has been expanded to a postgraduate Master of Science study program "Plasma and Aesthetic Laser Medicine - PALM" [3]. Intended first as a full-scope study program for doctors interested in the cross-disciplinary field of aesthetic medicine by noninvasive treatment procedures like laser and cold plasma, the curriculum can now be tailored as well to plasma medicine and the needs and interests of all members of the clinical plasma therapy and research team, the plasma doctors, the plasma nurses, the plasma natural scientists, and engineers. Standards of university education in scientifically based customized lectures and patient-related real-life training provide the most effective approach to assure GCP in plasma therapy.

21.2 Study Courses

21

21.2.1 Postgraduate M.Sc. "Plasma and Aesthetic Laser Medicine – PALM"

21.2.1.1 Target Group

The full postgraduate education program is targeted toward medical doctors and dentists, who are intending to gain expertise, especially in aesthetic medicine to clinically apply laser and cold plasma medical devices, or to start clinical research mainly in plasma and aesthetic laser medicine. A prerequisite for admission as a candidate to the PALM study program is a state-approved university degree with professional qualification in human medicine or in dental medicine.

> ❯ **Important to Know**
> This study program is intended to lead to a master's degree, at present the only available postgraduate university-based master's degree internationally concerning clinical plasma medicine.

21.2.1.2 Aims of Qualification

After having finished the postgraduate education, doctors will have interdisciplinary in-depth knowledge and skills across the area of aesthetic laser medicine and plasma medicine aligned with their individual priority setting. They will have the ability to critically assess in context, available methods, and techniques, and will also be able to investigate innovative questions that constantly arise in clinical medicine using scientific methods.

21.2.1.3 Curriculum

To take into account the different interests of clinical practitioners and medical doctors in research, the study program can be individually customized. The curriculum is based upon three types of learning and teaching events: on one hand, systematic learning with a scientific focus, called *dies academicus (lat.)*, on the other hand, case-related learning with treatment of patients, called *hospitatio (lat.)*, and additionally, independent self-studies according to individual learning objectives, called *studium generale (lat.)*.

> **Tip**
>
> Some teaching events are offered abroad. Participation means international networking within the global scientific community.

All teaching events are provided in a buffet system. Doctors have the free choice to select their menu of competing *dies academicus* and *hospitation* at different places, with different timing, held by different schools in Germany and abroad, presented in German or in English based upon the location of the teaching event.

The content of the full-scope PALM program comprises six thematic fields, supplied in six independent modules: principles of aesthetic medicine and laser medicine (module 1); laser treatment of typical indications in aesthetic medicine (module 2); laser treatment of rare indications in aesthetic medicine (module 3); laser treatment of difficult indications in aesthetic medicine (module 4); understanding and application of clinical plasma medicine (module 5); aesthetic medicine as a cross-disciplinary area (module 6). Each module contains three independent micromodules to be individually filled by the teaching staff with certain scientific or practical content as a complementing assortment following the guidelines of good clinical practice.

> **Important to Know**
> The content of micromodules in terms of scientific guidelines of the specialty and current literature is based upon this textbook.

The workload of the curriculum, expressed in credit points (CP) referring to the European Credit Point System, comprises the six modules with 6 CP each, one active participation at a scientific congress (1 CP), a master thesis (21 CP), and a master colloquium (2 CP) to a total of 60 CP. The master thesis concludes the scientific postgraduate education, a paper written in English or German. The content has to be related to aesthetic medicine in general and laser or plasma medicine in detail to prove compound knowledge in the cross-section of the specialty. The paper should not comprise fewer than 50 DIN A4 pages (approx. 1500 characters/page).

> **Important to Know**
> 60 CP means 1.800 hours of workload; however, preparation and follow-up of teaching events and every kind of self-study are included.

21.2.1.4 Examination

The master thesis has to be defended orally in English or German within a public master colloquium by means of a presentation in front of a board of examiners. Thirty minutes have been envisaged for the presentation and a subsequently following discussion. Furthermore, there will be a second oral presentation of three clinical cases treated by the candidate. Thirty minutes have been envisaged for this portion of the evaluation as well.

21.2.1.5 Degree

The study program is intended to lead to the "Post-Graduate M. Sc. in Plasma and Aesthetic Laser Medicine" that will be delivered by Greifswald University Medicine after completion of the full study program, in total 60 CP.

In case of an individually customized program with reduced workload and less than 60 CP achieved, the program can lead to the "Diploma Plasma and Aesthetic Laser Medicine" as a documentation of continued education.

On the basis of interuniversity agreements with partner institutions abroad, and in appropriate cases, the M.Sc. degree as well as the Diploma can be delivered

21

by Greifswald University Medicine in shared academic sovereignty as a double degree, together with the partner university abroad.

21.2.1.6   Tuition Fees and Study Service

Postgraduate education in Germany is connected with fees to pay the honoraria of the module/micromodule providers and cover the expenses of program administration. Tuition fees in principle are set by Greifswald University. However, tuition fees for modules/micromodules given in other countries might follow local customs and guidelines.

The study counseling of the PALM program takes place under the umbrella of the *Weiterbildungsbuero Universitaet Greifswald* (Greifswald University Office of Post-Graduate Education), the central organizing and administrative body. The PALM study service is the main contact for all aspects of content and student affairs in the program, if required, in consultation with the administrative offices of the partner teaching institutions abroad.

21.2.2   Postgraduate Education in Clinical Plasma Medicine for Doctors

21.2.2.1   Target Group

Doctors and dentists interested not so much in laser and aesthetic medicine, but especially in cold plasma therapy and research, are offered a section of the full PALM program, mainly dealing with plasma medicine. Prerequisite for admission as a candidate is a state-approved university degree with professional qualification in human medicine or in dental medicine.

> **Tip**
>
> This selected course will not lead to a master's degree but can be extended later on to the full master's study program.

21.2.2.2   Aims of Qualification

After having finished the plasma medicine part of the PALM program, doctors will have interdisciplinary in-depth knowledge and skills especially in the area of plasma medicine, based on their individual predetermined priority setting. They will have the ability to use plasma medical devices for treatment, the knowledge to assess critically the indication, to evaluate therapy results in context of available methods and techniques, and they will also be able to investigate with scientific methods innovative questions that constantly arise in clinical plasma medicine.

21.2.2.3   Curriculum

The study program will concentrate on the plasma medicine content and especially module 5: understanding and applying clinical plasma medicine (▶ Box 21.1). The

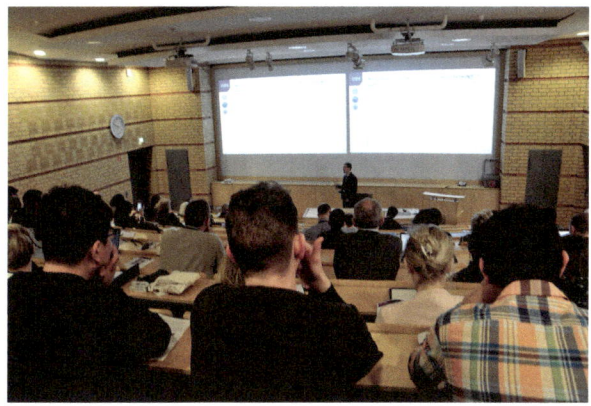

■ **Fig. 21.1** Participating at a scientific plasma-related conference like the international workshop on plasma in cancer treatment 2018 in Greifswald is an advantage in every aspect. Beyond gain in knowledge and mutually rewarding exchange, participation adds to the account of workload in *studium generale* (in total 4 CP), and taking part as a speaker or with a poster presentation will be honored with 1 credit point (CP)

curriculum is just as the full-scope PALM program based upon the three types of learning and teaching events, *dies academicus*, *hospitation*, and *studium generale* (■ Fig. 21.1), taking into account the different interests of clinical practitioners and medical doctors in research. The module contains three independent micro-modules to be individually filled by the teaching staff with certain scientific or practical content as a complementing assortment.

All teaching events again are provided in a buffet system. Doctors have the free choice of completing *dies academicus* and *hospitation* at different places, with different timing, held by different schools in Germany and abroad, presented in German or in English based upon the location of the teaching event.

The workload of this special curriculum, expressed in CP referring to the European Credit Point System, comprises module 5 of the PALM program with 6 CP (▶ Box 21.1), an active participation at a scientific congress with 1 CP (■ Fig. 21.1), a master-thesis equivalent written work (11 CP) and a master-colloquium equivalent oral examination (2 CP). The master-thesis equivalent written work concludes the scientific postgraduate education, a paper written in English or German. It should not comprise less than 25 DIN A4 pages (approx. 1500 characters/page).

The international cooperation in plasma research and the global community of doctors interested in plasma medicine calls for distance teaching by modern technology whenever feasible, not at least for ecological reasons. Distance teaching will strongly profit from 5G mobile connectivity. Doctors and teachers participating in joint study courses with remote partners should as soon as possible benefit from touchable holograms and instinctual interaction by, for example, Microsoft HoloLens 2 tetherless headsets.

21

Box 21.1   Module 5 is one of the 6 of the complete Master of Science study program to demonstrate the pattern of teaching events, and it is the main module of the focused plasma medicine courses, common to all degree programs. The box explains the organization of the module, the orientation of the teaching events (seminars and lectures (*dies academicus*) or practical training (*hospitation*)) the workload in total hours including self-studies, and the CP to be earned

Module 5
- Understanding and application of clinical plasma medicine
- In total 180 hours of workload; 6 CP to be acquired:

Micromodule 5.1
- Dies academicus I: Basic aspects of plasma physics, plasma biology and plasma technology
- Dies academicus II detailed aspects of plasma medicine and clinical plasma medicine
- In total 30 hours of lectures including preparation and follow-up; 1 CP

Micromodule 5.2
- Hospitation I: Observation of treatment procedures in clinical plasma medicine
- Hospitation II observing and assisting treatment procedures in clinical plasma medicine
- In total 20 hours of training including preparation and follow-up; 2/3 CP

Micromodule 5.3
- Hospitation I: Assisted treatment of patients with plasma devices
- Hospitation II: Treatment of patients with plasma devices under supervision
- In total 10 hours of treatment including preparation and follow-up; 1/3 CP

Self-study (◘ Fig. 21.1)
- Studium generale
- In total 120 hours of self-directed learning; 4 CP

21.2.2.4   Examination

The master-thesis equivalent written work, dealing with plasma medicine in general and a clinical aspect in detail to demonstrate compound knowledge in the cross-disciplinary field of applied plasma medicine, has to be defended orally in English or German within a public master-colloquium equivalent examination by means of a presentation in front of a board of examiners. Thirty minutes have been envisaged for the presentation and a subsequently following discussion. Furthermore, there will be a second oral presentation, this time about three clinical plasma medicine cases treated by the candidate. Thirty minutes have been envisaged as well.

21.2.2.5   Diploma

The study program is intended to lead to the "Diploma of Plasma Medicine" that will be delivered by Greifswald University Medicine according to a workload of in total 20 CP: completion of the selected module program, active participation at a scientific congress, presentation of a master-thesis equivalent written work and successful master-colloquium equivalent oral examination.

On the basis of interuniversity agreements with partner institutions abroad, in appropriate cases, the Diploma can be delivered by Greifswald University Medicine in shared academic sovereignty together with a partner university abroad.

21.2.2.6 Tuition Fees and Study Service

Postgraduate education in Germany is connected with fees to pay the honoraria of the module/micromodule providers and cover the expenses of program administration. Tuition fees in principle are set by Greifswald University; however, tuition fees for modules/micromodules given in other countries might follow local customs and guidelines.

The study counseling takes place in context of the PALM program under the umbrella of the *Weiterbildungsbuero Universitaet Greifswald* (Greifswald University Office of PostGraduate Education), the central organizing and administrative body. The study service is the main contact for all aspects of content and student affairs in the program, if required, in consultation with the administrative offices of the partner teaching institutions abroad.

21.2.3 Postgraduate Education in Clinical Plasma Medicine for Natural Scientists and Engineers

21.2.3.1 Target Group

Natural scientists and engineers coworking in clinical plasma medicine research groups or interested in identifying the doctors' perspective in plasma therapy are offered the section of the full PALM program that only deals with clinical plasma medicine (▶ Box 21.1). Prerequisite for admission as a candidate is a state-approved university degree at least at bachelor's level proving professional qualification in natural sciences, engineering, plasma technology, or any other scientific discipline related to plasma medicine and research.

❯ **Important to Know**
Clinical plasma medicine is applied plasma research, just to put an emphasis upon the need for looking beyond borders.

21.2.3.2 Aims of Qualification

After having finished the plasma medicine part of the PALM program, nonmedical scientists will have interdisciplinary in-depth knowledge aligned with their individual professional background and clear understanding of the doctors' view of plasma medical devices. In research groups they will be able to discuss on equal eye level expectations, limitations, and opportunities of the study protocol with the doctors involved, and they will be informed partners in discussing methods, techniques, innovative questions, and papers to be published.

21

21.2.3.3 **Curriculum**

The study program will concentrate on the plasma medicine content and module 5 (▶ Box 21.1): understanding and application of clinical plasma medicine. The curriculum is the full-scope PALM program based upon the three types of learning and teaching events, *dies academicus*, *hospitation*, and *studium generale* (◘ Fig. 21.1), taking into account the individual interests of different research projects and the expertise of the individual natural scientists and engineers involved. The module contains three independent micromodules to be individually filled by the teaching staff with certain scientific or practical content as a complementing assortment for the researchers' choice.

All teaching events are provided in a buffet system. Candidates have the free choice of completing *dies academicus* and *hospitation* at different places, with different timing, held by different schools in Germany and abroad, presented in German or in English based upon the location of the teaching event.

The workload of this special curriculum, expressed in CP referring to the European Credit Point System, comprises module 5 of the PALM program with 6 CP, one active participation at a scientific congress (1 CP), a master-thesis equivalent written work (11 CP), and a master-colloquium equivalent oral examination (2 CP). The master-thesis equivalent written work concludes the scientific postgraduate education, a paper written in English or German. It should not comprise less than 25 DIN A4 pages (approx. 1500 characters/page).

Tip

There is no requirement to adhere rigidly to *clinical* plasma medicine.

The international cooperation in plasma research and the global community of researchers interested in plasma medicine calls for distance teaching by modern technology whenever feasible, not at least for ecological reasons. Mixed reality is clearly supported. Distance teaching will strongly profit from 5G mobile connectivity. Candidates and teachers participating in joint study courses with remote partners should as soon as possible benefit from touchable holograms and instinctual interaction by, for example, Microsoft HoloLens 2 tetherless headsets.

21.2.3.4 **Examination**

The master-thesis equivalent written work, dealing with plasma medicine in general and a self-chosen nonclinical scientific aspect in detail, has to be defended orally in English or German within a public master-colloquium equivalent oral examination by means of a presentation in front of a board of examiners. Thirty minutes have been envisaged for the presentation and a subsequently following discussion. Furthermore, there will be a second oral presentation of a scientific paper related to plasma medicine and published as the corresponding author in a peer-reviewed journal. Thirty minutes have been envisaged as well.

21.2.3.5 Diploma

The study program is intended to lead to the "Diploma of Plasma Medicine" that will be delivered by Greifswald University Medicine according to a workload of in total 20 CP: completion of the selected module program, active participation including oral or poster presentation at a scientific congress, presentation of a master-thesis equivalent written work and successful master-colloquium equivalent oral examination.

On the basis of interuniversity agreements with partner institutions abroad, in appropriate cases, the Diploma can be delivered by Greifswald University Medicine in shared academic sovereignty together with a partner university abroad.

21.2.3.6 Tuition Fees and Study Service

Postgraduate education in Germany is connected with fees to pay the honoraria of the module/micromodule providers and cover the expenses of program administration. Tuition fees in principle are set by Greifswald University; however, tuition fees for modules/micromodules given in other countries might follow local customs and guidelines.

The study counseling takes place under the umbrella of the *Weiterbildungsbuero Universitaet Greifswald* (Greifswald University Office of Post-Graduate Education), the central organizing and administrative body. The PALM study service is the main contact for all aspects of content and participants' affairs in the program, if required in consultation with the administrative offices of a partner teaching institution abroad.

21.2.4 Professional Continuous Training in Clinical Plasma Medicine for Nurses

21.2.4.1 Target Group

Nurses carrying out wound care and management with plasma medical devices supervised by doctors need comprehensive introduction and practical instruction to plasma medicine. They are offered module 5 (▶ Box 21.1) dealing with clinical plasma medicine as professional continuous training [4]. There is no prerequisite for admission.

> **Tip**
>
> Clinical plasma teams may coordinate professional training and doctors' study program to participate at the same teaching events.

21.2.4.2 Aims of Training

After having finished module 5 of the PALM program, nurses will have interdisciplinary in-depth knowledge and skills especially in the area of plasma medicine, based upon their individual priority setting. They will have the ability to use plasma

21

medical devices safely and securely for treatment, and to contribute their sound practical experience to the plasma therapy and research team.

21.2.4.3 Professional Training

Nurses are invited to attend teaching events of module 5: understanding and application of clinical plasma medicine. They should participate in all the three micromodules, *dies academicus* as well as *hospitation*, with a special professional emphasis of nurses on wound care and wound management by plasma.

The workload of professional advanced training is not expressed by CP but by three certificates of attendance referring to each micromodule of module.

21.2.4.4 Examination

There is no active contribution required at the master or master-equivalent colloquium, but participation as an observing member of the plasma therapy and research team is required.

21.2.4.5 Certificate

The program is intended to lead to a "Certificate of Professional Advanced Training for Nurses, embedded in the Post-Graduate M.Sc. Program "Plasma and Aesthetic Laser Medicine – PALM," delivered together with the certificates of other members of the plasma therapy and research team.

21.2.4.6 Tuition Fees

There are no tuition fees.

21.2.4.7 Study Counseling

As for the full-scope and selected PALM study program, the study counseling of nurses as well takes place under the umbrella of the *Weiterbildungsbuero Universitaet Greifswald* (Greifswald University Office of Post-Graduate Education), the central organizing and administrative body. The PALM study service is the main contact not only for doctors and scientists, but for all aspects of professional advanced training for nurses, too.

21.3 Conclusion

The considerable demand, not only for qualified doctors and nurses, but also for scientific staff and research assistants in an extremely innovative field, calls for continuing and postgraduate education programs in plasma medicine as a matter of research quality assurance and of patients' safety matters. Greifswald University has developed since 2001 a university-based postgraduate medical education program focused upon clinical application of photonic energy devices. Recently this program has been expanded to a postgraduate Master of Science Study Program "Plasma and Aesthetic Laser Medicine - PALM."

> **Important to Know**
> The course program is inviting international cooperation within the scientific community.

Intended first as a full-scope study program for doctors interested in the cross-section field of aesthetic medicine by noninvasive treatment procedures like laser and cold plasma, the curriculum can now be tailored as well to plasma medicine by itself and the needs and interests of all members of the clinical plasma therapy and research team: the plasma doctors, the plasma nurses, the plasma natural scientists, and engineers.

Contact for further information and application: *Weiterbildungsbuero Universitaet Greifswald* **(Greifswald University Office of Post-Graduate Education, Email:** masterzahn@uni-greifswald.de**), PALM study service**

References

1. Metelmann HR, Waite PD, Hammes S. Quality standards in aesthetic medicine. In: Raulin C, Karsai S, editors. Laser and IPL technology in dermatology and aesthetic medicine. Berlin; Heidelberg: Springer; 2011. p. 377–81.
2. Hammes S. Qualitätssicherung in der ästhetischen Medizin durch universitäre Weiterbildung: Diploma in Aesthetic Laser Medicine. In: Metelmann HR, Hammes S, editors. Lasermedizin in der Ästhetischen Chirurgie. Berlin; Heidelberg; New York: Springer; 2012. https://doi.org/10.1007/978-3-642-17424-7.
3. Hammes S, Westermann U, Metelmann HR. Qualitätsmanagement durch postgraduale Weiterbildung. In: Metelmann HR, von Woedtke T, Weltmann KD, editors. Plasmamedizin. Berlin; Heidelberg: Springer; 2016. p. 201–7.
4. Kirschner S, Bethke B, Kirschner A, Brueckner S, Gostomski B. Training wound nurses in plasma medicine. In: Metelmann HR, von Woedtke T, Weltmann KD, editors. Comprehensive clinical plasma medicine. Berlin; Heidelberg: Springer; 2018. p. 473–81.

Suggested Reading

Metelmann HR, von Woedtke T, Weltmann KD, editors. Comprehensive clinical plasma medicine. Berlin; Heidelberg: Springer; 2016. isbn:978-3-030-09806-3.

What Are the Requirements of a Cold Plasma Medicine Clinic

Steffen Emmert, Lars Boeckmann,
Tobias Fischer, Thomas von Woedtke,
Klaus-Dieter Weltmann,
and Hans-Robert Metelmann

Contents

© Springer Nature Switzerland AG 2022
H.-R. Metelmann et al. (eds.), *Textbook of Good Clinical Practice in Cold Plasma Therapy*, https://doi.org/10.1007/978-3-030-87857-3_22

Core Messages

- A plasma clinic should provide all patient care settings: inpatient, day-care, out-patient, as well as home-care settings within a collaborative network that fits the patients' needs according to their individual disease situation.
- For the mere medical plasma application trained doctors, nurses, and a plasma physicist or biologist may be mandatory.
- For a comprehensive plasma clinic (CPC) further requirements in research, teaching, and development may be necessary.
- A CPC should provide research facilities including a phase I–II study center unit, lab space, as well as an animal research facility: an interdisciplinary research center.
- A CPC should provide teaching opportunities. Teaching should be offered to a wide range of specialists: medical doctors, dental doctors, natural scientists (physics, chemistry, biology), engineering scientists, as well as nursing and technical assistant personnel.
- As plasma medicine is still a thriving new field space for entrepreneurship may be also provided in a CPC.

22.1 Introduction

The introduction of cold atmospheric pressure plasma into medical applications can be regarded as highly innovational in medicine [1–3]. Through modulation of cellular redox chemistry cold atmospheric pressure plasma allows the modulation of signaling cascades to trigger cellular responses for medical treatment purposes. The spectrum of targets ranges from multi-resistant germs, fungi, and viruses, benign cells, and mechanisms involved in wound healing, to malignant cells and tumor immunology [4, 5]. How the utilization of cold atmospheric pressure plasma can be adjusted individually to the benefit of the respective patient is the main topic of plasma medicine, and, hence, a plasma clinic.

The research and development in plasma application in medicine currently passes a first milestone. Plasma physicists have developed several suitable plasma sources that generate cold plasma at body temperatures under atmospheric conditions. These plasma sources have been further refined by start-up companies according to structured application studies, mainly to accelerate wound healing, into certified medical products. Besides this, empiric research plasma biologists have elucidated the essentials of plasma effects to living cells (redox chemistry and cell signaling biology) [6, 7]. In many centers all over the world, further clinical studies are currently developed to broaden the field of plasma application beyond wound healing. This paves the way towards a second milestone: a comprehensive plasma clinic (CPC).

22.2 Requirements of a Plasma Medicine Clinic

As the plasma technology advances and several plasma devices have been developed for clinical use [6] it is obvious that plasma medicine takes the next milestone: Implementation in the clinic as a plasma medicine clinical section. To achieve this goal, plasma medicine needs to be integrated into the clinical routine on the administrative as well as scientific level. On the basis of the current state of the art of experimental and clinical plasma medicine, the implementation in three action fields seems realistic: Clinical Dermatology including tissue regeneration and wound healing [3, 4]; Microbiology and Hygiene and Dental Medicine including disinfection/antimicrobial treatments and implantology [6]; and Oncology, which might impose the most promising potential in the future [8–10] (■ Fig. 22.1).

Clinical Dermatology: This field of plasma application has advanced the most in the last years [3, 4]. Plasma devices are already in routine use for inpatient as well as outpatient treatment. As early as 2013 two different plasma technologies, a plasma jet (■ Fig. 22.2) as well as a dielectric barrier discharge (DBD) plasma device (■ Fig. 22.3) have been licensed for wound treatment. Based on the pilot studies for these device developments, basic standards in plasma application have been defined

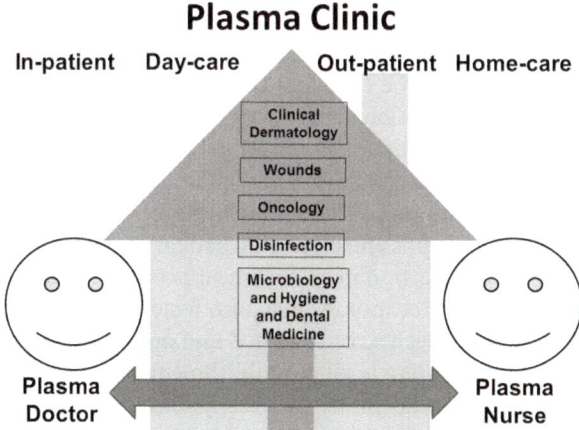

■ Fig. 22.1 Requirements of a plasma clinic: medical doctor, nurse, and a network of all patient care settings (inpatient, day-care, outpatient, home care)

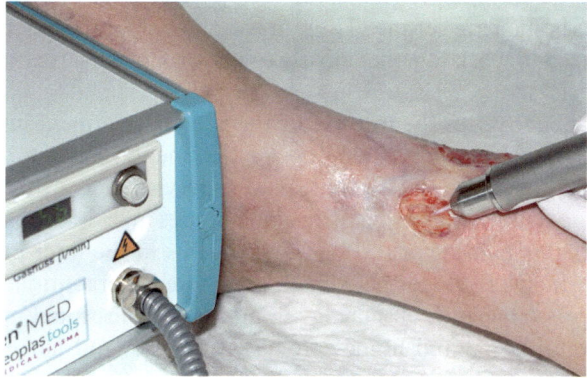

■ Fig. 22.2 Application of a plasma jet to a chronic wound

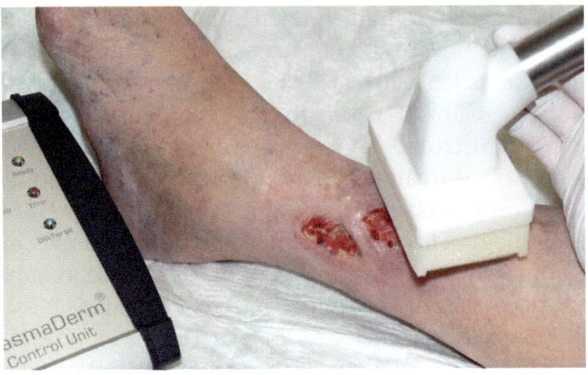

Fig. 22.3 Application of a DBD plasma source to a flat chronic wound

as outlined in previous chapters. Still, some questions on plasma wound treatment remain. These questions need to be addressed within the routine use of plasma wound treatment and include a more precise definition of the single plasma treatment duration depending on the type and condition of the respective wound, the frequency of treatment application, and the total duration of the plasma treatment. Plasma registries with clinical data in "real world plasma use" in dermatology will answer these questions. However, additional digital technologies such as teledermatological, digital documentation of the treatment processes as well as the treatment outcomes including wound apps and electronic patient-reported outcomes will facilitate and accelerate data collection in such clinical plasma registries. Artificial intelligence including blog chain technology may also foster the development of clinical treatment algorithms. With such a consolidated and optimized plasma use for tissue regeneration and wound healing a solid establishment of plasma treatment can be achieved in dermatology in a hospital as well as in an outpatient setting.

To this end, a comprehensive plasma management including all medical disciplines, doctors, nurses, and biologists/physicists is mandatory to raise the most benefit of plasma for public health. A modern wound management should incorporate novel treatment modalities like plasma to the already complex modern wound treatments and a close structured interplay between inpatient and patient treatments in a home-care setting. Thus, in the clinic doctors, nurses, and a biologist/physicist need to work together closely to perform plasma treatment and maintain plasma devices.

A great challenge poses the transfer of the plasma treatment into a home-care setting. Usually, nurses perform home-care treatments and the doctors, family practitioners, or doctors in the local hospital supervise such a treatment. At least in Germany, due to a strict division of responsibilities in hospital-based and home-care treatments this interplay calls for new concepts in the inter-professional collaboration of hospital-based personnel and family practitioners as well as home-care nurses. The solution may lay in an inter-professional networking concept with hospital-based and home-care-based doctors and nurses for a specific region to improve structural, process, and outcome quality of plasma therapy. Of course, new digital technologies may support such a network as mentioned above.

This said, such concepts result in a permanent and continuous optimization of plasma treatment parameters and a more individualized and personalized definition of treatment modalities. These concepts will also facilitate the integration of new plasma-technological developments into clinical practice and should also guide the continuous development and improvement of new plasma technologies.

In addition to Clinical Dermatology, new application fields of plasma can be envisaged in a hospital. This includes Microbiology and Hygiene and Dental Medicine [6]. These areas have also been heavily researched in the past. The step to clinical routine in these areas is near; however, this may need some more translational investigation compared with dermatological plasma wound treatment. The development of plasma towards skin disinfection, elimination of multi-resistant bacteria from skin and cavities, and implantology including avoidance of infections of indwelling cannulas or other transcutaneous drivelines (arterial, venous, cardiac, etc.) is of utmost interest. In the dental clinic, the body of preclinical experiences is on the way to be implemented in routine dental root infection and caries therapy as well as treatment for dental implant infections. Plasma may also be used in a prophylactic setting to avoid the aforementioned infections.

Based on in vitro investigations, the use of animal models and first clinical trials plasma application for the amelioration of oncological diseases may pose a very promising use in the future. Already, world congresses of plasma in oncology bring together doctors, nurses, biologists, and physicists to optimize plasma devices for oncological treatments. First results showed positive effects on decontamination of skin ulcerating head and neck tumors with respect to odor in a palliative setting. Currently, research is performed on the technical as well as the biological level to selectively kill tumor cells and induce immunogenic cell death in skin tumors like squamous cell carcinoma or melanoma [8–10].

22.3 Requirements of a Comprehensive Plasma Medicine Clinic: Research

In parallel with the establishment of comprehensive cancer centers (CCC), we propose the term CPC, if basic research and translational plasma research is performed at such a clinical center in addition to mere clinical application (◉ Fig. 22.4). Historically, cold atmospheric plasma was developed by physicists, and then biologists and chemists researched the biomedical properties of the plasma cocktail [11]. Finally, doctors performed clinical research for proper plasma applications. These days, as nursing develops towards an academic discipline with bachelor and master degrees in nursing and plasma medicine expands to a network-treatment including home-care application, again performed by specially trained nurses, new concepts in inter-professional co-working spaces need to be researched.

To this end, a CPC (◉ Fig. 22.4) should include an interdisciplinary research unit. Ideally, such a plasma research unit may contain a center to perform clinical phase I-II trials as well as investigator initiated trials (IITs). This is practically a special inpatient ward to monitor effects and potential side-effects of new treatments with specially trained doctors and study nurses in good clinical practice.

Comprehensive Plasma Clinic (CPC)

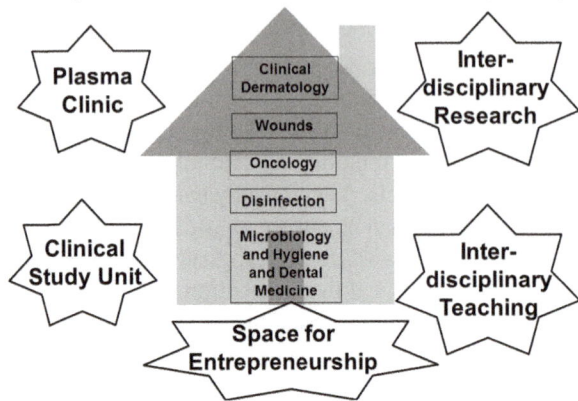

Fig. 22.4 Requirements of a comprehensive plasma clinic (CPC): clinical study unit, interdisciplinary research, interdisciplinary teaching, and space for entrepreneurship

Such a unit needs to be separated from other clinical activities as a special patient monitoring is mandatory. Such a clinical trial unit connects the clinic with translational research at the interface of bringing new devices or new combinatory treatments with plasma to first use in man.

Such an interdisciplinary plasma research center annexed to a clinic should also offer enough lab space to perform biomedical, chemical, and engineering research as well as offices as think-tanks for research beyond the wet-lab including nursing, administration, and health in a broader sense. This, of course, may also include public health economics and marketing research for start-up companies that may evolve from such research. Lab space may allow for the use of pathogenic substances and probes and, therefore, should be licensed according to biology safety levels I and II. In addition, the development of new treatment devices and substances (plasma treated liquids may be one example) still necessitates some in vivo testing of safety and efficacy. Despite enormous efforts to reduce, refine, or replace animal testing, it is still not possible to introduce new therapies for man without at least a minimum of testing in vivo in animals. To this end, an interdisciplinary research unit of a CPC should also offer the possibilities to perform the minimum of animal experiments needed to bring a new plasma treatment into human use.

22.4 Requirements of a Comprehensive Plasma Medicine Clinic: Teaching

Talking about research at a CPC (■ Fig. 22.4) inevitably also means that teaching is another prerequisite of an interdisciplinary research unit. Research without teaching and bringing new investigations to the attention of all the different specialties involved in plasma medicine is quite senseless. Therefore, a CPC teaching unit may be viewed as an integrative model for an internationally visible dermatological and plasma medical translational teaching in all plasma application fields including oncology, microbiology, hygiene, biology, chemistry, physics, engineering, and nursing.

Such a teaching unit also aims at all different levels of education. Already high school students may get acquainted with plasma medicine (e.g., within school rotation, girls days, or other training days). Then, special bachelor and master studies may be offered for university students in all aforementioned disciplines including human medicine, dental medicine, veterinarian medicine, nursing, natural sciences, engineering, and economics. However, training does not stop with a final university degree. Specialized training in subspecialties may be offered and already experienced people may have the opportunity to learn about plasma medicine or broaden their knowledge within congresses or training courses.

To this end, the University Greifswald offers as the first University in Europe a postgraduate study program for aesthetic laser medicine (► https://laserstudium. com/). This international study program results in the earning of the grade "Diploma in aesthetic laser medicine" (DALM). Quality assurance in aesthetic medicine guaranteed by University-guided advanced training is the main goal of this study program. The University of Greifswald, the German Dermatological Laser Society, and Leibniz Institute for Plasma Research and Technology e.V. joined together to foster clinical application, teaching, and research in aesthetic medicine under the motto beautiful health. So far, more than 140 doctors from Germany, Switzerland, Austria, India, Kuwait, and the USA have earned the DALM degree. Lately, it was decided to extend this study program to allow for the earning of a diploma in plasma medicine (DPM) by attending lectures (dies academicus), practical training in plasma clinics, and literature studies (► https://laserstudium.com/index.php?title=DALM_Struktur#Mit_Schwerpunkt_PlasmaMedizin).

See also ► Chap. 21.

22.5 Requirements of a Comprehensive Plasma Medicine Clinic: Entrepreneurship

It is obvious that in a comprehensive plasma medicine clinical center also the last puzzle piece shall not be missing: space for entrepreneurship (□ Fig. 22.4). This is the final step to bring new knowledge to routine clinical use. The successful cooperation and mutual understanding between the different disciplines within a CPC make it possible to understand and to use the full potential of the plasma medical applications. Such a center either generates from within or via industry-collaborations personnel who patent new plasma-technological innovations and devices and pursue to establish spin-off companies.

A perfect example is our excellence project ONKOTHER-H (► https://www.onkother-h.med.uni-rostock.de/). This cooperative network is funded by the European Social Fund (ESF) within the qualification program "Promotion of young scientists in excellent research networks – program for research excellence of the state Mecklenburg-West Pomerania." The goal of this network is to establish a developmental platform for new and innovative cancer therapies on the example of skin cancer – the most common cancer in man [12]. To this end, eight research groups work together on an interdisciplinary and trans-institutional level from two Universities and a Leibniz Research Institute. The goal is to understand the molecular mechanisms of plasma action to kill skin cancer cells and based on that to develop a new plasma device for skin cancer treatment. At the end of this project, it is a declared goal to patent this new plasma device and to establish a spin-off to market it.

22.6 Conclusion

Plasma medicine is a highly innovative and dynamic new field in medicine. Plasma devices for wound treatment have been medically certified according to clinical studies, however, could be improved for certain wound conditions. Secondly, further fields of plasma medicine including cancer treatment, dental applications, and cosmetics are currently explored. The development of new devices can be expected. To this end, a clinic for plasma application should provide trained doctoral and nursing staff. A plasma biologist or physicist may be helpful. Within a plasma care network inpatient, outpatient, day-care as well as home-care plasma treatment should be provided. The requirements for a CPC should additionally include a clinical study unit, interdisciplinary research and teaching, and space for entrepreneurship.

Acknowledgments   This work is partly supported by the European Social Fund (ESF), reference: ESF/14-BM-A55-0001/18, ESF/14-BM-A55-0005/18, ESF/14-BM-A55-0006/18, and the Ministry of Education, Science and Culture of Mecklenburg-West Pomerania, Germany. S.E. is supported by the Deutsche Forschungsgemeinschaft (DFG EM 63/13-1) and the Damp Foundation. L.B. is supported by the Dermatological Society of Mecklenburg-West Pomerania.

References

1. von Woedtke T, Schmidt A, Bekeschus S, Wende K, Weltmann KD. Plasma medicine: a field of applied redox biology. In Vivo. 2019;33:1011–26.
2. Emmert S, editor. Wound treatment with cold atmospheric plasma – examples and operation guidelines from clinical practice. Munich: Springer Medizin; 2019. p. 1–93.
3. Bernhardt T, Semmler ML, Schäfer M, Bekeschus S, Emmert S, Boeckmann L. Plasma medicine: applications of cold atmospheric pressure plasma in dermatology. Oxidative Med Cell Longev. 2019;3873928:1–10.
4. Boeckmann L, Bernhardt T, Schäfer M, Semmler ML, Kordt M, Waldner AC, Wendt F, Sagwal S, Bekeschus S, Berner J, Kwiatek E, Frey A, Fischer T, Emmert S. Current indications for plasma therapy in dermatology. Hautarzt. 2020;71:109–13.
5. Semmler MS, Bekeschus S, Schäfer M, Bernhardt T, Fischer T, Witzke K, Seebauer C, Rebl H, Grambow E, Vollmar B, Nebe B, Metelmann HR, von Woedtke T, Emmert S, Boeckmann L. Molecular mechanisms for the efficacy of cold atmospheric pressure plasma (CAP) in cancer treatment. Cancers. 2020;12:e269. (1–19).

6. Metelmann R, von Woedtke T, Weltmann KD, editors. Comprehensive clinical plasma medicine. Heidelberg: Springer; 2018.
7. Metelmann R, von Woedtke T, Weltmann KD, editors. Plasmamedizin: Kaltplasma in der medizinischen Anwendung. Heidelberg: Springer; 2016.
8. Metelmann H-R, Seebauer C, Miller V, Fridman A, Bauer G, Graves DB, et al. Clinical experience with cold plasma in the treatment of locally advanced head and neck cancer. Clin Plasma Med. 2018;9:6–13.
9. Witzke K, Seebauer C, Jesse K, Kwiatek E, Berner J, Semmler M, Böckmann L, Emmert S, Weltmann KD, Metelmann H, Bekeschus S. Plasma medical oncology: immunological interpretation of head and neck squamous cell carcinoma. Plasma Process Polym. 2020;17:e1900258. (1–9).
10. Berner J, Seebauer C, Sagwal S, Boeckmann L, Emmert S, Metelmann H, Bekeschus S. Medical gas plasma treatment in head and neck cancer – challenges and opportunities. Appl Sci. 2020;10:1944. (1–14).
11. Tiede R, Helmke A, Wandke D, Viölk W, Emmert S. PlasmaDerm®: kaltes Atmosphärendruckplasma als Spitzeninnovation. In: Spitzenforschung in der Dermatologie. Innovationen und Auszeichnungen 2015. Lampertheim: ALPHA Informations-GmbH; 2015. p. 70–80.
12. Böckmann L, Schäfer M, Semmler ML, Bernhardt T, Hinz B, Nebe B, Vollmar B, Langer P, Metelmann HR, Bekeschus S, Suhm C, Fischer T, Emmert S. Entwicklungsplattform für innovative onkologische Therapien am Beispiel des häufigsten menschlichen Krebses – Hautkrebs. In: Spitzenforschung in der Dermatologie. Innovationen und Auszeichnungen 2019. Lampertheim: ALPHA Informations-GmbH; 2019. p. 12–21.

Supplementary Information

Index